Hippocrates Now

Bloomsbury Studies in Classical Reception

Bloomsbury Studies in Classical Reception presents scholarly monographs offering new and innovative research and debate to students and scholars in the reception of Classical Studies. Each volume will explore the appropriation, reconceptualization and recontextualization of various aspects of the Graeco-Roman world and its culture, looking at the impact of the ancient world on modernity. Research will also cover reception within antiquity, the theory and practice of translation, and reception theory.

Also available in the Series:

Ancient Magic and the Supernatural in the Modern Visual and Performing Arts, edited by Filippo Carlà & Irene Berti
Ancient Greek Myth in World Fiction since 1989, edited by Justine McConnell & Edith Hall
Antipodean Antiquities, edited by Marguerite Johnson
Classics in Extremis, edited by Edmund Richardson
Frankenstein and its Classics, edited by Jesse Weiner, Benjamin Eldon Stevens & Brett M. Rogers
Greek and Roman Classics in the British Struggle for Social Reform, edited by Henry Stead & Edith Hall
Homer's Iliad and the Trojan War: Dialogues on Tradition, Jan Haywood & Naoíse Mac Sweeney
Imagining Xerxes, Emma Bridges
Julius Caesar's Self-Created Image and Its Dramatic Afterlife, Miryana Dimitrova
Once and Future Antiquities in Science Fiction and Fantasy, edited by Brett M. Rogers & Benjamin Eldon Stevens
Ovid's Myth of Pygmalion on Screen, Paula James
Reading Poetry, Writing Genre, edited by Silvio Bär & Emily Hauser
The Codex Fori Mussolini, Han Lamers and Bettina Reitz-Joosse
The Classics in Modernist Translation, edited by Miranda Hickman and Lynn Kozak
The Gentle, Jealous God, Simon Perris
Victorian Classical Burlesques, Laura Monrós-Gaspar
Victorian Epic Burlesques, Rachel Bryant Davies

Also published by Bloomsbury:

Greek and Roman Medicine, Helen King
Greek Medicine from the Heroic to the Hellenistic Age, James Longrigg
A Cultural History of Medicine in Antiquity, edited by Laurence Totelin

Hippocrates Now

The 'Father of Medicine' in the Internet Age

Helen King

BLOOMSBURY ACADEMIC
LONDON • NEW YORK • OXFORD • NEW DELHI • SYDNEY

BLOOMSBURY ACADEMIC
Bloomsbury Publishing Plc
50 Bedford Square, London, WC1B 3DP, UK
1385 Broadway, New York, NY 10018, USA
29 Earlsfort Terrace, Dublin 2, Ireland

BLOOMSBURY, BLOOMSBURY ACADEMIC and the Diana logo are trademarks
of Bloomsbury Publishing Plc

First published in Great Britain 2020
Paperback edition published 2021

Copyright © Helen King, 2020

Helen King has asserted her right under the Copyright, Designs and Patents Act, 1988,
to be identified as Author of this work.

This work is published subject to a Creative Commons Attribution Non-commercial
No Derivatives Licence. You may share this work for non-commercial purposes only, provided
you give attribution to the copyright holder and the publisher.

For legal purposes the Acknowledgements on p. viii constitute an extension of this copyright page.

Cover design: Terry Woodley
Cover image © yoeml/Shutterstock

All rights reserved. No part of this publication may be reproduced or transmitted in any form or by any
means, electronic or mechanical, including photocopying, recording, or any information storage or
retrieval system, without prior permission in writing from the publishers.

Bloomsbury Publishing Plc does not have any control over, or responsibility for, any third-party websites
referred to or in this book. All internet addresses given in this book were correct at the time of going to
press. The author and publisher regret any inconvenience caused if addresses have changed or sites
have ceased to exist, but can accept no responsibility for any such changes.

A catalogue record for this book is available from the British Library.

Library of Congress Cataloging-in-Publication Data
Names: King, Helen, 1957– author.
Title: Hippocrates now : the "father of medicine" in the internet age / Helen King.
Description: London ; New York, NY : Bloomsbury Academic, 2019. | Series: Bloomsbury studies in
classical reception | Includes bibliographical references and index. | Summary: "We need to talk about
Hippocrates. Current scholarship attributes none of the works of the 'Hippocratic corpus' to him, and the
ancient biographical traditions of his life are not only late, but also written for their own promotional
purposes. Yet Hippocrates features powerfully in our assumptions about ancient medicine, and our
beliefs about what medicine – and the physician himself – should be. In both orthodox and alternative
medicine, he continues to be a model to be emulated. This book will challenge widespread assumptions
about Hippocrates (and, in the process, about the history of medicine in ancient Greece and beyond)
and will also explore the creation of modern myths about the ancient world. Why do we continue to use
Hippocrates, and how are new myths constructed around his name? How do news stories and the
internet contribute to our picture of him? And what can this tell us about wider popular engagements
with the classical world today, in memes, 'quotes' and online?"– Provided by publisher.
Identifiers: LCCN 2019017436 (print) | LCCN 2019980524 (ebook) | ISBN 9781350005891 (hardback) |
ISBN 9781350005907 (epub) | ISBN 9781350005914 (pdf)
Subjects: LCSH: Hippocrates. | Hippocrates–Influence. | Hippocrates–In mass media. |
Physicians–Greece–Biography. | Medicine, Greek and Roman–In mass media. |
Medicine–Historiography. | Greece–History–To 146 B.C.–Biography–Sources.
Classification: LCC R126.H8 K56 2019 (print) | LCC R126.H8 (ebook) | DDC 610.938—dc23
LC record available at https://lccn.loc.gov/2019017436
LC ebook record available at https://lccn.loc.gov/2019980524

ISBN:	HB:	978-1-3500-0589-1
	PB:	978-1-3501-9318-5
	ePDF:	978-1-3500-0591-4
	eBook:	978-1-3500-0590-7

Series: Bloomsbury Studies in Classical Reception

Typeset by RefineCatch Limited, Bungay, Suffolk

To find out more about our authors and books visit www.bloomsbury.com
and sign up for our newsletters.

Contents

List of Figures		vii
Acknowledgements		viii
List of Abbreviations		x
	Introduction	1
	Receiving Hippocrates	2
	Looking like Hippocrates	7
	Hairs of Hippocrates	12
	Writing this book	14
1	What We Know About Hippocrates	17
2	What We Thought We Knew	19
	Hippocrates as God and Galen as his prophet?	22
	Finding a Hippocratic treatise	25
	Making a Corpus	29
	Authors and titles: What is a treatise?	31
	Creating the myths: Biographies and pseudepigrapha	35
	Being 'nice': The personality of Hippocrates	37
	Moving beyond the myths	39
3	Sabotaging the Story: What Hippocrates Didn't Write	43
	Writing new stories	44
	Wikipedia as a moving target	49
	Being the daddy	52
	Two decades in the slammer?	55
	Spreading the myths	57
	The Complicated Body	60
	From coercion to freedom	64
4	Needing a Bit of Information: Hippocrates in the News	67
	Taking and breaking: The Hippocratic *Oath*	68

	Imhotep and the power of Egyptian medicine	73
	Poop proof: Hippocrates' parasites	78
	Julius please her: Hippocratic hysteria	82
	A long history? Meanwhile in Babylon	88
	The Hippocrates detox diet	91
	Conclusion	93
5	Hippocrates in Quotes	95
	Flitting like a bee: Becoming a quote	97
	First do no harm	101
	Walking is the best medicine	105
6	Let Food Be Thy Medicine	111
	Back to the source?	115
	Which foods? Liver, garlic and watercress	123
	Death begins in the gut: Constipation and Hippocrates	127
	Conclusion	131
7	The Holistic Hippocrates: 'Treating the Patient, Not Just the Disease'	133
	The self-healing body	134
	Hippocrates in contemporary holistic medicine	138
	Invoking Hippocrates through history	145
	Hippocrates branded	149
	Conclusion	152
	Conclusion: Strange Remedies?	155
Notes		161
Bibliography		231
Index		255

Figures

1. Engraving: portrait of Hippocrates from Francis Clifton, *Hippocrates upon Airs, Water and Situation; upon Epidemical Diseases; and upon Prognostics, in Acute Cases especially* (London: J. Watts, 1734), frontispiece. Wellcome Collection. CC BY — 9
2. Portrait of Hippocrates from Johannes Antonides van der Linden, *Magni Hippocratis Coi opera omnia* (Lugduni Batavorum [Leiden]: Gaasbeeck, 1663), frontispiece. Wellcome Collection. CC BY — 10
3. Daniel Le Clerc, *The History of Physick, or, an account of the rise and progress of the art* (London: D Brown et al., 1699). Wellcome Collection. CC BY — 11
4. A fool is writing an insult on the pedestal of a statue of Hippocrates. Lithograph by Cham, *c.* 1850. Wellcome Collection. CC BY — 156

Acknowledgements

This book had its genesis in the conference organized by David Cantor at the College of Physicians of Philadelphia, which led to the publication of his edited collection of essays, *Reinventing Hippocrates*, in 2002. Having written for that collection a piece on the Renaissance Hippocrates, I continued to think about how the reception of this ancient figure is continuing to shift even now. Ten years after that book was published, the development of my project, 'Hippocrates Electric,' was supported by The Open University. Thanks to their generosity, Dr Joanna Brown was funded to help me scope the field, and I owe an enormous debt, particularly in Chapters 5 and 7, to her research and writing. Due to the pressures of the day job, the project then stalled until after my retirement in 2017, but writing the sections on 'How do we know what we know?' for The Open University's MA in Classical Studies made me think more deeply about how the internet has – and has not – changed the ways in which we do research and find information. As ever, questions and ideas from students have been important in thinking about the questions I am addressing here, and I would particularly like to thank all who have taken the FutureLearn MOOC I put together on 'Health and Wellbeing in the Ancient World'; for many of them, returning to education after many years away, the development of their internet literacy has been an important journey.

I would also like to record my thanks to those who generously helped me with specific queries on the material I am using here: they include Jacqueline Fabre-Serris, Mary Hague-Yearl (Director of the McGill Oslerian Library), Michael H. Malloy (John P. McGovern Chair in Oslerian Education) and Bahia Dawatly (Leverhulme Trust). In addition, the audiences to whom I have presented sections of this and the wider project have helped me think through the issues in different ways. Among these, I would particularly like to thank participants in the conferences on 'The Forgotten Other' and 'Ancient Holisms' at King's College London; those at my 2018 lecture to the Dutch Ancient Medicine Society, University of Utrecht, especially Aiste Celkyte and Anton van Hooff; and those at my 2019 Whitehead Annual Lecture in Manchester. Staff and students at Gustavus Adolphus College, MN, where I was a Rydell Visiting Professor in 2017–18, also shared my enthusiasm for the project, and I would like to record my thanks to Yurie Hong for the invitation. Laurence Totelin and Rebecca Flemming stimulated me to write an account of the events I describe in Chapter 3 while, towards the end of the writing process, a conversation with Alan Levinovitz helped me see the wood rather than the trees.

Abbreviations

BHM	*Bulletin of the History of Medicine*
BMJ	*British Medical Journal*
CMG	Corpus Medicorum Graecorum
DJR	Lesley Dean-Jones and Ralph Rosen (eds), *Ancient Concepts of the Hippocratic. Papers Presented at the XIIIth International Hippocrates Colloquium, Austin, Texas, August 2008*, Studies in Ancient Medicine 46, Leiden and Boston: Brill, 2015.
HHI	Hippocrates Health Institute
JHM	*Journal of the History of Medicine and Allied Sciences*
K	Carl Gottlob Kühn, *Claudii Galeni opera omnia*, 20 vols (Leipzig: Knobloch, 1821–33)
LFBTM	Let Food Be Thy Medicine
Littré	Emile Littré, *Oeuvres complètes d'Hippocrate*, 10 vols (Paris: Baillière, 1839–61)
Loeb	Loeb Classical Library (Cambridge, MA: Harvard University Press and London: Heinemann)
OUP	Oxford University Press
SDA	Seventh Day Adventist
WLGR	*Women's Lives in Greece and Rome*

Introduction

'Too bad Hippocrates didn't have Twitter 2,400 years ago, because he's a pretty quotable guy.'[1] This is how a 2017 article from the Australian Fitness Network by a sports nutrition specialist, aimed at those working in the fitness industry, summarizes the current value of Hippocrates to the modern world, before exploring various things he is supposed to have said; these include 'Let food be your medicine', 'Walking is the best medicine' and 'The natural healing force within each of us is the greatest force in getting well.' While he is by no means the only figure from the ancient world for whom there are lists of 'quotes' online,[2] whose 'words' are tweeted daily, who features as a common topic for secondary school projects, and for whom programmes, institutes, prizes, products and an online medical news service – the *Hippocratic Post* – are currently named, I believe that Hippocrates offers a particularly striking example of how the classical world is received outside the academy today.[3]

Hippocrates' role in medicine remains exceptional; as Julius Rocca noted, 'Few, if any other professional bodies today either lay claim to an abiding relationship to a figure from classical antiquity or attempt to make use of one.'[4] In the comparable case of Socrates, for whom there already exists a full study of his reception,[5] his name tends to feature in connection with various educational initiatives, such as the Aspen Institute's Socrates Program, 'a forum for emerging leaders (approximately ages 28–45) from various professions to convene and explore contemporary issues through expert-moderated dialogue'. The bilingual Socrates Academy in Matthews, North Carolina uses the Socratic method to teach the three Rs.[6] Socrates is known today for a method of 'moderated dialogue' as well as for his challenge to state religion, whereas the name of Hippocrates often carries a far more practical, material dimension: an electric juicer, a 'miraculous' face cream, a soup and a highly-controversial residential raw-food diet programme currently claim his authority, and what are assumed to be 'his' views feature extensively in support of both orthodox and alternative medicine.[7] In this book I shall mostly be using the term 'alternative', although I accept Robert Jütte's point on German uses, namely that alternative 'gives the twin mistaken impressions that there is a real alternative and that patients or clients really have a choice'; Jütte preferred 'nonconventional'.[8] As James Whorton has charted for the United States (and to a lesser extent for Britain), in the mid-1990s 'alternative' medicine became 'complementary' (suggesting its use alongside orthodox medicine) and then moved towards 'integrative' as a range of methods were employed together.[9] The warmth of that word 'integrative' is unusual in the history of the relationship between medical approaches because 'alternatives' tend to oscillate between trying to graft themselves on to the Hippocratic family tree and wanting to annihilate the established system. At a 1911 party in honour of Andrew Taylor Still, the founder of osteopathy, the toast included: 'The name that shall be blazoned out of the Skies of Science will not be Hippocrates, the Father of Medicine, but Andrew Taylor Still, the Father of the Healing Art.'[10]

Putting the Hippocratic *Oath* up in one's consulting room remains a way 'to let your patients know your role as a healer', in the words of the Christian Medical & Dental Associations, who sell a silver-framed version with the title 'A pledge to my patients'.[11] Pleas for other professions to construct an oath for themselves are widespread on social media. On the other side of the doctor–patient relationship, a site to which I shall return in Chapter 4 links to the *Oath* and exhorts readers to 'Download a copy prior to your next doctor or dental appointment and conduct a performance evaluation!'[12] Above all, however, Hippocrates' name still means compassion: 'The man who mends women: the wrath of Hippocrates' is a 2015 documentary film directed by Thierry Michel, and tells the story of Denis Mukwege and his work helping women who survived rape carried out during the violence in the Congo.[13]

Receiving Hippocrates

When I taught at the University of Reading, we offered a third-year classical reception course called 'Uses and Abuses of Antiquity'. It raised the question of where, if anywhere, we should draw the line between a valid 'use' and an invalid 'abuse'. Was the use of the Roman fasces, symbol of the power of life and death over citizens, on the Lincoln Memorial a 'use', and the presence of precisely the same symbol on door handles in a Vegas shopping mall a 'misuse'? What gives us the right to judge? More recently, teaching at Gustavus Adolphus College in Minnesota, I discussed the use of Classics as part of a course on 'Masculinities'. Should the references to the Caesars in a 1944 advertisement for Cannon bath towels and the parallels drawn there between American soldiers in Europe and the Roman army count as use, or abuse?[14] Classical reception looks at the ways in which successive ages have reinterpreted the ancient world across different media, introducing new meanings; it proposes that the meaning of a classical text always includes the response of the reader and, in the words of Charles Martindale, the 'text becomes not a fixed but a moving target, and so more difficult to hit'.[15]

But are there any limits on this movement? As a scholar of reception, I know that the professional and the lay reader of a text will read for different purposes and have different insights.[16] Yet, in responding to current receptions of Hippocrates, I also share the unease of Elizabeth Craik in her recent survey of the Hippocratic Corpus: 'Statements prefaced by "Hippocrates said ..." or "Hippocrates knew ...", all too common in general writing about early medicine, are fundamentally misplaced.'[17] In 2002, David Cantor noted that 'Until recently, most accounts of the Hippocratic tradition tended not to explain variety, but to consider whether or not the various visions and uses of Hippocrates captured something of the original figure or his insights.' The task was understood as being 'to identify the "true" Hippocrates and then to assess the authenticity of subsequent depictions of him and his medicine'.[18] What was missing, Cantor went on to argue, was any attempt to explore just why Hippocrates was shown in a particular way, at a particular time or by a particular group of people: the reception dimension. He noted the use of Hippocrates in late-1990s computer games, in which Hippocrates could be a character using medicine for world domination, or the name for a starship or an ambulance.[19] Since 2002, references to Hippocrates have continued to expand; social media and news stories have introduced him to new audiences, and in this book I shall be exploring how this happens. Many people today are not responding directly to actual treatises from the Hippocratic Corpus, but actively constructing their own Hippocrates from selected 'quotes'. This is a highly creative form of reception; it may owe nothing at all to what is in the Corpus, and in this it differs from the imaginative creations of biographies of Hippocrates which already existed from soon after his death.[20]

In many ways, 'Hippocrates now' is reminiscent of fan fiction, in which fans of a book, film or TV series write new stories using the existing characters. Yet even this is not an entirely free process: as one writer of such fiction, StillWaters1, comments, 'I write fan fiction because I love the challenge of immersing myself in established characters and worlds, and taking them to new places *while remaining true to their voices and actions* ... my goal is to sit back, get out of the way, and let the characters speak through my hands. I hope I do them credit [my italics].'[21]

The work of StillWaters1 includes a 2010 story called 'A Hippocratic Proof'.[22] In this, the original ship's doctor on the *Enterprise*, 'Bones' McCoy, is disturbed by evidence that Starfleet failed to act on evidence that a member of a survey team who rejected vaccination against pneumococcal meningitis had travelled on to another planet. He states, 'I will prevent disease wherever I can, for prevention is preferable to cure' and refers to his 'oath'; 'sometimes you wonder if you've ever been able to uphold it at all'. Mr Spock, as a Vulcan, does not understand that this comes from a modern version of the Hippocratic *Oath*, but Captain Kirk correctly identifies it as 'Not the ancient Greek version, but a more modern one adapted in the twentieth century.' Mr Spock then asks the computer to locate this version, correlates the clauses in it with McCoy's actions as recorded in the ship's log, and thus proves to McCoy that he is indeed remaining loyal to the *Oath*.[23] The story is consistent not only with the ways in which the characters speak but also with their personalities.

While fan fiction can be judged by other fans in terms of how far a writer has succeeded in 'remaining true to [the] voices and actions' of the fictional characters, this is more difficult for Hippocrates. My intention in this book is to explore further the 'visions and uses' to which Cantor referred, not across the entire history of Western medicine, but today: hence, *Hippocrates Now*. When Cantor recently revisited modern receptions of Hippocrates, he concluded that, other than in debates on ethics, he is 'no longer the point of reference in medical debates and training that he was in previous centuries.'[24] From my work on current receptions, I disagree. Hippocrates is still very much a point of reference in all sorts of medical debates, both within and beyond the mainstream. While my focus is on how he is used in medicine of all kinds, I shall also examine some of the current areas of popular culture from which people learn about Hippocrates.

Stories matter. A reviewer of a nineteenth-century work on Hippocrates noted that 'The severity of historical investigation, affords some degree of mortification to the lovers of agreeable anecdotes'.[25] In this book, I hope I shall not be unduly severe in discussing some of the stories about Hippocrates which currently circulate, because I believe that the ways in which they are told are themselves of historical interest. In his chapter for Cantor's 2002 essay collection, John Harley Warner noted 'the constitutive role that historical storytelling has played in medical culture', with retelling the story of medicine itself as 'a central ritual of professional culture'.[26] While there has always been an industry in telling stories about Hippocrates, I will investigate the extent to which the versions of Hippocrates that now surround us are specific to our age and its concerns. How do they help us to understand the uses of knowledge, specifically the uses of ancient Greek medicine, in the twenty-first century?

I am largely restricting my discussion to the English-speaking world, although there are also traditions of using Hippocrates as ancestor by alternative medicine groups in many parts of mainland Europe.[27] For each of these alternatives, just as for Western biomedicine with Hippocrates, the history was to a large extent 'the history of its founder', as Clemens von Bönninghausen put it in 1834.[28] However, alternative or non-conventional medical systems also included, and continue to include, Hippocrates in their histories. The German physician and historian Ernst-Günther Schink – the Waffen-SS's nutritional expert – was a co-author of a book on the medical value of fasting, tracing the practice, via Hildegard of Bingen, back to Hippocrates.[29] Hildegard, presented as an authentically German practitioner, still has her own internet life on the site 'Healthy Hildegard', crediting her with the 'origins of holistic health' and paying tribute to how 'a purpose-driven life can begin at 40'.[30] According to Oliver Micke and Jutta Hübner, around 3 per cent of all those living in Germany use the 'poorly defined overpriced preparations' of 'Hildegard Medicine', and 'Healthy Hildegard' also promotes the idea that Hildegard's remedies too can be traced back to Hippocrates.[31]

Nor is this just about alternative medicine: history remains important even today within Western biomedicine, whether that means creating a genealogy of continuity of practice, or evoking moral absolutes as suggested by the

Hippocratic *Oath*, to which I shall return in Chapter 4. John Harley Warner argues that, until the last third of the nineteenth century, history rather than science was the true source of orthodox physicians' authority; the power of 'two millennia of enduring tradition' summoned by the name of Hippocrates provided them with a lineage, which in turn gave them legitimacy over the various 'irregular' practitioners.[32] In this historical rewriting, Hippocrates was 'highly malleable'. Some praised him unconditionally, and others criticized him for ignorance – for example, in confusing veins and arteries – or for holding 'absurd' views, but such criticisms could be qualified on the grounds that things were different in Greece in Hippocrates' time and that perhaps a more interventionist medicine has become necessary 'now'.[33]

There also remains a thriving market for books about Hippocrates by and for orthodox medical practitioners; in the title of a 2011 collection of essays, *Hippocrates is Not Dead*.[34] He lives in Classics too: while I was completing this book, *The Cambridge Companion to Hippocrates* was published, aimed at providing 'the uninitiated reader with a first overview'. In the Introduction, the editor Peter Pormann began, 'Hippocrates remains a figure shrouded in mystery. We have next to no indubitable facts about his life' yet at the same time 'Hippocrates remains a hot topic of debate'.[35] The 1946 book *Hippocratic Wisdom*, by the biometeorologist and former professor of pathology at the University of Illinois, William Petersen, includes

> Why bother with Hippocrates when there is so much to learn in modern texts? Because today, as never before, knowledge of the historical continuity of the tradition that combines theory and practice is indispensable. The student obtaining knowledge and skill only at the top levels of the modern medical skyscraper should know something of the foundation structures and the service plants in the basement and sub-basement if he is to be something more than a technician.[36]

Petersen was drawn to Hippocrates because of passages suggesting the influence of the seasons and of weather, which resonated with his own views. *Hippocrates is Not Dead* focused on the *Oath*, taking a Roman Catholic perspective which 'explains the Hippocratic vision of medicine and its relevance to our times'.[37] The contributor John Brehany addressed his 2007 Catholic Medical Association audience as follows: 'I don't want to make the Hippocratic Oath and Tradition sound like a defensive strategy. I think they are better described as a positive and guiding resource for you in your career as physicians.'[38]

There are also recent books naming or alluding to Hippocrates which offer a more challenging call to action. For example, Michael Taylor's 2013 *Hippocrates Cried* focused on what he saw as the biggest problems in current US psychiatric medicine:

> Without thought, labels are applied and drugs with significant side effects but with only modest efficiency are prescribed. Various brands of psychotherapy are offered with little consideration of what actually helps and which patients are best suited to a particular brand. This is twenty-first century U.S. psychiatry. As a field we have in my view ignored the oath to first, do no harm.[39]

In a 2018 book entitled *Doing Harm*, Maya Dusenbery demonstrated how women are systematically left out of health care because of sex or gender bias, meaning that their symptoms are not taken as seriously as they should be.[40] The title is clearly a reference to that much-shared 'Hippocrates quote', 'First do no harm,' to which I shall return in Chapter 5, and an article mentioning Dusenbery's work opened with 'Hippocrates would be turning over in his grave. A man who admonished caregivers to do no harm, and to use food as our medicine as well to exercise regularly, has to be rather displeased with modern medicine.'[41] These claims about food and exercise will be discussed in Chapters 5 and 6.

Looking like Hippocrates

In addition to the uses of Hippocrates within mainstream and other medical systems today, there is also a much more personal connection which many who call on his name appear to feel. This connection is fed by the images of him which we see now, many of which go back to earlier generations' attempts to imagine him. Portraits and busts of Hippocrates, like framed copies of the *Oath*, are still considered appropriate ornaments for a doctor's office or consulting room. Susan Lederer has traced this trend in the construction of a medical space to the nineteenth century and cites the physician D.W. Cathell who recommended using such images as a reminder of the genealogy of medicine to which one belonged.[42]

But what should Hippocrates look like? Writing in the *British Medical Journal* in 1997, John Fabre commented that 'Many have seen a presumed likeness of "the father of medicine" – a sharp eyed, balding Greek in a toga, often under a tree'.[43] This is a reference to the very old plane tree on Cos, under which Hippocrates was supposed to have taught, and which has often been a place of pilgrimage for doctors, with seeds, leaves or branches being taken home as souvenirs; medical institutions have even cloned 'Hippocratic' plane trees, with one at the National Library of Medicine in Bethesda and another at the College of Physicians in Philadelphia.[44] Leaves from a tree at Glasgow University, grown from seeds of the one on Cos, were used by the artist Christine Borland for her 1999 works 'Spirit Collection: Hippocrates'; she was interested in the role of the family in passing on medical conditions.[45] More mundane is a gavel of wood made 'from the plane tree of Hippocrates' currently at the University Medical Center at Duke University.[46]

The tree also features in one of the four postage stamps chosen by J.V. Pai-Dhungat to illustrate a 2015 article. One of the others used a second-century CE tombstone of a physician called Jason examining a child,[47] while the other two were variations on the most famous image of all: a stone bust of Hippocrates, based on one from the Roman world, seen in the background of Rubens' portrait of his friend the doctor Ludovicus Nonnius (1553–1645) and dated to around 1627.[48] This image has an interesting history, which I have discussed in more detail elsewhere; it was used on the certificates issued to those men successfully completing his course in midwifery by William Smellie in the 1750s, an unusual move when midwifery is one of the few medical specialisms for which Hippocrates is not known.[49] Gerard Van der Gucht (1695 or 1696–1776) made an engraving based on one by Rubens in 1638, which was then used as the frontispiece to Francis Clifton's *Hippocrates upon Airs, Water and Situation; upon Epidemical Diseases; and upon Prognostics, in Acute Cases especially* (1734), a book owned by Smellie and in which he may have first seen this representation (Figure 1).[50]

In this image, Hippocrates has a receding hairline and is bearded; his forehead is lined, suggesting both thought and concern for his patient. Many current comments on his appearance reproduce images of this bust and base their written descriptions on it; for example, 'Hippocrates embodied the perfect doctor: kind, wise, old, knowledgeable, with a long beard and profound

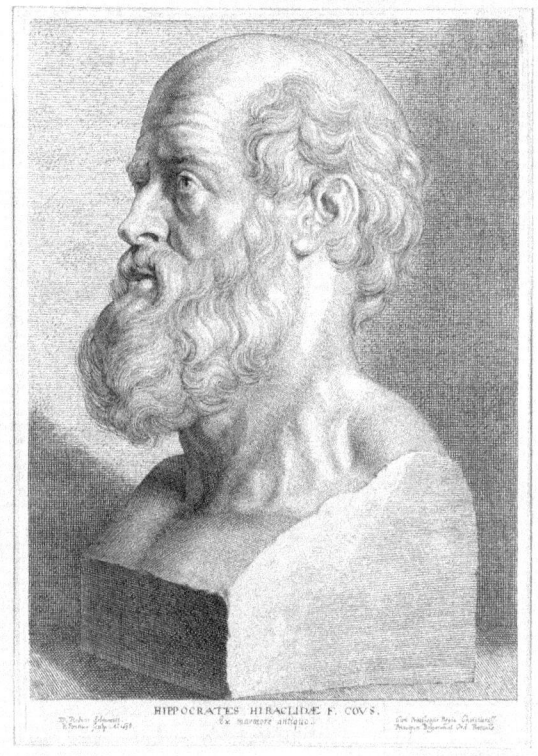

Fig. 1 Engraving: portrait of Hippocrates from Francis Clifton, *Hippocrates upon Airs, Water and Situation; upon Epidemical Diseases; and upon Prognostics, in Acute Cases especially* (London: J. Watts, 1734), frontispiece. Wellcome Collection. CC BY.

wrinkles around perceptive eyes. At least that is what we'd like to think.'[51] While scholars have noted from at least the end of the nineteenth century that the representations of Hippocrates 'are all without authority',[52] this does not stop people viewing them as potentially, or actually, realistic.[53]

The Rubens Hippocrates was not, however, the only option available to those who wanted to know what the great man looked like. Other images available to writers in the eighteenth century showed him with a full head of hair, as in Linden's *Magni Hippocratis Coi opera omnia* of 1665, where he is shown writing; a herb and some surgical instruments complete the picture (Figure 2).[54]

This claimed to be a 'genuine' representation, based on an old coin from Constantinople, although of course that made it no more genuine than any other; nothing survives from Hippocrates' own time.[55] The iconography of

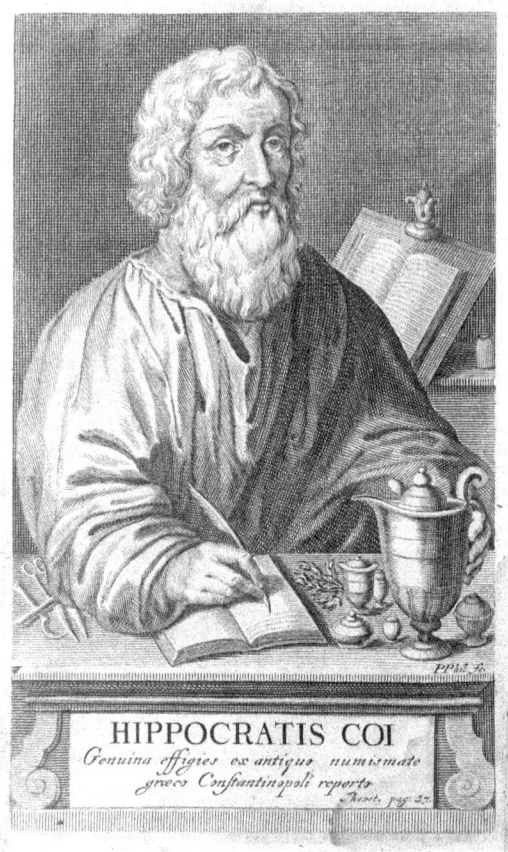

Fig. 2 Portrait of Hippocrates from Johannes Antonides van der Linden, *Magni Hippocratis Coi opera omnia* (Lugduni Batavorum [Leiden]: Gaasbeeck, 1665), frontispiece. Wellcome Collection. CC BY.

Hippocrates interacts with the texts in the 'Hippocratic Corpus'; one of these, *On the Physician*, describes how a doctor should look healthy, and an image that probably originated in the late third century BCE represented him to match this text, as 'a well-fed, confident, partly bald elderly man'.[56] In Benjamin Rush's 1806 lecture 'On the opinions and modes of practice of Hippocrates,' he was envisaged as 'Mild in his appearance, and dignified in his deportment, with gray hairs loosely flowing over his shoulders.'[57]

The balding Hippocrates, however, remains the dominant image, even today. Some images still identified as 'Hippocrates' show him with very little hair at all.[58] In *Assassin's Creed: Odyssey*, released in summer 2018, the character Alexios even makes a joke about how Hippocrates doesn't like anyone to mention his lack of hair.⁵⁹ The idea that he was bald goes back to the biographies that circulated in the ancient world, one of which claims that this is why he was shown with his cloak pulled over his head, as in this image from Daniel Le Clerc's 1699 *The History of Physick* (Figure 3), but there were other explanations given; for example, that his head was weak, a claim based on another early biography which stated that he had a rather small body and a weak head, possibly derived from Aristotle's comment that Hippocrates did not owe his title 'the great' to his physical size.⁶⁰ Other explanations for the head-covering were: because he had been initiated into the Mysteries at Eleusis; because the head is the seat of the soul; or simply that pulling it over his head meant 'that it might not hinder him in his business'.⁶¹ Le Clerc's Hippocrates is leaner and more hungry than the 'well-fed, confident, partly bald elderly man' with whom we are familiar today.

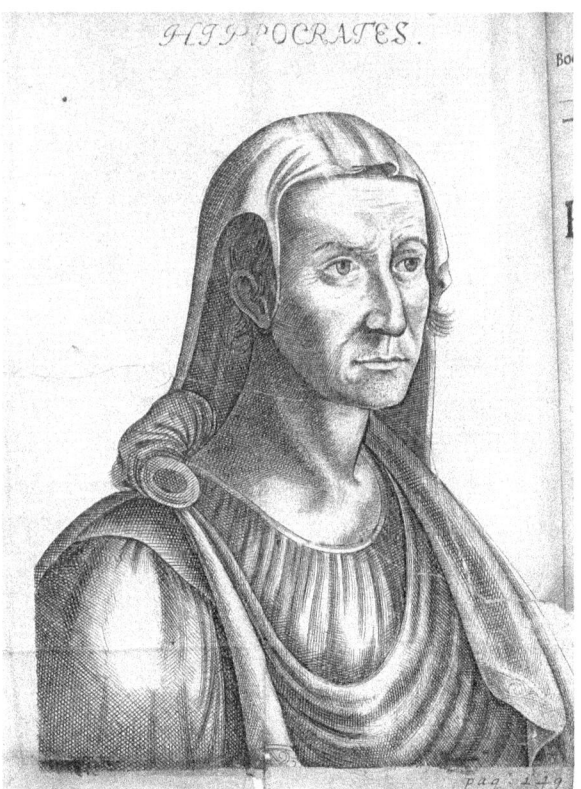

Fig. 3 Daniel Le Clerc, *The History of Physick, or, an account of the rise and progress of the art* (London: D Brown et al., 1699). Wellcome Collection. CC BY.

Hairs of Hippocrates

Exploring current variations on the historical baldness theme provides a good introduction to how we construct Hippocrates now. He must – of course! – have known how to look after himself, simply because he was the Father of Medicine: 'He did live a healthy life to about (estimated to be around 115 years of age) and was considered one of the greatest physicians of his time.'[62] The baldness has historically been one of the unusual situations in which the normal 'Hippocrates was right' trope does not apply; the other is, of course, his death. On the answers.com site, a suggested answer to the question 'What was Hippocrates [sic] cause of death?' is 'He died of natural causes he tried to cure himself but the medicine he took just was not strong enough so he passed away.'[63] With baldness, the message may be that Hippocrates could cure it, so we should look to Hippocrates, but instead it is more commonly that, despite the 'fact' that even Hippocrates couldn't find a cure for it, there may be one now; the story usually leads up to a claim for the efficacy of a new treatment being advertised or to a news report of such a treatment.

The Linden image with a full head of hair is used on a Belgian site promoting hair loss prevention, 'a battle as old as history itself': here, Hippocrates is a hero of hair loss, who came up with his own formula to prevent it and who was the first to observe that eunuchs did not suffer from it.[64] On the Wikipedia English-language Hippocrates page – something to which I shall return throughout this book, and particularly in Chapter 3, because it remains the main source for other online and print stories – a claim was added on 1 October 2011 by user 'Doctor ash karen' that 'The most severe form of hair loss and baldness is called the Hippocratic form.' The source given was a dead web link, to 'The dilemma of balding solve [sic] by father of medicine Hippocrates. Healthy Hair Highlights News. 15 August 2011'.[65] While this may count as advertising, something forbidden on Wikipedia, it was not identified as such; instead, user 'WANAX' simply moved it within the article to what he or she thought was 'a more fitting place'.[66] The original link was reported as dead in April 2012,[67] but it is reasonable to suppose that it originally went to a variant on the very common online story to the effect that 'Hippocrates had a personal interest in finding a cure for baldness as he suffered from hair loss. He developed a number of different treatments including a mixture of horseradish, cumin, pigeon droppings, and nettles to the scalp. This and other treatments failed to work and he lost the rest of his hair.'[68]

This is from 'Alopecia World'; in other sites, both in the 'weird and wacky facts' genre and in advertising for private medicine, he 'was plagued by' or 'personally grappled with' male pattern baldness.[69] It is interesting that the 'Alopecia World' version does not have Hippocrates 'solve' balding; on the contrary, his self-treatment makes it worse. Elsewhere, 'He prescribed himself and fellow chrome domes a topical concoction of opium, horseradish, pigeon droppings, beetroot and spices. It didn't stop anyone's hairline from receding.'[70] A similar story is that the 'potion' 'Containing beetroot, horseradish, pigeon droppings, spices and opium ... was an abject failure.'[71] The pigeon droppings aspect remains most striking to modern readers, but in the ancient world these were known as a form of animal excrement with no bad smell.[72]

In Chapter 4 I shall focus on how Hippocrates plays out in news stories today. The story of his baldness is regularly retold to preface any apparent breakthrough in treating male pattern baldness, and in contrast to these modern developments the ancient remedy may be presented not only as ineffective, but as positively harmful. For example, a 2005 discussion on a hair loss forum repeated an article from *The Independent* to the effect that his 'concoction proved disastrous. Hippocrates became ever balder, so much so that, even now, extreme cases of hair loss are referred to as "Hippocratic baldness".'[73] In 2007, *The Times* described Hippocrates' remedy as 'a blend of pigeon droppings, cumin, horseradish and beet-root'; an earlier story on the same topic in the same newspaper – 'Then and now: Baldness' – instead had Hippocrates 'slapping on a mixture of opium, horseradish, pigeon droppings and beetroot. It didn't work. He got so sparse that hairlessness became called "Hippocratic baldness".'[74] In addition to showing how dependent on each other these stories are, this also demonstrates the variation in the ingredients named; opium often replaces cumin. Sometimes some perfumes are added to the mix; for example, in some versions he uses 'an ointment of opium and essence of roses. His hair failed to grow back. He then tried a formulation of acacia oil and wine. Again, no luck', a version which featured in a 1982 medical book as 'opium with the essence of lilies or roses, mixed with wine and olive oil'.[75]

Perhaps unexpectedly, this remedy does indeed originate from the Hippocratic Corpus. Historically, the use of irritant substances – usually combined with something to make the whole thing smell more appealing – has been standard for hair regrowth remedies across the ages, whether for men or for women.[76] But this particular remedy has nothing to do with male pattern baldness, let alone with Hippocrates himself, and it does not include opium. It comes from the gynaecological treatise, *Diseases of Women* (2.189), where it sits between recipes for face packs and freckle removal. Laurence Totelin translates this recipe for hair loss in women as 'If she loses hair, apply as a cataplasm: cumin or excrement of pigeons, or crushed radish, or <rub?> with crushed onion, or beet, or nettle.'[77]

Writing this book

I regard this book not only as a study of the contemporary Hippocrates, but also as a case study in how classical studies plays out in news media, social media and the internet more broadly. Because of users' personal engagement with Hippocrates and because of the invocation of his name to support claims made for modern methods of healing and promoting wellbeing, it is an extreme example, but no less valuable for that.

The way we do history has changed completely in the last decade or so. When writing my earlier books, I spent many days travelling to many libraries, but for this my main resource has been the internet, supplemented by the Wellcome Collection in London. Even where I am citing books, for those published before 1923 I have more likely than not read them in full-text online, for example through my access to the superb library of The Open Library but also through open-access projects such as the Internet Archive.[78] For what is not available online, I have expanded my personal collection of books by purchasing second-hand copies sourced online: often cheaper than the fare to a library holding a copy. I have used a range of search engines, joined social media platforms, blogged, commented on other blogs and become a Wikipedia editor. For the last five years or so, I have also had a range of Google alerts giving me weekly summaries of where key terms like 'Hippocrates' have featured. For any scholar today, social media provide wonderful opportunities not only to keep up with what is happening in the field but also to interact with other academics. I have gained enormously from the community of scholars of medieval medicine on MEDMED-L, founded in 2008 and moderated by its founder, Monica Green. At points when I have been stuck on a particularly annoying question – such as whether a quote widely attributed to Sir William Osler is authentic – Twitter rapidly connected me with the best possible library and, in this instance, with its supportive librarian, Mary Hague-Yearl.

There are many hazards to this sort of approach. Not everyone who knows about a topic is on social media. The quantity of what is digitized does not yet even match what is not, and I shall discuss this further later in this book when looking at specific examples. Web searches are, of course, fallible. One of the reasons why errors about ancient and medieval medicine persist in work written by those in the field of medicine is that they rely on searching for key words in PubMed and Medline, which do not include work from history journals, and therefore miss the most recent research.[79] My earlier experiences of using databases like Early English Books Online (EEBO) or Eighteenth Century Collections Online (ECCO) taught me the hazards of spelling, which the feature of 'fuzzy search' cannot resolve; in some earlier research, I realized that searching for the character 'Phaethousa' was never going to work when she was called 'Phetula' by some seventeenth-century writers, while others told her story but completely omitted her name![80] Searching for sources for this book, it was clear that looking for the complete phrase 'First do no harm' would not only miss those who simply quote 'Do no harm' but would also pass over those who reverse the image, as in the title *Doing Harm*, used for a 2014 thriller by Kelly Parsons set in a hospital[81] and also for a 2018 book by Maya Dusenbery exposing sex and gender bias in modern biomedicine today which I have already mentioned.[82] Google Books has rightly been compared to reading tea-leaves, not just because of its missing pages but because claims that it can be used to track the changing popularity of key terms or the emergence of words and phrases simply do not understand the nature of its materials.[83] Many of my references are to websites, and by the time you read this book some will have died; I apologise now for this, and searching for keywords will often bring you to a site's new location online.

Bearing in mind my subject, it is worth clarifying here that I am not medically-trained, although I worked for nearly a decade as a visiting professor at what was then the Peninsula Medical School in Truro, where I taught a special subject group on the history of dissection. I am, however, as we all are, a patient. As such, I have benefitted from half a dozen or so surgical procedures, some of them major. I have also used a range of alternative medicines, including homeopathy and osteopathy. The polite way of putting this would be to say that my approach to medicine is 'eclectic', but I have no particular axe to grind.

In the rest of this book, I want to begin by looking at what we know about Hippocrates, before addressing what we used to think we knew. After establishing the current status of Hippocrates in the study of ancient medicine, I will look at the other places where we meet him today. This will include a detailed study of a particular story which was spread by Wikipedia – the main authority for anyone wanting to learn the basics about him – as well as news stories which illustrate how we veer from regarding him as the Father of Medicine who was by definition 'right', to using him to set up a gulf between the weird ancient and the entirely sensible and properly understood modern. I shall then focus on the short quotes which are the main means of spreading his alleged message today, before looking at the broader picture, through the current focus on him as holistic. The reception of Hippocrates today goes beyond what Cantor called 'playful flexibility' or Michel de Certeau called 'the reader's impertinence', and into matters of life and death.[84] All of these are 'Hippocrates Now'.

1

What We Know About Hippocrates

Hippocrates lived in classical Greece and was associated with the island of Cos. He gained a reputation as a writer and a medical doctor.

2

What We Thought We Knew

I was tempted to start this book with a blank sheet because it would represent, more vividly than words could ever do, our lack of knowledge about the historical figure behind this book, and of the sort of medicine he advocated.[1] Yet we still need to talk about Hippocrates. His name holds power; any internet search for 'Hippocrates quotes' will reveal many aphorisms and passages being attributed to the Father of Medicine, imparting his 'wisdom' for today while using him to support a range of medical practices. Not necessarily even deriving from what we call the 'Hippocratic Corpus' – the collection of ancient Greek treatises traditionally associated with his name – these phrases and sentences draw on an image of Hippocrates as 'a good practical physician', the voice of reason, a sympathetic observer, a careful recorder of experience, courageous and honest, and a patriot; character traits which themselves come out of those treatises which different historical periods have chosen to include in the Hippocratic Corpus.[2] In the 1950s, he was even seen as morally at 'the level of the greatest Christian', a view shared by Herbert Ratner, for whom 'Hippocrates comes closer to God in his vision of medicine' than did contemporary medical education.[3]

To quote from a popular history of medicine, '"In truth we know little or nothing of Hippocrates," says one historian, preparatory to writing of him at length': I am aware that the number of pages in this chapter suggests that I have fallen into this trap, as described by the late poet and satirist Richard Armour.[4] But it is important to realize that the invocation of the name of Hippocrates is far from new. A Latin treatise based on sections of the Hippocratic *Diseases of Women 2*, preserved in two French manuscripts from the ninth century, raises the value of what follows by adding a prologue that hails him: 'Herald of truth and master who does not lie, as if made out of the seed of the gods, unique in the world, Hippocrates illuminated the art of medicine and provided good health to the human race.'[5] What is perhaps most surprising is the longevity of this inspiring and positive image. Patients today, apparently, even 'wonder aloud at how nice it might be to have Hippocrates as their doctor.'[6] Why? Perhaps because the other options are so unattractive, as in a 1991 book title, *Hitler or Hippocrates?*[7] More commonly, however, Hippocrates is contrasted with mainstream medicine in a series of binaries, summarized here by David Newman:

> Hippocrates was a holistic practitioner intent on treating the complete person, whereas today we tend to specialize in exquisitely narrow fields of anatomic and physiologic knowledge, leaving the balance of the human body to our colleagues. Hippocrates was a devoted and objective empiricist, while most modern doctors spend so little time with each patient that it's absurd to claim serious observational skills. Hippocrates was a consummate communicator, while today's doctors (ask our patients) are walking communication nightmares. Hippocrates felt and demonstrated sympathy, while we've chosen a colder, more 'scientific' model for doctor-patient interaction...[8]

This summary already takes us into the central aim of this book: to explore the versions of 'Hippocrates' which are dominant at present, considering why so many variations are possible, and discussing what they tell us both about how the internet does history and also about our continued need for a 'Father of Medicine'. Even that title is controversial, and not just because of other claimants, an aspect to which I shall return in Chapter 3. In language that resembles the wording of those ninth-century gynaecological manuscripts, a letter which forms part of the very earliest Hippocratic tradition describes him as 'father of health, saviour, soother of pain . . . leader in the divine science'.[9] So, which is he to be: saviour or scientist, Father of Medicine or Father of Health? Although it is rarely used today, 'Father of Health' seems more appropriate for the current association of Hippocrates with holistic medicine, to which I shall return in Chapter 7.

Not only the first and the best, Hippocrates is real, and his authority depends on this.[10] Suggestions that perhaps he did not really exist are labelled in religious terms as 'heresy' or 'sacrilege'.[11] Since at least the early Roman empire, the underlying message of almost – but not quite – all users of the name of Hippocrates is not just that he was real, and great, but that 'Hippocrates was so spot-on', 'Smart man he was', and 'Hippocrates was right'.[12] This last statement has been chosen for titles of articles promoting allegedly Hippocratic aphorisms such as 'walking is the best medicine' or 'all disease begins in the gut', to which I shall return in Chapters 5 and 6.[13] Why do we so badly want to believe in an omniscient Hippocrates today?

Before focusing on 'Hippocrates now', however, we need some sense of the basics. In this chapter, I shall consider not only some answers that are now being given, but some which have historically been offered, to the question of what, if anything, Hippocrates wrote: something we need to think about if we are to decide whether or not he was 'right'. Most probably, in my view, nothing that survives can be attributed to him but, while my virtually-empty Chapter 1 will be controversial, this is hardly a new stance to adopt: this was also the position taken by Ludwig Edelstein in 1939.[14]

The absence of any words which we can confidently attribute to Hippocrates himself does seem odd, bearing in mind his fame, and living with this absence can be painful. In 1939, Edelstein warned that 'The longing to read Hippocrates' own writings, the difficulty of becoming reconciled to the fact that they are not extant, should at any rate be no reason for setting up the methodological postulate that they must have been preserved.'[15] Here, Edelstein correctly identified the extra dimension of 'longing', also noted by Jaap Mansfeld in a 1980 article in which he described the 'emotional' reasons why we would like to attribute certain treatises to Hippocrates himself.[16] This is never just about the head: in the afterlife of Hippocrates, the heart too plays its part.

The translator of the earliest volumes of the Loeb Classical Library edition of the works of the Corpus, W.H.S. Jones, wrote in 1923 that 'Ignorance and uncertainty seem to be the final result of most of the interesting problems presented by the Hippocratic collection.'[17] However, none of this closes our questions down, because we still need to know why, over the course of two and a half millennia of Hippocratic reception, some treatises have been considered his own work. I shall outline this here, and also address the further question of who Hippocrates was, or at least what he has represented to those invoking his name to claim his authority for what they say. Some scholars of ancient medicine consider that 'even if some measure of doubt inevitably remains, the personality of Hippocrates himself no longer remains blurred as it once was'.[18] Is that the case? Who was Hippocrates?

Hippocrates as God and Galen as his prophet?[19]

There is one person whose contribution to what we thought we knew about Hippocrates deserves special attention: Galen, the great second-century CE physician who claimed to be Hippocrates' true interpreter and heir, and who selected Hippocrates 'to personify medical authority'.[20] In his McGovern lecture of 1998, Paul Potter, who translated a number of the most recently published volumes of the Loeb Classical Library Hippocrates, argued that the proposition that Hippocrates wrote none of the treatises in the Hippocratic Corpus was as improbable as the claim that he wrote them all.[21] But which treatises, if any?

The sixty or so treatises included in the Hippocratic Corpus remain, as Wesley Smith put it, 'stubbornly anonymous'.[22] Ann Hanson goes further: 'there is nothing to connect "Hippocrates", the famous physician from Cos mentioned by Plato and Aristotle, with any single medical treatise in our present Hippocratic *Corpus*'.[23] As summarized by Geoffrey Lloyd in 1991, when he revisited his 1975 article on the historic 'Hippocratic question' – which if any of the treatises is by Hippocrates? – 'the evidence we have allows us in *no* case to be confident that a work is by Hippocrates himself' [author's italics].[24] In a later work he reiterated the point that 'None can reliably be attributed to Hippocrates himself, the famous doctor mentioned by both Plato and Aristotle ... Many treatises are, in any case, compilations, the work of several different writers.'[25]

When it came to the big picture Galen, while he agreed that one treatise may contain the work of more than one author, thought very differently: work attributed to Hippocrates could be authentic. He not only wrote commentaries on the many treatises he attributed to the great man but also a work, now lost, entitled *On the Authentic and Spurious Writings of Hippocrates*.[26] Over the many centuries in which people have asked the 'Hippocratic question', the only part of the Corpus which has been given a firm author of any kind is the third section of one of the treatises in the Corpus, and that attribution was on Galen's recommendation. In his commentary on the treatise *On the Nature of Man*, Galen argued that the first section was by Hippocrates himself, the second part was anonymous (and wrong; although perhaps his logic is rather that it is wrong, and therefore anonymous), and the third part was by Polybus, disciple and sometimes also named as son-in-law of Hippocrates.²⁷ There has been widespread acceptance of this Polybus authorship, but not of Galen's views on the earlier parts of this treatise.²⁸

As Eric Nelson has recently pointed out, nobody whose work is in the Hippocratic Corpus used the word 'Hippocratic' of a person or of an idea; 'Hippocrates, after all, might have been no more aware that he was Hippocratic than Jesus might have been aware that he was "Christian"'.²⁹ By the time of Galen, the label had come into use: what did it mean? Véronique Boudon-Millot has examined Galen's use of the adjective ἱπποκράτειος and has shown that, when he applies this word to a person, it is usually to criticize 'Hippocrateans' for failing to understand the text or the doctrine of Hippocrates; or, to put it another way, to show that not everyone who announced they were Hippocratic should be taken as such.³⁰ In his approach to Hippocrates, Galen thus presented himself as the true prophet.

None of this, however, is straightforward, and it is clear that Galen drew on his own beliefs about medicine as the yardstick by which to measure which works from the Corpus he would dignify as being by Hippocrates himself.³¹ This made the creation of Galen's Hippocrates into a circular process: to quote Geoffrey Lloyd, 'it is not just that Galen agrees with Hippocrates: it is rather that Hippocrates serves as a key authority for the views that he, Galen, favours', with the four-humour theory of the earlier part of *On the Nature of Man* conveniently forming the basis of Galen's own medical theories.³² So Galen's version of Hippocrates is, in the words of Ann Hanson, 'an Hippocrates who is very much like Galen himself', even though his uses of Hippocrates are so various that Jacques Jouanna comments 'Galen's Hippocrates is frankly puzzling at times'.³³ To quote Rebecca Flemming, 'For Galen the "divine Hippocrates" was a key figure in the construction of his own medical authority, as he laid claim to be the true heir of the founding father of Greek medicine' and 'it is his version of the Hippocratic tradition, his interpretation of Hippocratic thinking, which has transmitted itself most effectively down the ages.'³⁴

What was this interpretation? Most important to Galen as truly 'Hippocratic' were ideas about the innate/acquired heat of the body, and the four elements, humours and qualities. According to him, *On the Nature of Man* should be seen as the 'foundation' for all that Hippocrates discovered.³⁵ Yet, within the

Hippocratic Corpus, the four-humour theory of *On the Nature of Man* is only one option on offer, for both the number and the identity of the humours (here, blood, phlegm, black bile and yellow bile); however, because of Galen's elevation of this treatise the other models, in which there were different numbers of fluids or simply fire and water in opposition, had no future.[36] In the popular imagination, Hippocrates remains all about the humours: in one quest in the game *Assassin's Creed: Odyssey*, when Hippocrates visits a patient the woman who has called him in confidently tells him that the problem here is 'phlegm'.[37] As well as four humours, there were also four elements (earth, air, fire, water), four qualities (hot, cold, wet, dry), four age groups (infancy, youth, maturity, old age) and four temperaments (sanguine, phlegmatic, choleric, melancholy), and these could be mapped on to each other, a process which began with Galen but which was elaborated in subsequent medicine.[38] The relationship between Galen and his 'Hippocrates' has recently been revisited by Jim Hankinson, who comments on the role of the four elements that 'in fact Galen and "Hippocrates" have rather different views about both the nature and identity of the elements, even as Galen seeks to elide that fact'.[39]

Galen's 'Hippocrates' is not always what he seems, part of the wider issue that he works with a 'peculiar version of medical history'.[40] Boudon-Millot has asked 'To what extent did Galen himself believe in the Hippocrates whom he had thus created?' and Hankinson concludes that '[Galen's] Hippocrates is, in a sense, a construction. But he is, I believe, a legitimate interpretative construction.'[41] This raises the question: who determines legitimacy? Galen decided what the historical Hippocrates had written, by prioritizing the treatises that matched his own views, so that if any of his contemporaries were to challenge Galen, they would also be starting a fight with Hippocrates. Like many doctors in more recent history, Galen wanted Hippocrates on his side, and was prepared for a certain amount of massaging of the evidence in order to keep him there. His influence is far-reaching, and not just on our views of what Hippocrates wrote and believed. As Wesley Smith has demonstrated, where he tells us something about ancient medicine – for example, that doctors used to be educated by family members and this training included dissection – 'it has been taken as primary evidence about the Coan school. People cite it, and they do not cite anything else, *because there is nothing* [my italics].'[42]

Finding a Hippocratic treatise

If we try to forget the many centuries dominated by Galen's view of what was really by Hippocrates, what other contenders are there in the Corpus? While modern authors still pursue the 'Hippocratic question', the most ancient biographers of Hippocrates showed no interest in coming up with lists of what he really wrote.[43] Even as far back as the first century CE, it was at least clear to those who worked on the Hippocratic Corpus that it could not all be by a single author, because different medical theories, practices, behaviours and styles exist among those anonymous treatises which have at some time carried his name.[44] For example, the *Oath* prohibits abortive pessaries, while *Generation/Nature of the Child* sees a doctor encouraging a slave girl to dislodge her pregnancy by jumping up and down. In a work dedicated to Nero's doctor, Andromachus, the first-century CE Greek lexicographer Erotian gave a list of what he considered authentic works by Hippocrates, based in turn on a third-century list by Bacchius of Tanagra; the aim of both writers was to explain unusual words, and the Hippocratic texts provided plenty of examples of those. Erotian's list remained the basis of editions of the Corpus made in the nineteenth century.[45] However, as Pilar Pérez Cañizares recently noted, there are treatises which we now consider 'Hippocratic' but which are mentioned by neither Erotian nor Galen.[46]

Despite the lack of any firm evidence, there has long been a scholarly industry based on trying to show that one or more of the extant treatises is by Hippocrates himself. In the second half of the sixteenth century, the 'Paris Hippocratics' favoured the treatises *Coan Prognoses* and *Epidemics*; the case history format of much of the *Epidemics* sits particularly easily with a Hippocrates who is all about observation and a good bedside manner.[47] At the same time, Petrus Severinus was challenging Galen's claims for Hippocratic authorship of part of *On the Nature of Man* while attacking Galen's followers as having 'placed Hippocrates's name on their ignorance'. For him, occult philosophy and the chemical ideas of Paracelsus were closer to true Hippocratic medicine, and *Ancient Medicine* and *Regimen 1* had better claims to Hippocratic authorship.[48] In the seventeenth century, Thomas Sydenham, who studied epidemic disease, presented an empirical, theory-averse Hippocrates and favoured not only *Epidemics* but also *Prognostics* and *Aphorisms* as genuine works, so that – recalling Galen – 'the Hippocrates that Sydenham perceived in those works was the Hippocrates most like himself'.[49] In the nineteenth century, Houdart argued for *Prorrhetic* and *Coan Prognoses*, with their inclusion of named patients, as preceding *Prognostics*, because the latter moved beyond these individuals to become 'a much more finished production'; on this argument from style and from assumptions about how science develops, the first two must predate Hippocrates with *Prognostics* being by the great man himself.[50]

Turning to a more recent period, and to classicists rather than practising physicians, in the 1980s Mansfeld supported the authenticity of *Airs Waters Places*: Wesley Smith, of *On Regimen*.[51] All such attempts are a matter of arguing a case, made more difficult by the lack of external evidence, and so far – even with several decades of computer analysis of word frequency and vocabulary choices – the scholarly jury has remained out.[52] Without internal evidence from the Corpus stating what Hippocrates' own views were, it is always going to be difficult to reconstruct the historical Hippocrates. The danger remains that we simply follow Galen by picking a treatise we like, and deciding that this must be by Hippocrates.

Sometimes, the reverse happens: a treatise in the Corpus is so poorly written, or proposes such an implausible theory, that its readers decide it cannot be by Hippocrates, but then discovery of new evidence means that what was previously dismissed needs to be re-evaluated. The outstanding example was the discovery in 1890 of the first- or second-century CE *Anonymus Londinensis* papyrus, which probably relates to a previously-lost book which Galen described; a work by a disciple of Aristotle called Menon, summarizing ancient medical theories. *Anonymus Londinensis* may be 'a later abstract' based on Menon's work: it does not quote from it verbatim, and it may be influenced by Stoic philosophy.[53] When giving the beliefs of Hippocrates, the writer of the text on the papyrus reports that he thought changes in 'breaths' – gases left over from the process of digestion – cause disease. This meant that the Hippocratic treatise *On Breaths* (or *On Winds*), usually dismissed as 'the work of a second-rate Sophist, indeed of a mere gossipmonger', started to look like a truly Hippocratic piece; although, for those who were not happy about attributing these ideas to him, there was always a let-out clause by saying it was by a different 'Hippocrates', by arguing that Menon 'distorts the material he excerpts in the direction of his own ideas', or by suggesting that the original of Menon has here been 'rather seriously rewritten'.[54]

David Wootton, in *Bad Medicine: Doctors doing harm since Hippocrates*, acknowledges that 'modern scholars argue that these works were written over a period of two hundred years or so, and that it is quite possible that none of them are actually by Hippocrates', but also asserts that the treatise *Fractures* has one of the best claims to be by Hippocrates himself; his source for this view is not given.[55] However, ultimately it must be Galen, who wrote one of his earliest commentaries on it, his purpose in these being to explain anything unclear in the original Greek: the series of commentaries began with those works he thought most likely to be by Hippocrates himself, which were the surgical treatises.[56]

This tradition of *Fractures* as the real thing was picked up in 1849 when Francis Adams was asked by the Sydenham Society to produce an English translation of 'the genuine works of Hippocrates': the title of the two volumes he went on to publish.[57] He aimed to translate only 'the whole of those Treatises which are now regarded as genuine'; even the use of 'now' reveals the continuing disagreement on what was by Hippocrates. Adams considered he was translating a single author whose work was a model of 'excellence' and who had brought the medical art to 'perfection'.[58] Like everyone else, he interpreted the history of medicine in terms of the context of his own world – what else could he have done? – referring to 'many intelligent Mesmerists of the present day', and to the principle of 'Animal magnetism'.[59]

Adams expressed his 'enthusiastic admiration' for Hippocrates as a 'bold operator', making *Fractures* a 'genuine work' because of the similarities between the treatments offered with those of his own time: on club foot, Adams believed that 'In a word, until the days of Delpech and Stromeyer, no one entertained ideas so sound and scientific on the nature of this deformity as Hippocrates'.[60] In her recent excellent survey of the Hippocratic Corpus, Elizabeth Craik answered her own question, 'Who wrote the surgical works, and for whom; why, when and where?' with 'We can only guess.' In addition to echoing Adams' admiration for the clinical knowledge shown, she points out that the Greek prose style of *Fractures* and *Joints* is 'remarkable'; they were 'surely written for posterity'.[61] She therefore concludes that here 'Perhaps indeed we have the words of Hippocrates.'[62]

I have already mentioned the lack of external evidence for Hippocrates' ideas, the *Anonymus Londinensis* papyrus being a rare exception. As a reviewer for the *Edinburgh Medical and Surgical Journal* put it in 1839, 'It is certainly a remarkable circumstance, that Hippocrates should have been so little mentioned, either by contemporaries, or by the principal historians, for a long period after his time.'[63] In the search for the authentic Hippocrates, many have tried to find such evidence in Aristotle and Plato, whose mentions of him are the closest literary evidence to the supposed lifetime of the man himself.

The fame of the name can be traced back to two brief references in Plato's dialogues, in which Socrates helps people to understand a topic by questioning them on it; however, Plato never quotes directly from any Hippocratic treatise. In the *Protagoras*, set in around 433 BCE but written over thirty years later, there is a reference to 'Hippocrates of Cos the Asclepiad' who teaches medicine for a fee, just as a famous sculptor like Phideas of Athens teaches his apprentices: in *Phaedrus*, set in the period between 411 and 404 BCE but again written over thirty years after its dramatic date, we are told that the way Hippocrates 'the Asclepiad' studies a part is by understanding the whole, and then that anything complex is best understood by first understanding its constituent parts. It is not clear, however, whether the medical application of this would be needing to know about the whole body in order to understand its parts, or understanding the body only by understanding 'nature' as a whole.[64] In both references, Plato uses Hippocrates for his own purposes; for example, studying the part by understanding the whole is also how Plato's character of Socrates thinks the soul should be approached. Plato is just the first of many to interpret 'the available information about Hippocrates's method on the basis of his own system of thought'.[65]

As I mentioned in the Introduction, Aristotle also mentions Hippocrates, in a very casual way that suggests his audience would know of him as someone 'great by reason of his science rather than of his size'; does this imply that Hippocrates was unusually small in stature, or is that pushing it too far?[66] None of these snippets, other than the parts/whole one and the labelling of Hippocrates as an 'Asclepiad' – perhaps as a claimed descendent of the semi-divine Asclepius, famous for his healing skills, or perhaps by then merely a generic word for 'healer' – offer much help to those trying to find a genuine treatise in the Hippocratic Corpus.[67]

Making a Corpus

And what about the Corpus and its relationship to Hippocrates? Who put these texts together under his name? Was their collection haphazard, or focused? The individual treatises of the Hippocratic Corpus represent some of the very earliest ancient Greek prose writing, and their merger into a corpus began at the end of the fourth century BCE.[68] In 1990, Wesley Smith stated that 'It remains a mystery how and over what period of time the Corpus itself, so heterogeneous and of diverse qualities and points of view, came into being.'[69] Overall, Lesley Dean-Jones memorably suggested that the Corpus grew 'more like an octopus than a snowball' while Pilar Pérez Cañizares characterized its contents as 'haphazard and probably based more on chance than on any sort of intended quality control'.[70] Others would change the emphasis. Jacques Jouanna proposed 'an ancient and globally coherent core that can be seen as constituting a distinctly Hippocratic style of thought'; because Hippocrates was from Cos, this would be a Coan core, to which treatises from Cnidos – once considered the rival medical establishment to that of Hippocrates – were then added, with various others coming in after the first century CE.[71]

For anyone wanting to create a narrative about how these texts came to cluster together, the Great Library at Alexandria – object of many scholarly and not-so-scholarly fantasies about a past in which all knowledge was to be found in one place – was an obvious venue to select. The idea of a library founded to 'collect, if possible, all the books in the world' comes from what may be the earliest extant source for the library: a letter claiming to be by a second-century BCE writer, Aristeas, which stated that the library holdings had already passed 200,000 books.[72] However, this letter appears to be Jewish propaganda for the translation of the Hebrew Bible into Greek; it has many factual errors and there is no reason to believe what it says about either the purpose or the size of the library. Roger Bagnall has pointed to 'the unreal character' of much of what has been written about the library, here and subsequently: the library has achieved what Susan Stephens labelled 'almost mythic status . . . in Western discourse'.[73]

In *The Hippocratic Tradition*, first published in 1979, Wesley Smith picked up Max Wellmann's 1929 suggestion that a 'careless librarian' in Alexandria had 'indiscriminately lumped the most discrepant works together under

Hippocrates' name and in the process effectively effaced any evidence for attributing them correctly'.[74] And this was not the only 'lost library' speculation. The great nineteenth-century French editor of the Corpus, Emile Littré, also looked to Alexandria for the origin of the Corpus, but suggested that the texts were mostly from a single family's library.[75] One of the few things we know about Hippocrates, via Plato, was that he came from/worked on Cos. In the 1920s, Johannes Ilberg suggested that there had been a library there, and that this was merged with the library from Cnidos and moved to Alexandria, where all the treatises were considered to be by Hippocrates.[76] Jones, too, thought that the Hippocratic collection as we now have it looks exactly like a modern medical school library – or at least what one would have looked like in the 1920s – and 'indeed a school of medicine, like that which had its home at Cos, could not well have done without one'. This would account for some treatises which are not very impressive – they could be books 'of no great interest or value, presented to the library or acquired by chance'.[77] One myth about Hippocrates is that he burned the library on Cos (or, in a variant, on Cnidos!), 'presumably so that he could take credit for inventing the treatments themselves'; the earliest evidence for this is the mid-third century BCE Andreas, *On Medical Genealogy*.[78] Burning, rather than collecting, books seems an unlikely move for a hero; but, while Jouanna dismissed the story as 'malicious' and 'slanderous' and suggested that it 'scarcely deserves attention', Pinault suggests that an unflattering story like this could have been told to make Hippocrates look human.[79] If the Corpus was originally a library or family collection, it no longer needs to be 'by Hippocrates', so Smith argued that 'It is likely that the works that became the Hippocratic Corpus did not arrive in Alexandria as Hippocratic writings, but became so there ... The works of the Corpus are therefore simply anonymous pre-Alexandrian medical works.'[80] Julius Rocca proposed that their merger around the name of Hippocrates relates to a wider tendency in the Hellenistic period to have an 'authority figure' for each discipline, so Hippocrates could be seen as the medical equivalent of Euclid for mathematics, or Plato or Aristotle for philosophy; and, of course, both Plato and Aristotle mention Hippocrates in positive terms.[81]

We receive the ancient world as fragments; whether of papyrus, stone, words quoted in later ancient sources or isolated texts. One way of managing this fragmentation is, paradoxically, to break our material up into different fragments and then try to 'recover a lost unity'.[82] Philip van der Eijk has argued that we should dismember the Hippocratic 'body' – the meaning of 'Corpus', of course – by contextualizing and understanding the individual texts with a view to regrouping them later.[83] Are those included in the Corpus simply there by chance; linked because of their shared use of Ionian dialect, because commentaries were written on them from an early date, or because they conform to Plato's view of the medical art and of Hippocrates as the model for physicians?[84] Hanson too has identified the commentary tradition, which began in the third century BCE possibly with Bacchius of Tanagra, as very important in the creation of 'Hippocrates': 'Explaining what "Hippocrates really means" refashioned the Father of Medicine into an authority figure in the present among the doctors the commentator was addressing.'[85]

A further question concerns whether the label 'Hippocratic' still has any value, particularly as we are increasingly aware that there were medical works which did not make it into the Hippocratic Corpus. The 2002 International Hippocrates Colloquium, 'Hippocrates in Context', included a thread on authors not included in the Corpus while the proceedings of the 2008 Colloquium were dedicated to 'Ancient Concepts of the Hippocratic'. In the 2008 Colloquium, Ann Ellis Hanson explored the many papyrus fragments mentioning medicine which have languished in the 'unidentified' pile while experts have concentrated on literary pieces.[86] Van der Eijk noted that much of the evidence for writers whose work was not included in the Corpus was already discussed in 1840 and 1856 by M.-S. Houdart, now a forgotten name; it was Emile Littré who wanted to trace the medical science to Hippocrates alone, but this was accompanied by rejecting the various myths about his life.[87]

Authors and titles: What is a treatise?

The Corpus is made up of a number of treatises, but that number fluctuates. Most recently, Craik lists only fifty-one treatises, while in 2003 Geoffrey Lloyd had 'some seventy treatises'. Popular histories of medicine suggest there are even more: for example, Kenneth Walker's 1959 *The Story of Medicine* has 'about a hundred volumes'.[88] Why such imprecision even on basic facts? Partly this is the result of issues of authenticity: the invaluable list compiled by

Gerhard Fichtner has 170 items because it includes all those attributed to Hippocrates during the medieval period, most of which are clearly just cashing in on the name.[89] However, another factor is that it can be far from obvious how we should divide up the texts that form the Hippocratic Corpus. Were some texts which have been transmitted separately through the long centuries of copying and recopying of manuscripts originally part of a single treatise? For example, *Generation/Nature of the Child* seem to be parts of one work, with *Diseases IV* and possibly also *On Glands* then being by the same author.[90] Should *Fractures* and *Joints* be seen as part of a longer treatise on surgery (as some people in Galen's time thought) and, if so, were any other Hippocratic treatises once in that?[91] It is also unclear whether some texts we have represent fragments of otherwise lost treatises (for example, *Diseases of Young Girls*, which seems very short considering its grandiose opening comments about medicine and 'the eternal').[92] Furthermore, from the ancient world onwards it has been believed that some 'treatises' were formed by merging previously separate works by different writers (for example, the components of *On the Nature of Man*, as already mentioned).

An even more fundamental question is what, in this context, is a treatise? A written work, certainly, but there are issues around the titles under which those works have been transmitted to us, about whether any had just a single author, and whether such written works are original compositions or bring together earlier knowledge. The term 'author' itself is problematic and Craik suggested that the word 'redactor' is often more appropriate; Volker Langholf, however, went further:

> the person who gave the treatise its shape ... was free to blend his own texts and other people's texts, he was 'author' and 'redactor' at the same time (so that these conventional philological terms may be inappropriate), he could reformulate and adapt texts taken over, he could present new messages in new or in conventional stylistic forms, and traditional messages likewise.[93]

The Hippocratic gynaecological treatises can help to illustrate some of these issues. Generally known in English as *Diseases of Women* 1 and 2, and *On Sterility*, even these titles are questionable. In the Corpus as a whole, titles are not part of the originals, so they do not necessarily reflect the content.[94] For example, *On Bones* mostly concerns vascular anatomy, while *On the Excision of the Foetus* bears this title based on its first chapter only.⁹⁵ In addition, references in some ancient authors suggest further works, now lost; Erotian mentioned one called *Wounds and Traits*.⁹⁶ In *Affections*, the advice to readers to 'use one of the remedies from the *Pharmakitis*' or 'from *Ta Pharmaka*' could be understood as suggesting there is a lost work on drugs available to which those who put together the treatises had access, and which they expected their readers to know; although it could represent an intention to compile such a work in the future, or could simply envisage the reader resorting to their own private recipe collections, on the assumption that any doctor would have one.⁹⁷ Many other collections of material which do not survive, such as 'lists of diseases, lists of prescriptions, lists of anatomical features', may have been available to those who put together the treatises in the versions in which they have come down to us.⁹⁸

The *Diseases of Women* treatises include material which overlaps with *Nature of Woman* and with *Epidemics*.⁹⁹ Who is copying whom, or are they all drawing on a common source? A further problem relates to translation: the first two *Diseases of Women* treatises come to us under the label of *Peri gynaikeiôn*, 'Concerning *gynaikeia*', a Greek word meaning 'diseases of women' but also used for 'remedies for diseases of women', 'menstruation', 'women's genitalia' and just 'women's things' in general. Our usual English translation fails to capture this complexity. The title of *On Sterility* (*Peri aphorôn*), a treatise sometimes seen as the third volume of *Peri gynaikeiôn*, has a different feel if we translate it instead as *Barrenness*; somehow less medical and more 'biblical'. *Barrenness* was the option chosen by Paul Potter in his 2012 English translation for the Loeb Classical Library; he glossed it as 'Literally the title means: "On those who do not bear"'.¹⁰⁰

As for any 'author' for these treatises, Hermann Grensemann studied the three major gynaecological works and attempted to pull out of them various 'strata', from 'A1' – which at one point he argued was the earliest Greek medical prose that survives – up to 'D', then going on to recreate what he presented as the original, early fourth-century gynaecological text 'C'.¹⁰¹ Whether or not we agree with his conclusions about the relative dates, it is clear that even one 'treatise' may contain traces of several earlier pieces of writing. Looking at the wood, rather than the trees, Elizabeth Craik has recently suggested that not only these three treatises, but also *Nature of Woman* and *On Glands*, are – in the forms in which they have reached us – the work of a single writer, making him 'responsible for more of the "Hippocratic" Corpus than … any other writer'.[102] Once again, a writer seems to emerge from the confusion, whether or not he can be identified with Hippocrates.

Was there any stage at which any treatises were attached to names? Pérez Cañizares regards anonymity as part of the original Corpus, and Craik speculates that 'medical collegiality' may have stopped anyone claiming authorship.[103] In contrast, and on the grounds that anonymity was rare in ancient Greek culture, van der Eijk has come down in favour of the treatises having been anonymized at some stage of their transmission; he cites the prominence with which both Herodotus and Thucydides introduced their own names at the beginning of their texts, and makes the point that some Hippocratic treatises are written by strong personalities making liberal use of the authorial ego.[104] The gynaecological treatises include phrases like 'there are some who think this, but I think the opposite' and 'this is what I have to say about these matters'.[105] With such a strong authorial voice, would there not have been names attached to the original versions?

A further question is whether we can go back even further, before the time when the texts were written down, either as the works of the Hippocratic Corpus or as the raw materials on which they were based. Did they emerge from an oral tradition? In 2005, Volker Langholf made a strong case for the Hippocratic Corpus having drawn on 'oral or performative' sources in 'medical lore and common knowledge'.[106] In the 1980s, Aline Rousselle had famously claimed that the gynaecological texts represented female traditions, taken over and written down by men: 'All the explanations given are women's explanations. The doctor repeats them', and 'It is "women's knowledge", based on observation, which the Hippocratic doctors have copied'.[107] Her contemporary Paola Manuli instead regarded the origins of these texts as lying in punitive male fantasies.[108] Why the difference? Rousselle's view derives from practice; from the large number of recipes in these texts, which she linked to an image of the kitchens of the ancient world, where women chat and learn. In contrast, Manuli focused on theory, and in particular on those elements of the theory of the female body which to us seem bizarre – the wandering womb, and treatment by fumigations in which smoke is passed in through the vagina. She found it difficult to believe that women would think about their bodies in this way. In the mid-1990s, compromises were suggested: Nancy Demand proposed that women created the knowledge and men then transmitted it, while Lesley Dean-Jones noted that the texts claim to contain 'privileged information available only from women'.[109]

My own contributions to this debate were twofold. First, I took up the point that medicine in the ancient world was considered a *technē* (Greek) or an *ars* (Latin), summed up by Ferrari and Vegetti as 'any practical activity that required intellectual competence as well as manual dexterity, was based on scientific knowledge, produced results that it was possible to verify, and was governed by well-defined rules that could be transmitted by teaching'.[110] I suggested that the creation of gynaecological knowledge was seen as combining women's experience and men's reason; women were graded by Hippocratic writers according to their level of 'experience', with 'experience of the diseases arising from menstruation' as one of the key factors.[111] One passage of the gynaecological texts presents women's medicine as a specialism, on the grounds that the treatment of men's diseases differed significantly from the healing of those of women.[112] Ten years later, I added a more radical suggestion that, when the male writers claimed that they knew something because women had told them, this could be a strategic move to show the superiority of their evidence-base, rather than an honest statement.[113]

This example shows that, at the very least, it's complicated. A Hippocratic treatise is unlikely to be a discrete text with a single 'author'. It may never be possible to uncover the relationship between these treatises and the lost texts and oral traditions from which they originated.

Creating the myths: Biographies and pseudepigrapha

Many of the myths about Hippocrates derive from the tradition of creating family trees and biographies for him; the earliest biographies date to around 500 years after he was first mentioned, but they drew on earlier stories. This was a 'myth-making process' rather than fact-finding.[114] One way to account for the obvious variations within the Hippocratic Corpus was to attribute some – whatever counted as the 'best' – treatises to Hippocrates, and others to members of his family. This conveniently built on a section in the Hippocratic *Oath* which described medicine as being taught by a man to his sons and to the sons of his own teacher 'without fee and written covenant', and could also be linked to Plato's reference in *Protagoras* to Hippocrates normally teaching medicine for a fee.[115]

It also fitted in with the treatises known as the 'pseudepigrapha'; letters and decrees concerning Hippocrates created probably from the mid-third century BCE. Francis Adams accepted that these biographical traditions were relatively late 'and of little authority', but they have proved seductive.[116] The picture they give of Hippocrates as a person shows the virtues traditionally associated with him, alongside more questionable stories. Nelson comments on one of these texts, in which Hippocrates appeals to the Thessalians to have his family lands returned to him, that 'the *Epibomios* ['The Speech at the Altar'] seems more like an embarrassing picture of one's parent that, with all due respect, ought to be discarded from the family photo album', and suggests that the coming together of the earliest texts of the pseudepigrapha both 'helped imprint Hippocrates' name on an anonymous collection of medical texts and sparked the creation of other Hippocratic pseudepigrapha'.[117] Wesley Smith pointed out that some of the pseudepigrapha 'show no consciousness of the Corpus', while others do, and suggested that this could help indicate when the Corpus was formed.[118] Nelson argued that two different versions of Hippocrates exist in the pseudepigrapha: the member of a healing clan, and the individual hero. One of the pseudepigraphic texts, *Decree*, took on the role of merging the traditions and inching them closer to the individual hero.[119]

As Edelstein was already well aware in 1939, there is the danger that all this can all be very circular, with the authors of the biographies picking up details from the treatises in the Corpus to strengthen their stories; more recent scholarship has demonstrated further how such biographies were written for their authors' own promotional purposes.[120] Our desire for a biography can be illustrated by Jouanna; he commented that these sources should mostly 'be used with the greatest caution', yet he also continues to believe that they give us 'information about the family background and life of Hippocrates that is either certain or probable'.[121] Amongst the more reliable information, he included the biographical tradition's year of birth for Hippocrates as 460 BCE, but even this is dependent on when he needed to have been born in order to have been old enough to have made a name for himself by the time Plato's *Protagoras* mentions him as a famous doctor: the date of 460 conveniently places him in his late twenties at the time when the dialogue is set. While today the dates most commonly given for Hippocrates' life are 460–370 BCE, there is even less ancient evidence for his date of death; different traditions put his age at death at anything between 85 and 109.[122] One of the most extreme variations online puts the dates of 'the acknowledged Greek father of medicine, Hippocrates' at 460–337 BCE.[123]

Thomas Rütten has pointed out that the most ancient biographies, those of Soranus[124] (early second century), the *Suda*[125] (tenth century) and John Tzetzes[126] (twelfth century), tell us far more about the history of medicine than about Hippocrates. The *Suda* singles out as the 'foremost' works *Oath*, *Prognostics* and *Aphorisms*, followed in fourth place by 'sixty books' which 'encompass the whole medical science and wisdom'; doctors, we are told, honour the works of Hippocrates 'like utterances from a god and not as coming from a human mouth'.[127] Tzetzes has 350 'books' (Greek *biblia*) as by Hippocrates, which presumably relates to the use of book rolls.[128] A further biography is the 'Brussels "Life"', an anonymous twelfth-century manuscript, which speculates that Hippocrates had 'a rather small body and a weak head'; this recalls – and presumably is based on – Aristotle's remarks on Hippocrates not being 'great' in stature.[129] Rütten notes that any biography of Hippocrates, including those created or repeated today, is a way to 'give concrete form to the concerns of professional politics and religion, to theoretical concepts, and to ethical-moral claims', so that Hippocrates becomes 'the projection screen for all the medicinal utopias that since the Roman Republic have taken him and his writings in tow'.[130] Everyone – in biomedicine and in various branches of alternative medicine – wants Hippocrates on their team.

Being 'nice': The personality of Hippocrates

At the beginning of this chapter I mentioned the claim that patients today think that it would be 'nice' to have Hippocrates as their doctor and, 'If you were *really* lucky, you had access to a doctor like Hippocrates'.[131] In the history of medicine – book-burning aside – Hippocrates almost always comes out as a much 'nicer' person than Galen, who was presented in twentieth-century histories of medicine as 'conceited, dogmatic and abusive of those who disagreed with him', or as 'forceful and opinionative', 'not nearly so great a man as Hippocrates'.¹³² Partly this is about Hippocrates' supposed methods, but even more it is about his character.

In the game *Assassin's Creed: Odyssey*, which will define him for a new generation, the scenario involves the theft of his notes on 'diseases of the mind'; Hippocrates states his methods as 'observation, experience and experimentation'.¹³³ These are entirely consistent with a tradition going back several centuries. In ante-bellum America, 'representations made him stand above all else for empiricism and against rationalism … "he showed that observation is the only true guide to those truths, which nature permits the human mind to reach"'.¹³⁴ In 2000, two doctors praised the way Hippocrates 'insisted on careful observation and the keeping of notes'.¹³⁵ In an earlier book published in a series aimed at grammar school sixth forms, technical college students and undergraduates, as well as the 'general reader', Poynter and Keele stated confidently that 'Hippocrates founded the method which we call "clinical observation" … This method is logical and its discoveries were so true that every doctor uses them at the bedside even today.'¹³⁶ A further element, the absence of any emotion in reporting that patients died, was singled out by Stubbs and Bligh in their 1931 *Sixty Centuries of Health and Physick*: the physician is 'no longer healer but the detached scientist'. They interrupt two passages giving case histories from the *Epidemics* to remark, 'Could anything be more modern in feeling, i.e. permanently true in tone and character, than this and the following set of calmly observed bedside records?'¹³⁷ For them, this is not the ancient world: it is 'the youth of our modern world'.¹³⁸ However, as Vivien Longhi has shown, 'Hippocrates the clinical observer' is yet another myth, one created by eighteenth-century medicine.¹³⁹

'Even today', and 'could anything be more modern?' It is clear that the desire to claim Hippocrates has not died away. Hippocrates' character is the object of even more admiration for what William Osler referred to in 1913 as 'the note of humanity', which he ranked even above accurate observation, with the *Oath* as 'the high-water mark of professional morality'.¹⁴⁰ Fielding Garrison's much-reprinted history of medicine puts it as follows: 'It is the method of Hippocrates, the use of the mind and senses as diagnostic instruments, together with his transparent honesty and his elevated conception of the physician's calling, his high seriousness and deep respect for his patients, that make him, by common consent, the "Father of Medicine" and the greatest of all physicians.'¹⁴¹

Yet there are moments in the Hippocratic Corpus where the doctor seems far from honest. In *Epidemics* 6.5.7, to treat a painful ear, the doctor should wrap wool round a finger, add some warm oil and then pass it over the ear so that the patient thinks something has been removed from it. The wool is then thrown in the fire, 'presumably destroying the evidence'.[142] Amneris Roselli characterizes Galen's Hippocrates as 'lover of truth', a view also found in Apollonius of Citium.[143] It is not surprising, then, that Galen disliked the blatant deception recommended by this *Epidemics* passage, which is underlined by the final word of the passage being ἀπάτη, 'deceit', and so he labelled it as spurious. This was the only way to save Hippocrates' reputation, as 'It is better to suppose that this sentence was not written by Hippocrates'.[144] Dioscorides took a different approach, removing all text after the doctor holds his hand over the ear. In their edition of *Epidemics* 6, however, Manetti and Roselli argued that all but the final word is authentic, so the doctor is without doubt being described as actively deceiving the patient.[145]

Many claims about Hippocrates' character derive from – or are reinforced by – the pseudepigrapha. These include nine letters in which he is invited, but refuses, to help Artaxerxes, the Persian king, to deal with a plague ravaging his territory; the three main biographies also contain this story.[146] Hippocrates states both that he has enough money already, and that he will not help the enemies of the Greeks. In its form, this story mirrors others in which a wise man refuses the gold of the East.[147] In 1792, the artist Girodet painted Hippocrates rejecting the gifts of the king. The various Persians around Hippocrates showed different expressions as the great doctor refuses to help them: angry, amazed, or sad. Meanwhile, Hippocrates' foot was shown pushing away the pile of money on the floor. When this was painted, Hippocrates' patriotism and his disdain for wealth were as important as his 'scientific' medicine in making him so great; the contrast between Hippocrates 'as the representative of Western civilization' and the 'Oriental stranger' is also significant in Girodet's painting.[148]

Moving beyond the myths

Once we lose our reliance on the myths surrounding Hippocrates, we become free to examine the Hippocratic texts not as 'the work of a single great man' but as something far more interesting. For example, as Lloyd observed, we can become more aware of the inconsistencies between treatises, or within one treatise, and we can consider them more as 'practical handbooks, not works of grand literature'.[149] While the personality of Hippocrates has been largely consistent over time, there have always been differences in how he has been characterized and which treatises are assigned his name. Does the existence of different versions of 'Hippocrates' really matter, and are there limits to the versions that should be created?

Modern presentations of Hippocrates are – like Galen, but without the philological skills – claiming Hippocrates as an ally in medical realities now. This goes beyond simple 'reception' and into something far more active, picking and mixing from classical texts but also creating entirely new stories about Hippocrates which then take on a life of their own; I shall be introducing a particularly striking story of this kind in the next chapter, where I shall be focusing on Hippocrates as what David Cantor memorably described as 'not so much as a "real" person [but] as a malleable cultural artefact, constantly moulded and remoulded according to need.'[150] Throughout the rest of this book, I shall be looking at both mainstream and alternative/complementary forms of medicine, since 'even branches of healing which consciously locate themselves as "alternative" to orthodox medicine have been only too keen to "discover" the principles of their own approach in the *Corpus*'.[151] Like Rosalind Coward, who wrote about the ideology of the alternative health movement in 1989, my intention here is not to come to conclusions about 'the efficacy of alternative medicine, but instead ... to "unpick" the meanings which cluster around' the movement.[152]

It remains the case that, as Benjamin Rush perceptively put it back in 1806, the power of Hippocrates' name may still be 'perpetuating many of the most popular and destructive errors in medicine'; Rush also went on to claim that 'it is remarkable that when he is quoted, it is chiefly to support a fact or an opinion that was discovered or suggested without the aid of his works'.[153] We could go further, and suggest that – with the exception of his alleged baldness – when he is quoted it is almost always to reinforce an argument, enlisting his support for what one wants to say. Thomas Rütten put it like this:

> As a timeless ideal, Hippocrates is ... always just ahead of reality and epitomizes whatever the current 'progressive' trend proclaims as its goal: be

it the power of eloquence or virtue, scholarliness or experience, the one proper method or comprehensive knowledge, genuine faith or true morality, Hippocrates can be seen to stand for any or all of these.

This means that Hippocrates is 'prone to any number of rejuvenations that ultimately dehistoricise him'.[154] How is he being reborn today? We have always made Hippocrates in our own image: what does the Hippocrates promoted today tell us about ourselves?

3

Sabotaging the Story: What Hippocrates Didn't Write[1]

Hippocrates now belongs to everyone: mainstream medicine, alternative and complementary medicine, advertisers and the general public. This was not always the case. Writing about medicine in the United States in the period before the Civil War, John Harley Warner describes a key benefit of invoking Hippocrates as being that, 'At a time when a multitude of irregular healers were competing successfully for recognition and clients, recounting an historical story that displayed two millennia of enduring tradition was a tool that orthodox physicians could use to set themselves apart.'[2]

Today, however, many other forms of medicine claim Hippocrates as part of their family trees, showing a high level of confidence that Hippocrates would be one of their number; if Hippocrates 'were living today, no doubt he would be labelled a Naturopath'.[3] Others fully accept that Hippocrates did not do what they are recommending, but are convinced he would have approved: he lived before the electric juicer, so 'it is doubtful that he was ever a "juice faster" in the present sense of that term. But I'll bet that he would be if he were alive in the 21st century – and reasonably so, given his philosophy of diet and medicine.'[4] This is not a new phenomenon. In the late nineteenth century, when dosimetry was invented by Adolphe Burggraeve at Ghent, it was placed 'under the protection of a great name' by being associated with Hippocrates; 'had he had the benefits of modern medical knowledge, Hippocrates *would have been favourable*' to it (author's italics).[5] 'No doubt', 'I'll bet that he would be' and 'would have been': perfect examples of how we think we know this man without a face and without a secure text to his name.

To return to one of my original questions, is there a point of reception, of recreation, of reimagining, beyond which he ceases to be Hippocrates? Does it matter, as long as someone can cite a text – even one, isolated phrase which has at some time been associated with him – to support what they say about him? Not for the first time, the interpretations of the Hippocratic Corpus and the biographies here seem to me to resemble fundamentalist approaches to the Bible; everything depends on whether one can produce a verse in support. It is no coincidence that this is the language of alternative medicine, as in the title of Sandra Cabot's *The Juice Fasting Bible*.[6] There is often a religious idiom used in alternative medicine, one which references the discourse of purity. Alan Levinovitz has observed that the language of sin and guilt, and of good and evil, is often applied to food today, and I shall return to this point in Chapter 7.[7] As we shall explore further in this chapter, for Hippocrates, as for God, individuals can be comfortable going beyond the texts and into their own imaginings. If they place their story cleverly or have sufficient charisma to carry a crowd with them, their followers will believe their gospel.[8]

In the rest of this book, I shall explore some contemporary uses of Hippocrates, as well as looking at specific 'verses' from the holy scriptures that are the Hippocratic Corpus, usually pithy aphorisms which he is supposed to have 'said': for popular tradition, the focus is normally on speech, not writing.[9] Among those currently most widely shared on the internet and via social media and memes are 'First do no harm', 'Let food be thy medicine', 'Walking is the best medicine' and 'All diseases begin in the gut'. Before that, however, in this chapter I want to explore in some detail a particularly striking example of a complete story about Hippocrates; an entirely new one, with no roots in any line of any text either of the Hippocratic Corpus or of the ancient biographical tradition. The creation and, even more, the later development of this story will introduce some of the specific roles Hippocrates has come to play in the early twenty-first century.

Writing new stories

Making up titles for 'Hippocratic treatises' is nothing new: the satirical writer Richard Armour came up with *The Cos and Effect of Disease*.[10] In addition to the many medieval treatises which claimed to be by Hippocrates (above, p. 32), mentions of other fictional treatises, including their contents, appear on the internet from time to time: for example 'In the fifth century BC, the Greek physician Hippocrates — namesake of the Hippocratic oath — wrote a thesis called "Natural Exercise" that references the therapeutic value of horseback riding.'[11] Since one of the few mentions of horse-riding (Greek *hippasiê*) in the Corpus is in *Airs Waters Places*, which offers as a reason for the infertility of the Scythians the 'constant jolting' of riding, this is an odd connection to make.[12] The treatise *Fistulas* also mentions horse-riding as a cause of fistulas, 'where blood collects in the buttock near the anus': no therapeutic value here.[13] *Natural Exercise* is as imaginary, although not as amusing, as *The Cos and Effect of Disease*.

More seriously, however, I was recently able to document entirely new myths about ancient medicine, including an imaginary Hippocratic treatise, being created on Wikipedia and then spreading far beyond it. In the modern market of knowledge, Wikipedia still holds the key position, and what is posted by editors is regulated by other editors, although they are unlikely to have specific subject knowledge.[14] Whether we are school students or general readers or journalists, it is the Wikipedia page that is likely to top our search lists and be our first destination in finding out the basics about Hippocrates. On 4 October 2014 I was looking at the Wikipedia article, 'Hippocrates', a 'Featured Article' (FA), meaning that it 'has been identified as one of the best articles produced by the Wikipedia community'.[15] This status guarantees its 'accuracy, neutrality, completeness, and style', and only around 0.1 per cent of articles are included in this category.[16] Those discussing the article 'Hippocrates' on its talkpage say things like 'the article seems so high-quality now that I am afraid to touch it'; the response from editor Rmrfstar posted on 28 February 2008 was 'You shouldn't ever be afraid to edit an article; any change can be easily undone. You are right, though, in the case of a Featured Article, it's probably better to ask first.'[17]

Despite its status, the page as it stands today is by no means one of the best in the English-language version of Wikipedia. The material mostly comes from tired secondary sources and histories of medicine by non-specialists, including outdated references to the supposed Coan/Cnidian split in Greek medicine and uncritical acceptance of material from the biographical tradition; it also has a very poor prose style.[18] Yet it is very heavily used. Created in May 2001, the page is currently running at a daily average of over 1,900 hits.[19] One user was Ian Learmonth ('MBChB(Stell), FRCS, FRCS(Ed), FCS(SA)Orth, Professor Emeritus'), whose opening address to the European Hip Society Meeting in 2010 began with 'Hippocratic medicine was humble and passive. Treatment was gentle, kind to the patient, and emphasized the importance of keeping the patient clean and sterile'.[20] Every word there is taken straight from the Wikipedia Hippocrates page.

In some cases, those who maintain the 'Hippocrates' article challenge claims without citations, and intervene with comments that show how cautious they are being; for example 'no way in hell is that illustration 2nd century AD', from Peter Isotalo after an attempt was made to insert a caption to a drawing of the 'Hippocratic bench' on 31 March 2014.[21] However, contrary to Wikipedia editing guidelines, the Hippocrates page includes many unreferenced sentences, such as 'The drink hypocras is also believed to have been invented by Hippocrates. Risus sardonicus, a sustained spasming of the face muscles may also be termed the Hippocratic Smile'. The first sentence is dubious: while spiced wine was known in the ancient world, the drink is usually associated with the medieval period, its name possibly derived from draining the spiced wine through a *manicum Hippocraticum* or 'Hippocratic sleeve' and, not surprisingly, that filtering method has also been seen as 'invented' by Hippocrates.[22] The *risus sardonicus*, a distorted grin caused by spasm, is one of the prognostic signs of imminent death, but the connection with Hippocrates in the wording of the second sentence seems to originate in Sir Arthur Conan Doyle's *The Sign of the Four*, when Sherlock Holmes discusses the likely cause of death of a character as poisoning; a novel should not count as a reliable source by Wikipedia standards, but there is no other evidence.[23] The use of the term 'Hippocratic smile' is reminiscent of the 'Hippocratic face', the *facies Hippocraticus*, based on the list of indications that death is approaching which is given in the treatise *Prognostics*, a list still used in medicine today.[24] The list does not include the facial feature of the *risus sardonicus*, but ends with 'It is also a deadly sign when the lips are loose, hanging, cold and very white.'[25]

Even the presence of citations is no guarantee of accuracy, as they may serve as a screen disguising poor material. For example, on 29 December 2010 a user successfully added

> In general, the Hippocratic medicine was very kind to the patient; treatment was gentle, and emphasized keeping the patient clean and sterile. For

example, only clean water or wine were ever used on wounds, though "dry" treatment was preferable. Soothing [[balm]]s were sometimes employed.²⁶

Despite its poor English, this is still there at the time of writing.²⁷ Indeed, it was copied verbatim, along with the Wikipedia reference to Hippocratic medicine as 'humble and passive', in one of the 'A Closer Look' textboxes punctuating Ben Witherington III's 2012 novel *A Week in the Life of Corinth*.²⁸ Its stated source, the 1966 reprint of the fourth edition of Garrison's *An Introduction to the History of Medicine*, is responsible not for all three sentences, but only for the second of them; Garrison does indeed say that Hippocratic medicine claimed wounds 'should never be irrigated except with clean water or wine, the dry state being nearest to the healthy', but he never mentions soothing balm or balms.²⁹ Adopted from Wikipedia, these 'balms' feature widely in recent popular works; for example, in MacLeod and Wishinsky's *A History of Just About Everything*, Hippocrates' favoured treatments are, 'cleanliness, diet, sleep and soothing balms', while Steve Parker's *Kill or Cure* includes, 'Bandaging, massage, and soothing balm might be required now and then.'³⁰

Sometimes this Wikipedia page is clearly being hijacked for marketing purposes; for example, the citation of an article on curing male pattern baldness, discussed in the Introduction. Even more striking is the revision which, in the version visible in mid-February 2019, read 'Generalized treatments he prescribed include fasting and the consumption of a mix of honey and vinegar. Hippocrates once said that "to eat when you are sick, is to feed your sickness."'³¹ Despite having no references, this entered the article on 17 March 2014, but originally as 'apple cider vinegar' rather than 'a mix of honey and vinegar'.³² Over the recent history of the page, 'a mix of honey and vinegar' keeps being reverted to 'apple cider vinegar'.³³ Examination of the contributions of the anonymous user who originally inserted the reference to apple cider vinegar shows them enthusiastically promoting the virtues of this product; the 'Vinegar' page was amended, also in March 2014, to state that apple cider vinegar is 'sweetened (usually with honey) for consumption as a health beverage'.³⁴ While there are many references to vinegar in the Hippocratic Corpus, acknowledged in modern medical articles, this is generic vinegar rather than apple cider vinegar specifically.³⁵

I am far from the first to observe that the page has been used to sell a particular kind of vinegar. Furthermore, an excellent discussion of 'Apple cider vinegar in ancient Greece' initiated by user 'ScottOden' on an Alexander the

Great discussion board on 22 April 2012 predates the Wikipedia insertion, and was based instead on a commercial site: Bragg Live Foods, who stated that Hippocrates was using this type of vinegar 'in 400 B.C.'. Oden looked for references to apple cider vinegar in the Hippocratic Corpus, but found only vinegar, sometimes with 'white vinegar' specified. He ended his post with 'My question is: am I missing something? Is Hippocrates' use of ACV just an urban legend given long legs by the health and fitness industry? Any help or insight would be greatly appreciated!'[36] A week later, he shared the response of the company: they replied simply that 'You can find it in the actual book of Hippocrates'! Recoiling from this level of ignorance, Oden asked 'why no one has called them on it, before' and wondered where the original claim originated.[37] Bragg Live Foods continue to repeat the wording Oden read, that 'Apple Cider Vinegar has been highly regarded throughout history', and the advertising for their book on the product still claims that 'Hippocrates, the father of medicine, treated his patients with Apple Cider Vinegar'.[38]

The claims certainly go back long before 2012, at least in the USA. A typical late-twentieth-century example would be an article in a University of Pittsburgh at Bradford online journal in 1998, where first-year student Bonnie K. McMillen wrote on ACV, repeated the Hippocratic origin claims and then went further: 'This naturally occurring germ killer was one of the very first medicines.'[39] Her source here appears to be the widely-used *The Vinegar Book* by Emily Thacker, first published in 1994 with several subsequent editions.[40] A 2015 story on a natural health site stating that 'all doctors still take the Hippocratic Oath' – a common error which will be discussed in Chapter 4 – comments that Hippocrates 'was a huge fan of what's now called "lifestyle medicine". He prescribed apple cider vinegar mixed with honey for coughs, colds, and even for treating diabetes – in the 4th century B.C.!'[41] On another site by an alternative health specialist, this vinegar is a 'forgotten ancient remedy' and 'a holy grail for the fountain of youth'; 'Hippocrates treated his patients with apple cider vinegar and honey for all sorts of ailments.'[42] The specific focus on vinegar made from apples is an American feature, based on American traditions. The claim that 'Hippocrates used vinegar as a medicine' was used to introduce the various ingredients of vinegar production around the world in a 1924 United States government publication for farmers aimed at avoiding perceived wastage of 'apples, peaches, grapes, and other fruits.'[43] In a study of the industry published in 1912,

J.J. Schommer had noted that apple cider vinegar 'forms the bulk of the table vinegar of the United States and Canada', simply because of the amount of windfall apples and apple peelings available.[44]

Wikipedia as a moving target

Despite the many acknowledged failings of this Wikipedia 'Featured Article' page, when I returned to the Hippocrates article in October 2014 I was nevertheless surprised to see the following:

> Historians agree that Hippocrates was born around the year 460 BC on the [[Greece|Greek]] island of [[Kos|Cos]], and became a famous ambassador for medicine against the strong opposing infrastructure of Greece. For this opposition he endured a 20-year prison sentence during which he wrote well known medical works such as "The Complicated Body", encompassing many of the things we know to be true today. Other biographical information, however, is likely to be untrue.
>
> (viewed 4 October 2014)[45]

I had a moment of extreme unease. Was my knowledge of the Hippocratic Corpus defective? Was this a known fake, like *On the Anatomy of the Veins*, which I had never encountered?[46] Had I somehow managed to miss a medieval text once attributed to Hippocrates? There were plenty of them, for example the *Astrology* with its confident opening: 'Hippocrates who was the best doctor and teacher said...'[47] After a few minutes, I realized that this section described an entirely imaginary incident and an entirely imaginary text. But how did it come to be there, especially bearing in mind that this article is monitored by many different editors? And how had these additions remained on the page for what the History feature of the page revealed was a period of four years?[48]

The Wikipedia talkpage reveals many of the other pressures on the Hippocrates page. Silly insertions, such as changing a spelling, or adding obscenities, simple 'I was here!' statements or adding 'was infact [sic] gay', are common but are automatically picked up and corrected, as are uses of the page as a site on which to declare one's love.[49] At one point, a suspect for some inserted errors was even named by an editor posting that 'There are NUMEROUS vandalisms here, even after some reversions. Why is it that whenever I type

"Hippocrates" into the Wikipedia Search it comes up with an article saying, "Why do I hate Canada so much?"'[50]

By its very nature, Wikipedia never stays still: like the internet as a whole, it is in what David Crystal called a 'permanent state of transition, lacking precedent, struggling for standards, and searching for direction'.[51] The movement of apple cider vinegar into and out of the page illustrates P.D. Magnus's point that 'One important difference between Wikipedia and traditional media, however, is the dynamic nature of its entries. An entry assessed today might be substantially extended or reworked tomorrow',[52] although in this particular case the movement is a pendulum swing rather than a reworking. Furthermore, the internet is both permanent and temporary: every piece of information posted there is stored indefinitely, available for those who know how to find and retrieve it.[53] On the other hand, comments and texts on the internet date quickly and fade from its collective memory; blog posts, comments on social networking sites, entire articles disappear from view as they are displaced by the new. The surfer is always a click away from the 'item not found' page, symbol of the transitory nature of the World Wide Web.

Experiments have been carried out to see how quickly errors inserted into Wikipedia are corrected. The additions I noticed had been on the page for four years, but those who have deliberately made false claims in order to see how quickly they were 'reverted' to the original wording have usually reported responses within hours or days. In 2004, Alex Halavais made thirteen changes to Wikipedia and left them there for two weeks.[54] A week later, he posted a piece on his blog entitled 'Please don't do this', because other people were trying it as well and he believed that there was a real risk that the potential destructive power of an 'online mob' 'could ruin a beautiful thing'.[55] He used the same username and IP address for all his changes, which made it easier for both bots (automated tools which do much of the basic maintenance) and real people to find and undo the edits.[56] In November and December 2007, P.D. Magnus inserted what he called 'fibs' – very short fictitious biographical claims – into well-tended entries on famous philosophers, using different IP addresses; for example, on John Stuart Mill, 'Following the death of his wife, Mill had a series of mistresses who helped him prepare manuscripts as well as sharing his bed.' If the fib had not been corrected within forty-eight hours – and between a third and half of them were – then Magnus removed them.[57]

Teachers at various levels of education sometimes change a Wikipedia article as a way of checking whether their students are developing the ability to evaluate what they find online: others change a page in order to give students live experience of editing.[58] In May 2018, Charles West, 'Wikipedia Advocate' at the University of Sheffield, published an important piece on 'Wikipedia in the History Classroom'.[59] He pointed out that the place of Wikipedia has been enhanced by the role it now plays as 'the go-to for Amazon's Alexa smart speaker', and contrasted the increase in Wikipedia's authoritative status outside the academy with 'official' history as performed in universities. For him, the key issue is that any encyclopaedia – online or otherwise – gives the impression that there are 'facts' on which all agree, whereas history is about teaching people to argue from evidence. West also discussed his own teaching and how he integrates digital literacy by asking his medieval history students to improve or create Wikipedia pages, assessing not the changes they make – which can rapidly be reverted – but their subsequent reflection on the experience. One of his students traced an error in dating a church council to other websites, and 'potentially from there into print'. There is still a misguided belief that 'the scholarly tradition of reporting back to published, print-on-paper sources' is somehow superior to using the internet, even though books and articles in print may take seriously something thoroughly untrustworthy which originated on the internet: for example, Hippocrates' time in prison.[60]

When I spotted the insertions on the Wikipedia page, in my Wikipedia and Twitter identity as 'fluff35', I immediately contacted a Wikipedia administrator and master editor, Yun Shui,[61] who shared my concern, replying that

> The text appears to have been in the article for quite some time without a source, but has not been questioned until now. However, I've been unable to locate any scholarly sources that confirm Hippocrates (sic?) incarceration (there are a number of instances where the claim is repeated, but nothing that would constitute a reliable source by Wikipedia's standards).[62]

Yun Shui then posted a notice on the article's talkpage, asking for a source, heading the discussion 'Hippocrates: Two decades in the slammer'.[63] He noted here that the only places he could find references to the imprisonment were 'just a couple of children's history books (not reknowned [sic] for their factual accuracy) and a self-published self-help book, together with a couple of websites with unknown levels of fact-checking'.

On 9 October Yun Shui returned to the talkpage to say,

> The more I look at it, the more I'm convinced this was a very successful hoax. The information was added by an anonymous IP back in 2010 with this edit, and has never been sourced. The only references I can find which report this information about Hippocrates writing a book called The Complicated Body while in prison post-date that addition (and almost all of them use remarkably similar wording, suggesting that they took the information from this article in the first place). Like Fluff35, I can't find any other reference to The Complicated Body, nor does it appear to be extant in any form. People, I believe we've been hoodwinked – I'm removing the segement [sic] in question from the article.
>
> Yunshui 雲水 08:30, 9 October 2014 (UTC)

Being the daddy

The removal of the story from the main Wikipedia page was not enough to kill it; it remains in its pre-October 2014 form on the Wikipedia for Schools page, but that is not the only problem.[64] Before going on to describe the subsequent life of these two Hippocratic myths, however, I would like to pause to examine the title 'Father of Medicine'. The various interventions on the Wikipedia Hippocrates page reflect wider disputes in the scholarly literature over how best he should be labelled: 'Father of Medicine', 'Father of Clinical Medicine', 'Father of Western Medicine' or 'Father of Modern Medicine'?[65] Beyond this page, he has also been claimed as 'the Father of Holistic Medicine'.[66] Claims of connection and fatherhood continue to be found today, particularly in the writing of medical practitioners, who want to construct a long and unbroken lineage for what they do; like American practitioners in the first half of the nineteenth century, by paying tribute to Hippocrates as the Father of Medicine they are 'confirming participation in a learned tradition and identity as a professional'.[67]

On the Wikipedia page, where Hippocrates is currently simply 'Father of Medicine', a link takes the reader to a list of fathers (and mothers) of various branches of science, with three options for this global title: Hippocrates, Charaka and Imhotep.[68] What does it mean for anyone to be the 'father' of any sort of medicine? The early-twenty-first century slang phrase, 'Who's the daddy?', was used to assert dominance ('Who's the best?'), and has also been adopted as the name of a DNA-testing service.[69] Both senses are relevant to this title of Hippocrates – superiority, and direct connection – but in the earliest tradition the title went to the god Apollo or to his semi-mortal son, Asclepius.[70] Jan Sapp's classic article on Mendel's role in the history of genetics shows how a founding father tends to be one whose ideas are at first rejected as 'ahead of his time', dies without recognition, but is then rediscovered during a later priority dispute, in which the solution to two scientists proposing the same thing at the same time is to project it back on to a previously-unrecognized 'founding father'.[71] Mendel, he suggested, is a useful 'father' because he published so little that it is easy to construct stories about him: in contrast, I would argue that Hippocrates is useful instead because there are so many texts that anyone looking for a foundation document for their medical approach will find something that fits.

There is, however, an important proviso here. Those who have called Hippocrates the Father of Medicine over the centuries have had very different ideas about what even biological fatherhood means, as beliefs about generation and reproduction have changed. In the modern period, a common model for science has a feminized Nature on whom the male scientist imposes his will; in Sapp's words, '"the founding fathers" penetrate Mother Nature to leave a child destined for greatness. However, the child is born "premature"...it is left to die because no one is prepared or willing to take care of it.'[72] In ancient Greek medicine, different models of the respective contributions existed. The woman may be a passive field in whom the father plants his seed; male seed may impose its form on blood, the raw material supplied by the woman; or both sexes may contribute to the sex and the qualities of the new being.[73] The male element in generation was particularly associated with the qualities of strength and speed. When the writer of the Hippocratic treatise *Generation/Nature of the Child* discussed 'quickening', the point at which the foetus first moves in the womb, he stated that this was generally at three months for a male and four months for a female because the male is 'stronger', formed from seed that is both thicker and stronger.[74]

I find it interesting that the fatherhood of Hippocrates dominated in the era after the discovery of ovum and sperm, when users knew perfectly well that generation 'takes two'. But if Hippocrates is the father of medicine, who is its mother? Jonathan Sawday has argued that the Western medical tradition even operates with 'twin fathers', Hippocrates and Galen. For him, this double paternity was combined with a view of Eastern medicine as unfathered, something which devalued it by feminizing it as a vessel passively 'carrying' Western medicine through the centuries.[75] Arabic translations of Hippocratic treatises and of Galen kept alive those ancient Greek works lost in the West, but only in the eleventh century was Eastern medicine able to 'give birth', when Constantine the African arrived in Italy with a cargo of books and proceeded to translate the lost works of Galen from Arabic into Latin. Here, fatherhood means priority, authority and – potentially – identity with the traits of the parent, characterized by being strong and moving quickly. In the terms of classical medicine, to have no father recalls the phenomenon of the 'uterine mole', a shapeless object formed from the mother's blood but with inadequate contribution from the father; it has no power of movement.[76]

In the many twentieth-century popular histories of medicine, no explicit attempt was made to explain what is implied by Hippocrates' 'fatherhood': for example, the elision of royal and paternal power in Macfie's 1907 *The Romance of Medicine*, where 'The king of the physicians of the period of Greek philosophy was undoubtedly Hippocrates, who is usually called the Father of Medicine'; Withington's 1921 'He is universally known as the Father of Medicine' and that title is 'well deserved'; or, in 1931, Stubbs and Bligh's confident (but mistaken) presentation of 'for over two thousand four hundred years Hippocrates has been acknowledged as the Father of Medicine' as 'incontrovertible fact'.[77] Sometimes, however, attempts made to justify the title reveal what was then considered important in medicine. For Guthrie in 1945, it was the 'spirit of scientific inquiry which dominated all the work of Hippocrates, the Father of Medicine, whose leadership, undimmed throughout the centuries, remains unchallenged to this day': the theme here is authority.[78] Poynter and Keele suggested that the title was due to the combination of 'careful observation of the symptoms and signs of disease' and 'a systematic study of the structure and function of the human body in health and disease': the implication here is that the father and his sons – the current medical profession – share the same qualities.[79]

What about Galen? Galen was never the Father of Medicine, but the 'Prince of Physicians', 'prince' not in the sense of 'heir to the throne', but a Roman *princeps*, 'first among equals', accepted by his peers as most fully embodying those qualities which they themselves share. Hippocrates, too, could be a *princeps*, as in the prefatory material to the 1525 Latin translation of the Hippocratic Corpus by Calvi where he is 'without dispute, of all physicians, the *princeps*' while in the 1546 translation by Stephanus we find 'Hippocrates and Galen, the *principes* of the best medical sect, namely the rational sect'.[80] Whatever we want medicine to be – rational, empirical, scientific, natural – that is the sort of medicine Hippocrates practised, and he transmits his own qualities to its later practice by 'fathering' it.

Two decades in the slammer?

No matter how flexible we believe the reception of Hippocrates can be, for me the Wikipedia claims for Hippocrates' prison term and his treatise fall into a category all of their own. Other than a correction – 'ambassador' was originally spelled 'embassador' – an attempt to change 'The Complicated Body' to 'The Complicated boy', a short-lived piece of vandalism in replacing 'ambassador for medicine' with 'ambassador for bullying', and an (unfortunately) unsuccessful attempt to make 'Historians agree that …' into 'Historians don't agree that …' they survived unchallenged from their insertion on 12 December 2010 to their deletion in October 2014.[81] One attempt was made to delete the whole section, but this was purely to replace it with the words 'Paige Durkin', and the section was back online within four hours.[82] An addition was made on 15 November 2012 to the effect that Hippocrates was given his 'twenty-year prison sentence for sodomizing his mother and killing his family', but that was deleted and reverted in less than an hour.[83] There was also an unsuccessful attempt to add to this section 'Hippocrates had sex with Dora the explorer every night'.[84]

Most significantly, during their four years on the page, the claims for the prison term and the treatise were widely repeated online and, despite their deletion, the nature of the internet means that they still survive: I shall discuss some examples in the next section. Not surprisingly, I have not found the claims cited in print media before 2010, but after the creation of these myths on Wikipedia they spread beyond the internet as well; for example Volume 1 of *The Puffin History of the World* (2013) tells children that Hippocrates 'wrote a book, *The Complicated Body*' while another children's book published in the same year states that Hippocrates spent twenty years in prison because his 'medical ideas contradicted many of the beliefs of his time'.[85] Children's books are not the only places to find these myths; they also feature in work for an adult audience that one would expect to have been through peer review. For example, the preface to Michael A. Taylor's *Hippocrates Cried: The Decline of American Psychiatry*, published by OUP in 2013, presents the familiar Hippocrates who argued that disease arose from 'environmental factors, poor diet, and unhealthy living habits' rather than the gods, before stating 'Hippocrates' novel opinions about disease and treatments got him into hot water with the Hellenistic powers that were and he was imprisoned for 20 years. He did not waste this time, however, and spent it writing several of his most famous treatises such as *The Complicated Body*.'[86]

No time wasting: while in the Wikipedia original, Hippocrates merely 'endured' his jail sentence, here he becomes a role model for the Protestant work ethic, as in a similar comment in an online biography, 'In fact, he used his time in prison productively as he wrote "The Complicated Body".'[87] Here, the message becomes how an initial obstacle proves to be a benefit. This 'productive' approach perhaps suggests one possibility for the origin of the prison story; Hippocrates' older contemporary Anaxagoras was imprisoned for denying that the sun was a god, and continued to work while in prison on the mathematical problem of 'squaring the circle'.[88] This puzzle was also attempted by Hippocrates' namesake, the mathematician Hippocrates of Chios. Perhaps somehow the names of the mathematicians have been swapped?

Another myth in Taylor's brief preface to *Hippocrates Cried* is that Hippocrates died 'in his 80s, probably at the hands of another physician'.[89] I have not located this story anywhere else; it is possible that it represents confusion with yet another Hippocrates, the Spartan governor, killed by Alcibiades according to Plutarch's biography of the latter.[90] Murder features in a further medical Hippocrates story, but with Hippocrates as criminal not victim: in a medieval legend, with a delightful disregard for around 700 years of history, Galen is Hippocrates' nephew, and Hippocrates murders him when he becomes too successful as a doctor.[91] As for Hippocrates' own death, Wikipedia currently restricts itself to 'Several different accounts of his death exist.'[92] The year given for Hippocrates' death has varied on this page; changed from *c.* 370 BCE to *c.* 377 BCE on 13 December 2010, this was rapidly changed back to the original. A further attempt on 13 January 2011 also failed, briefly reverting not to 370 but to 369, until 370 was reinstated on the following day.[93] There have been subsequent attempts to insert 377, but 370 remains the default position. As for the cause of death, another 'conspiracy theory' – 'some believe the government killed him' – was inserted on 9 September 2011 but rapidly removed.[94]

Spreading the myths

As Schultze and Bytwerk showed in the case of a fake Goebbels quote, 'The originator, whoever he or she was, lost all control over the original fabrication once it first appeared online. Originals can easily beget more copies of the fabrication no matter what the first author later intends.'[95] As with other Wikipedia articles, this Hippocrates story is widely copied by other websites. Answers.com, with its over-optimistic tag line, 'Making the world better, one answer at a time,' includes the question 'Did Hippocrates get put in prison?' and gives the answer 'He was in prison for twenty years.'[96] Another question there, 'How important was the influence of Hippocrates on Roman and medieval medicine', receives one answer copied straight from the Wikipedia entry:

> Historians agree that Hippocrates was born around the year 460 BC on the Greek island of Kos (Cos) and became a famous ambassador for medicine against the strong opposing infrastructure of Greece. For this opposition he endured a twenty year prison sentence during which he wrote very well known medical publications such as "The Complicated Body", encompassing many of the things we know to be true today.[97]

In another variant on this site, the Wikipedia wording on the prison sentence and the new book is followed immediately by the multiple anachronism that 'During medieval times the church was the main medical care and because of this Hippocrates theories were taught because Hippocrates had the church in mind at all times and his treatment usually involved God or the bible.'[98] This mixes Wikipedia with something entirely incomprehensible, as well as chronologically impossible.[99] It recalls another, but more elegant, chronological mishmash described by Vivian Nutton; the *Oath* as taken in Basel from 1570–1868, sworn before 'God the One and Three, the father of Hygieia and Panacea'.[100] In the ancient Greek version of the Hippocratic *Oath*, the doctor swears by Asclepius and his daughters, Hygieia (Health) and Panacea (All-Heal).

While the original Wikipedia phrasing, that Hippocrates was imprisoned because he was a 'famous ambassador for medicine against the strong opposing infrastructure of Greece', is often repeated verbatim, many users find this wording so opaque that they modify it. For example, 'Plato' posted in 'Classical Wisdom Weekly' on 12 March 2013, moving the words around so that Hippocrates 'was a strong proponent for medicine, even when it was opposing the infrastructure of Greece. As a result he endured a period of twenty years inside a prison where he authored many famous medical works, such as The Complicated Body.'[101] In another variant, it was 'his opposition against prevalent beliefs in Greece at the time regarding medicine' which led to his prison sentence.[102] Others have tried to combine the support for medicine and the 'infrastructure' with what they think they know about Hippocrates as an opponent of religion; he was 'jailed for 20 years' 'because he was a strong proponent of medicine being separate from religion'.[103] Again, this would resonate with the imprisoned Anaxagoras being punished for accounting for the sun in entirely natural terms.

In this story, then, Hippocrates is a rebel, not the voice of medical orthodoxy. Yet popular receptions are here very far from current scholarly views on what the Hippocratic texts say on religion. Did 'Hippocrates' fight against superstition, or religion, or both? The presentation of Hippocrates (historically, known as 'the divine Hippocrates') as the rational opponent of anything supernatural ignores the place of 'the divine' in the Hippocratic Corpus; Philip van der Eijk noted that the author of *On the Sacred Disease* shows 'a sincere religiosity in his vigorous defence of religion and his combat against magic and superstition', a key plank of which is that it is impious to accuse the gods of causing a disease.[104] Isabelle Torrance described the *Oath* – which calls on all the Greek gods as witnesses – as 'a religious text which binds the medical student to his craft through the invocation of a series of divinities'.[105]

The popular tradition much prefers simple dualisms here: light and dark, clean and dirty, science and religion. Nuland, for example, claims that

Hippocratic medicine 'provided the clear light which led Greek medicine out of the mire of theurgy and witchcraft'.[106] Bringing witchcraft into the mix is an odd move: the default position of the tradition has long been that not witches but priests are Hippocrates' rivals, as in the ancient stories that he himself had once been a priest, that his treatments were based on the inscriptions in the temple of Asclepius on Cos which described what the god had ordered patients to do, and that he burned a temple library to disguise his reliance on what he had learned as a priest.[107] Temkin rightly described this as 'The fable of the development of clinical medicine from temple medicine', but it remains alive and well, particularly among medical writers.[108]

In October 2012, on his website *Weeks* MD, Bradford S. Weeks repeated the twenty years in prison story. He used the usual dualistic language in describing Hippocrates as someone 'credited with bringing medicine out of the realms of superstition and into the light of science' who

> did some serious time. In his day, illness was understood to derive from Gods who were displeased and the remedy was delivered by the priest (after receiving adequate payment). Whether the cure worked or not, depended upon your degree of sin and the priest kept the payment regardless. If disease persisted, the only option was to go back to the priest and pay more ... The priests, their status and livelihood threatened, conspired with their political cronies to imprison their competition, Hippocrates, for 20 years.[109]

Whodunnit, here? The priests: their motive for silencing Hippocrates, financial. For many readers of the Wikipedia prison story, the priests represent the 'strong opposing infrastructure' and they work with their friends in politics, meaning that 'the establishment' more generally can be seen as responsible for Hippocrates' unjust treatment. In the way Hippocrates plays out on the internet, the message of money is often near the surface, recalling the story of him refusing the gifts offered by the Persian king in return for his services.[110] The priests are venal and value money: Hippocrates is honest and values something higher. This can be read as saying that modern medicine is ruled by the attempts of the pharmaceutical industry to sell its products: Hippocrates offers a simple, cheaper and more 'natural' solution to illness.

Other non-fiction (if that is the right word here) interpretations of the prison story have been created. Sean Patrick's 2013 motivational book, *Awakening your Inner Genius*, was marketed *inter alia* by telling potential readers that they can discover 'How Hippocrates' epic quest to reform medicine in ancient Greece was fueled by his unparalleled judgment, and how you too can sharpen your ability to make the right decisions at the right times.'[111] Here, Hippocrates becomes a sort of proto-Socrates. Using Hippocrates, you can learn 'how to sharpen your judgement to a razor's edge'.[112] In Chapter 9, Patrick added yet more to the original Wikipedia prison story, stating that the 'governing authorities – who claimed they were the spokespeople for the gods of health' resisted Hippocrates' 'reform'. They

> ordered Hippocrates to cease his teachings at once . . . Arriving in small rural city to treat citizens, he was arrested for disrespecting the gods. He was quickly sentenced to indefinite detention in state prison . . . while incarcerated, he wrote one of his most famous works, *The Complicated Body*, which contains many physiological conclusions that we know to be true today. Hippocrates spent nearly two decades in prison before finally being released.

Here Hippocrates is condemned by a coalition of the state and religion. He has already been warned not to teach; he goes on treating patients, but avoids the big cities (perhaps because he is more likely to be noticed if he goes there); the original sentence he receives is longer (does he have time off for good behaviour?); and, once again, *The Complicated Body* is 'true'.

The Complicated Body

Turning now to this written product of Hippocrates' incarceration, what precisely is this imaginary text thought to contain? Described – in a strange irony – as the only one of Hippocrates works not 'lost to history',[113] in its post-Wikipedia life it has become not just 'very famous', revolutionary and 'true', but also – as in *Awakening your Inner Genius* – a treatise on physiology.[114] Hippocrates 'wrote *The Complicated Body* while in prison, a work dealing with human mechanics'.[115] 'Most information in the book was verified by modern science', according to a 2014 account of a visit to Cos by Sylvie Halouzková.[116] It was not merely theoretical in approach, because the incarcerated Hippocrates had continued to see patients: 'During those 20 years, in addition to treating other prisoners (and visiting dignitaries – including, one supposes, numerous priests!) Hippocrates wrote his revolutionary medical text "The Complicated Body."'[117]

In late 2017 it featured in a historical novel ('a riveting medical romp through the War of the Roses') by Ornsby Hyde: *Dr William Hobbys: The promiscuous king's promiscuous doctor*.[118] The eponymous hero corrects another character with

> Hippocrates was born some four and a half centuries before Christ, and I am sure we are all familiar with his texts, *On the Physician* and *The Complicated Body* in which he also described the swelling of the terminal digit of the fingers called drumstick fingers, which you may perhaps have noticed the Queen also shows. Hippocrates thought this was due to chronic suppuration.

There is no mention of this symptom or its causes in *On the Physician*.[119]

For some, it is a general medical textbook. For example, *The Health Moderator* stated 'While in prison Hippocrates wrote a number of medical treatises such as The Complicated Body, encompassing many of the things about the body we know to be true today. Medicine at the time of Hippocrates knew little about anatomy and physiology because of the Greek taboo forbidding the dissection of humans.'[120] Another site invites us (how?) to 'review' it for ourselves:

> he wrote 'The Complicated Body,' a treatise that was many centuries ahead of its time. A great deal of what we know today to be true in modern medicine can be traced to the material in this work. Upon reviewing it, most will agree Hippocrates truly does deserve the title of being the "Father of Western Medicine".[121]

However, some people on the internet think they know even more about the specific contributions of this non-existent treatise. In 2012 one blogger developed the Wikipedia article to the effect that:

> Hippocrates was imprisoned for 20 years over his belief that diseases had natural causes rather than as the result of superstitions and gods. While he was in prison, he wrote a paper called 'The Complicated Body' and included his belief in the healing power of nature and that the body could heal itself. His writing encompassed many things about the body that we know to be true today.[122]

The Complicated Body must contain whatever is considered the essence of Hippocratic medicine; here, Nature as cause and as healer, a view commonly attributed to Hippocrates, as in Wikipedia's 'Hippocrates is credited with being the first person to believe that diseases were caused naturally, not because of superstition and gods' or its source, Nuland's 'the human body tends to heal itself'.[123]

In 2011, 'Sara C.' created a photo-book on mixbook.com called 'Hippocrates. The Pursuit to the Truth'.[124] Here we are told a lot of 'facts' about Hippocrates; he learned to read, write, spell, and play music at the young age of nine. Soon after, he went to a secondary school where he had two years of thorough athletic training. This is based on the online *Encyclopedia of World Biography*: 'After nine years of physical education, reading, writing, spelling, music, singing, and poetry, he went to a secondary school, where he spent two years and had very thorough athletic training.' In Sara C.'s interpretation, however, he must have started his education at birth.[125] The *Encyclopedia of World Biography* mentions neither the prison sentence nor *The Complicated Body* – probably this entry was created before the Wikipedia page was enhanced – but Sara C. naturally also drew on Wikipedia, particularly for her section 'Jail Time'. She picked up Hippocrates as 'the first person to believe that diseases were caused naturally, not because of superstition and gods' and the twenty-year imprisonment, but also incorporated further elements into the myth of *The Complicated Body*, explaining:

> As Hippocrates continued to pursue his career in medicine, it was realized that his ideas and theories were contradicting the Greek politics and governance. He believed that diseases were prevalent due to natural cause not as a result of superstition and gods. For this very reason, the physician spent twenty years in prison. While in jail Hippocrates wrote the well-known book of medicine, The Complicated Body. This book discusses many of the well-known ailments of the human body such as asthma and allergies. However, during his time the anatomy and physiology of the human body was not perfected, due to the Greek taboo forbidding the dissection of humans.[126] Hippocrates pursed his idea of how diseases occur and his belief is his pursue to find truth.

So Sara C. assumes the opposition to Hippocrates was due to his support of natural causes at a time when 'Greek politics and governance' (a gloss presumably based on looking up 'infrastructure' in a dictionary) supported the gods as cause. But 'asthma and allergies' are new to this myth, and pick up other internet sources including asthma sites and answers.com which state that

Hippocrates 'was the first person to describe the symptoms of asthma', that 'it was Hippocrates, particularly in his *Corpus Hippocraticum*, who made asthma a household name', or that he 'defined the disease asthma for the medical community'.[127] In a version of the story created in early 2019, the text includes remedies: 'In *The Complicated Body*, written by Hippocrates, he writes about the medicinal properties of willow bark and how it could be used to ease pain and reduce fevers.'[128]

One aspect still baffles me: the title. Was *The Complicated Body* chosen entirely at random? Searching online may suggest that the person who created the story based it on a Master's thesis by Nikolaos Angelou on healing from Hippocrates to the Christian Fathers: 'Each humour is tightly related to the corresponding basic elements (fire, air, earth and water) and qualities of matter as well as to a season of the year and particular diseases, all of which are also related to each other forming a complicated body of interdependence.'[129] However, the timing does not work; the thesis was submitted in August 2012 and the change to the Wikipedia page occurred on 12 December 2010. I have also found one attempt to present 'Corpus' as the author, not the texts. An online biography of Hippocrates with a particularly strange mixture of material that is presented as factual alongside comments that are supposed to be humorous states that 'despite his overwhelming fame there is actually very little we know of the man himself. This is because most of his work we know from the writings of Corpus, a practitioner under Hippocratic medicine and not from Hippocrates.'[130] Later in the short biography, however, its writer Kevin Lepton reverts to 'the Hippocratic Corpus' as a collection of medical works by several authors.

A post-doctoral researcher from Utrecht, Aiste Celkyte, suggested another possibility after I spoke there in June 2018. She wondered if the title *The Complicated Body* could somehow be a mistranslation of 'Hippocratic Corpus'. While I could see how 'corpus' could become 'body', how could 'complicated' enter the picture? She pointed out that in the period around 2010, when she was an undergraduate and when the insertion to the page was made, there were some unreliable Latin–English dictionaries online which gave what she described as 'very strange and elaborate translations of even simple words'.[131] While the dictionaries now available online are very different to what was available in 2010, she noted that the dictionary Ultralingua gives as their final translation of the word 'corpus' 'a whole composed of parts united, a body, frame, system, structure, community, corporation'.[132] This suggests that the word implies some complex structure, so the author of that paragraph from Wikipedia might have found the phrase 'Corpus Hippocraticum', assumed it was the name of a single treatise, googled for a Latin dictionary and then chosen 'a more flowery translation' from those offered. We can only speculate as to the editor's original intention. Others who have heard me speak on the topic have also noted possible links in the story to Socrates, as an imprisoned visionary, and to Adolf Hitler, who wrote the first part of *Mein Kampf* in prison.

From coercion to freedom

There is, however, one more question to consider: why does the story of Hippocrates in jail resonate so powerfully on the internet? Many modern reworkings contain a negative message about mainstream medicine today, often building on the themes addressed by the satirist Richard Armour: 'There are some fascinating legends about Hippocrates. One is that he never gave a thought to money. Another is that he admitted his errors. The reader should keep in mind that these are legends.'[133] Here, Hippocrates stands for a better past which did not really exist, characterized by no concerns for payment and honesty about results. Commonly, as well as being the Father of Medicine, he also represents active resistance to medicine today. In *Assassin's Creed: Odyssey*, when the Spartan soldier Alexios meets Hippocrates, he knows it is him because he doesn't follow 'tradition': 'Challenging tradition … you must be Hippokrates'.[134] This is the Hippocrates who is the first, who is not held back by the past, and who resists 'the authorities' or 'the infrastructure'. It is not the Hippocrates who himself became 'the tradition'.

The main critiques of modern medicine contained in retellings of Hippocrates now are that it is all about money, controlled by the government, and refuses to accept it is wrong. *The Health Moderator* likes the story of Hippocrates in prison because the site stands for 'health freedom issues that affect our right to choose our own pathway to health'; for protecting the individual against 'governmental restrictions and regulations that affect our ability to practice our "health beliefs" as we see fit'.[135] This Hippocrates, therefore, was 'opposed by authorities, who considered themselves mediators and spokesmen for their many gods, including those who ruled health ... Now all we need to do is de-fang the profiteering pharmaceuticals, the Monsantos and their GMOs—along with their coercive handmaidens among the government agencies—and return to genuine choice and food freedom.'[136]

The use of Hippocrates not as representative of current medicine but as a challenge to it is not new. As John Harley Warner pointed out in his study of the Hippocrates of antebellum America, this is a complex manoeuvre; there too, the stories told about him 'called for revolt while invoking the theme of return'.[137] For British medicine in the interwar period, Hippocrates 'offered an ideal to invoke against specialism and some forms of state medicine' as part of a move back to the individual doctor and the individual patient.[138] In an article predating the Wikipedia insertion, Wesley J. Smith (not to be confused with the scholar of ancient medicine, Wesley D. Smith), a lawyer and activist against abortion, euthanasia and cloning, and an opponent of 'scientocracy' – the situation in which scientists determine what is ethical – argued in favour of 'Defending the *Hippocratic Oath*,' and for 'the importance of conscience in health care'. He stated that what he called the 'coercive trend' in US medicine dates from the Mayor of New York City 'mandating abortion training for all OB/GYN residents working in the city's public hospitals' other than those who could assert their conscience.[139] Since then, he claimed, conscience clauses across the world had been dropped, with doctors who refuse to perform abortions being compelled to refer a woman to a doctor who will.[140]

Hippocrates provides a rallying call not only to resist the state and its demands, but also to fight back against 'Big Pharma', the derogatory term for the global pharmaceutical industry and for what is perceived as its infiltration of all areas of our lives. For the US, Rebecca Carley, an anti-vaccination and alternative medicine provider who will be discussed further in Chapter 7, made the following claim: 'Note that it is actually illegal to use the "cure" word when using natural therapies due to the corrupt influence of Big Pharma on lawmakers.'[141] As is the case here, criticism of Big Pharma is often linked to the promotion of an anti-vaccination agenda. In April 2014, the US satirical site GomerBlog posted 'New Medical Graduate Takes Hippocratic Oath, Followed by Big Pharma, Government Vaccine Oath', a story in which a medical graduate takes in quick succession his public *Hippocratic Oath* and a secret oath 'To forever hold the true knowledge of toxic vaccines and all the dangers that accompany them, a secret forever'.[142] A discussion of the situation in the Philippines, where a Traditional Alternative Medicine Act was passed in 1998 and promoted various medicinal plants, argues that the Food and Drug Administration (FDA) there is not actively encouraging this, speculating: 'Sometimes I wonder whether FDA's passivity on its obligation to promote the aforesaid plant cures is proof its officials' "golden fidelity" to the Big Pharma.'[143]

Developing the themes of resistance to the state and to Big Pharma, the story of Hippocrates in prison can become one of his many areas of appeal to alternative and complementary medicines. For example, it accounts for an article on 'Who was Hippocrates?' appearing on the website 'Rethinking Cancer', run by the Foundation for Advancement in Cancer Therapy, which promotes 'non-toxic biological approaches' to cancer treatment and prevention; if Hippocrates 'were living today ... he would be disregarded or limited in his work by those who now claim him as their patron saint and swear to the oath that bares [sic] his name'.[144]

Using the word 'Hippocratic' or 'Hippocrates' may be about distinguishing one type of medicine from others, or about promoting a particular approach to the body – the holistic Hippocrates, or the natural foods Hippocrates, both of whom will be discussed later in this book. It also claims a connection with the idealized 'Father of Medicine'. Hippocrates is 'timeless' but he wrote within a particular context. In the Wikipedia myth of Hippocrates in prison, he becomes a role model for hard work and for altruism: he can make the most of a bad situation, and he treats both prisoners and visiting dignitaries. He did not accept the status quo, particularly in religion. The imaginary treatise *The Complicated Body* reinforces the message that what he wrote is still true today. The book is about physiology, or about physiology and anatomy, or lists diseases including asthma and allergies. It is revolutionary: it can still be read: indeed, it is the only one of his works that survives.

For the users of Hippocrates described here, he remains a force for good, and an ideal to which to aspire. In the words of Dr Weeks, 'So, now you know the true history: Hippocrates spend [sic] two decades in the slammer for practicing above the standard of care.'[145] Only he didn't.

4

Needing a Bit of Information: Hippocrates in the News

While those deliberately looking for information on Hippocrates will head for Wikipedia, basic knowledge of him comes to many via press coverage of new medical stories although, of course, Wikipedia may still be the journalists' source. There is something about the coverage of the ancient world in the press in particular which seems to bring out the Indiana Jones in us. Whether this is about 'decoding' a text, finding something 'lost' or 'solving' a mystery, the way to attract a reader in the age of Dan Brown and the *Da Vinci Code* is to present a story as a puzzle that has at last been unravelled, preferably as a result of the wonders of modern technology which – like Alexander the Great slicing through the tangled Gordian Knot – takes a different approach to an established problem.[1] A recent textbook on medical Greek even riffed on the Dan Brown phenomenon by publishing under the title *The Hippocrates Code: Unravelling the Ancient Mysteries of Modern Medical Terminology*, but it correctly tells its readers that Hippocrates is 'a shadowy and semi-legendary figure, and none of the dozens of surviving medical tracts linked to his name can be definitively proved to have been written by him'.[2] The reception of the myth of Hippocrates in prison, discussed in the previous chapter, suggests that Hippocrates plays particularly well into conspiracy theories, so if a news story also includes a sense of a conspiracy, that is all to the good; and, continuing my conclusions from Chapter 3, in the case of Hippocrates, that conspiracy can be modern medicine as experienced by the reader.

In theory, current news stories should be one of the contexts in which modern scholarship on Hippocrates and the Corpus now has some influence, as complete treatises from the Corpus, and extracts from others, are increasingly available online; however, there are obstacles here.[3] Medical writers producing historical studies often use only PubMed, Medline and Scopus, none of which currently takes the user to journals in history (other than medical history) or classical studies, let alone to the monographs and chapters in edited volumes which are often more important to classical studies than are journal articles.[4] Possibly the rise of open access articles and academic blog posts will help, but only if journalists can locate them easily.

I suspect, however, that the short deadlines of the media militate against accuracy. So does the nature of the internet, where 'the online communicator is more likely to simply want to make a point in order to participate; he or she needs a bit of information, a quotation, or a turn of phrase'.[5] The 'impact agenda' of the UK Research Excellence Framework exercises puts an increasing premium on achieving reach (how many people?) and significance (did the research have a demonstrable effect?).[6] This encourages universities to issue press releases making claims which, perhaps, the research itself does not fully support, or which are written by the press team with insufficient input from the researchers themselves.

What do current news stories show about our continued need for Hippocrates? In this chapter I shall explore the press reactions to four research discoveries announced at the end of 2017 and in 2018, which I think illustrate the main ways in which Hippocrates is currently being used to sell stories: these involve three of the most important sources of new information for classical studies, namely archaeology, papyri and manuscripts. By the time you read this book, of course, those stories may have developed further; such is the nature of scholarship.

Taking and breaking: The Hippocratic *Oath*

On 21 May 2012, at the start of the project which has led to this book, my research assistant Joanna Brown collected all mentions of Hippocrates on Twitter from the previous week. Starting with Gaea Products selling balsamic vinegar with thyme honey as 'first used by the famous Greek medical legend Hippocrates!', this list featured many of the 'quotes' most popular today; short sayings attributed to him which have taken on a life of their own, which will be the subject of later chapters here.[7] Other tweets included the claim that

Hippocrates named cancer, and that his method of diagnosis was 'face reading' – as was that of Imhotep. Amidst the general enthusiasm for him, there was just one derogatory tweet: a political group, The People's Cube, commented on the hashtag #obamainhistory 'Hippocrates performed needless surgeries to get rich. Obama put an end to abuse and gives patients painkillers instead'. This developed their website's encouragement to members to publicize that 'Hippocrates created the Hypocrite's oath which requires doctors to perform needless surgeries so they can buy luxury cars and large homes. President Obama created the Independent Patient Advisory Board which prevents doctors from doing this and gives patients pain pills instead.'[8] While the common Hippocrates/hypocrites link is obviously very deliberate here, as it was in a US police operation targeting illegal drug prescriptions called 'Operation Hypocritical Oath', online invocation of Hippocrates also includes numerous but inevitable accidental confusions of the words, often with one person tweeting 'I hate hippocrates', followed by the intervention, 'Hippocrates was a Greek physician. I think you meant hypocrite.'[9]

Later in that month, some specific medical claims were also shared; for example, that Hippocrates cured Alzheimer's disease in 400 BCE by placing a 'copper top head its energy heals' [sic] and that 'Hippocrates' writings also contain the first references to proctoscopy for rectal examination. Boldly going etc etc'.[10] By then, however, many tweets were trying to link Hippocrates to an emerging news story: the British Medical Association had announced industrial action for 21 June, under which doctors would only be providing urgent and emergency care. Twitter's responses mostly referenced the *Oath*, including 'It's violating the Hippocratic oath', 'Where in the Hippocratic Oath does it say "Thou shalt not work to rule?"' and 'All doctors should be made to work for free, else they are sacrificing their Hippocratic oath.' During the BBC Question Time programme addressing the strike announcement, several people tweeted the comment of an audience member that 'The doctors' strike is breaking the Hippocratic oath for the sake of greed', but one person asked 'Do doctors actually "take" a Hippocratic oath these days? I didn't think they did?'[11] A good question, and a very good answer.

As we saw in Chapter 2, the *Oath* has long been regarded as 'the high-water mark of professional morality'; in 1921, Withington wrote that the *Oath* 'in dignity of tone and high morality . . . is well worthy of its supposed author' and in 1931 it was normal to describe it as 'genuinely Hippocratic'.[12] Writing in 2004, Steven Miles describes physicians taking part in policy debates who wave the *Oath* 'around like a censer'.[13] Studies of ancient medicine have moved on: 'no one now would attribute the oath to Hippocrates or say that it represents the generality of the medical profession, on Cos or elsewhere'.[14] Outside the academy, however, the continued widespread belief in the *Oath* as ubiquitous strengthens claims such as those mentioned in Chapter 3, that the Hippocratic *Oath* now exists alongside a secret oath to Big Pharma. In a 1995 episode of *The Simpsons* the unethical Dr Hibbert, who performs unnecessary operations, shows his lack of commitment to the *Oath* by saying 'Hippocrates, schmippocrates'.[15]

The *Oath* is widely mentioned in news stories. I remember in 2000 watching the trailer for a BBC *Panorama* documentary on Harold Shipman, the British GP who murdered at least 250 elderly patients before suspicions were raised in 1998: slowly zooming in on Shipman's face, the trailer included the words 'He broke the Hippocratic Oath.' This angle is still repeated; for example 'It's clear that the Hippocratic Oath meant nothing to Dr. Harold Shipman – he did not work for the well-being of patients and most certainly took the role of God when deciding their fate' or 'certainly, none of his patients questioned his adherence to the Hippocratic Oath, pledging to do everything in his power to prolong and save life'.[16] The words 'Hippocratic *Oath*' are often used for the version of the *Oath* written by Louis Lasagna, Dean of Tufts University's School of Medicine, in 1964, and the reference to the 'role of God' derives from Lasagna's 'Above all, I must not play at God'.[17] I find it noteworthy that, in a story about serial murder, anyone should even care about the Hippocratic *Oath*: murder is wrong in any case. Yet the references to the *Oath* suggest that the public at large does care, and that people believe they know what is in it. They want their doctor to be 'the kind of person who could swear an oath to uphold the highest possible professional aspirations'.[18] While this is not the place for a full discussion of the various clauses of the *Oath*, it is worth discussing the persistence of some errors about who takes it, in any of its current versions.

In a 1995 article, Vivian Nutton definitively demolished two myths: first, that the *Oath* is a 'fixed and unalterable document of medical ethics' and, second, that all doctors in the Western medical tradition have taken, and continue to take, it.[19] Different versions have been written, but none has ever been taken by all doctors. Published in a medical journal, Nutton's conclusions have still not reached the general reader. For example, the most recent version of *The Hutchinson Unabridged Encyclopedia with Atlas and Weather Guide* (widely used online in schools and colleges, and claiming to give 'an authoritative insight') tells us that the *Oath* is 'Taken by all doctors on qualifying'.[20] Those searching online may find 'All newly qualified doctors take what is called the *Hippocratic Oath*', the less dogmatic 'Most doctors still swear the *Hippocratic Oath* today' which still suggests that in the past all doctors would have taken it, or even references to 'the Hippocratic oath which all newly qualified doctors in the west have been required to swear since the 4th century'.[21] In fact, it is only in the last decades of the twentieth century that the use of the *Oath* – or, at least, some version of it – increased.[22]

A third myth that is still common is that Hippocrates wrote the *Oath*. In his *Bad Medicine: Doctors doing harm since Hippocrates*, first published in 2006, the intellectual historian David Wootton explicitly wrote the history of medicine 'against the grain' by foregrounding progress and 'distinguish[ing] good medicine from bad'.[23] For him, Hippocrates 'founded a tradition of medical education that continues uninterrupted to the present day'. Although he went on to acknowledge that the Hippocratic *Oath* does not have an unbroken tradition of being taken by doctors, claims that it does owing more to attempts to 'foster a sense of continuity', nevertheless he considered that 'The oath was written by Hippocrates'...'almost certainly'.[24] He used phrases like 'Hippocrates would have recognized', 'Hippocrates thought that', 'Hippocrates believed that' and 'Although Hippocrates had no way of knowing'.[25]

So why do the myths that there is just one *Oath*, written by Hippocrates and taken by all doctors, surface as soon as a medical issue comes up in the news, rather than die the death they deserve? Partly because we need an ideal against which to measure our response to ethical issues, even if that ideal never existed. The *Oath* remains 'the physician's calling-card', defining his character and that of his medicine as 'devoted to the care of his patients'.[26] Another aspect is that works of reference, perhaps inevitably, are largely parasitic upon each other; they remain in a closed world, rarely meeting new research and, just as in the early modern period, 'The printed books most likely to cite reference books were other reference books.'[27] Historically, such books have long been criticized for encouraging errors to proliferate and for encouraging superficial knowledge rather than real knowledge.[28] Furthermore, biomedical journals are very casual in the accuracy of their quotations and in their referencing of their sources, as can be seen by the way in which wording not in the *Oath* – such as 'First, do no harm,' an example to which I shall return in Chapter 5 – is persistently attributed to it.[29] Here, as elsewhere in the reception of Hippocrates, it is always difficult to correct 'a major inaccuracy that may well become "accepted fact"'.[30]

But, in medicine as elsewhere, there is also a strong element of emotion behind attempts like this to create continuities with the classical past. Nutton suggested that the revival of the *Oath* at the end of the last century was akin to the rise of the school prom, reflecting a renewed interest in formal ceremonies.[31] He also observed that oaths both bind and exclude. While citing the 1995 article as evidence for the *Oath* only having 'become a standard part of a formal medical school graduation ceremony' in 1804, and rightly noting that 'the tinkering with Hippocrates' oath began soon after its first utterance', Howard Markel described how he still feels an emotional reaction when standing to recite a version at commencement ceremonies.[32] Here, he echoed many others, such as J. Aaron Johnson, editor of the *Journal of the Medical Society of New Jersey*, who in 1964 described his own experience of such a ceremony as 'the solemn and moving high spot of the doctor's career' in which the 'incantation' of the *Oath* 'symbolized crossing of the bridge into a kind of priesthood – and this too was part of our heritage'.[33] In view of the popular image of Hippocratic medicine as opposed to that of 'the priests', this is a particularly ironic sensation. Other medical professionals, however, see no value in the *Oath*, and comment for example that they have become 'incredulous that the archaic text was still read at all'.[34]

In an article published a year after Nutton's 1995 piece, Dale Smith noted that, in a sense, it matters little what the actual content of any version of the *Oath* may be; just as in linking anonymous ancient Greek medical texts to Hippocrates, so in taking the *Oath* what matters most is 'the claiming of a dynamic heritage in medicine'.[35] For doctors, then, the *Oath* is about this heritage as well as marking their own transition to a new and honoured status. Johnson also proposed that an early 1960s decline in holding ceremonies in which the *Oath* was taken reflected then-changing views of the medical profession: 'There is some evidence that the public views doctors, as a group, with less enchantment than they did a half century ago ... Of course, the slow atrophy of the traditional *Oath* is not the cause of this; but it could be a symptom.'[36]

Imhotep and the power of Egyptian medicine

The regular return to the *Oath* in discussions of medical ethics is an important aspect of the way in which we learn about Hippocrates, but this document also features in challenges to his authority. In Chapter 3, when discussing his role as 'Father of Medicine', I mentioned other contenders from other cultures. One of the pressures on the Hippocrates Wikipedia page comes from attempts to take away this title and bestow it on Imhotep; for example, the talkpage comment that 'The article is bogus and based on an illusion in it's [sic] opening' (Tljackson224).[37] Tweeting on 31 May 2012, The Astrochologist, a professional astrologer, stated simply 'Imhotep predates Hippocrates'.[38]

Hippocrates has more to do with Imhotep than rivalry for the title of Father of Medicine, as websites and articles in medical journals regularly repeat a direct connection between them because 'Hippocrates visited Egypt to study and understand medicine'.[39] This myth has even been phrased in terms of Hippocrates travelling to use the library of Imhotep, dismissed by the classicist Jacques Jouanna as an 'impossible hypothesis'.[40] Yet the absence of any evidence for such a journey does nothing to prevent belief in it. In January 2019 @siliconenozzles asserted on Twitter:

> Enemas date all the way back to ancient Egypt, not to mention many different cultures. Hippocrates spent seven years in Egypt learning from the physicians, then brought these practices back to Greece, and they then slowly spread around the world.[41]

The claims for Imhotep's priority are worth examining not just in terms of how the history of ancient medicine responds to political pressures, but also because they demonstrate what we want medicine to be. Who was Imhotep? Or, more importantly, who do people think he was? A popular online ancient history site gives a timeline including: '2667 BCE–2648 BCE Imhotep in Egypt writes medical texts describing diagnosis and treatment of 100 diseases and 48 injuries.'[42] These medical texts are supposed to be those of the Edwin Smith Papyrus, one of the key sources for Egyptian medicine, dated to around 1600 BCE; its translator, James Breasted, speculated that the material could have been written by Imhotep then copied again and again over many centuries, a claim found widely on the internet.[43] Imhotep is described as being 'recorded in history as the world's first physician, a title that was later bestowed upon a Greek named Hippocrates who was born some 2,200 years later'; the same website states that Imhotep was 'referred to as Asclepius, the god of medicine, by the Greeks'.[44] Yet even the Wikipedia page dedicated to him admits that claims for him being a doctor are unreliable, with sources from his lifetime hailing him only as chancellor to the Pharaoh, Djoser, and architect of the step-pyramid; the first mention of his healing powers dates from 2,200 years after he died.[45] Within Egyptian studies it is acknowledged that, although his statues were eventually used in healing – for example water poured over them was used to treat various conditions – 'There is no information whether he was also a physician.'[46]

Whoever was Father of Medicine, Imhotep or Hippocrates, the myth takes a similar form. Hippocrates is believed to have shone the light of reason on the darkness of superstition, and those who want Imhotep to be the author of the Edwin Smith Papyrus play up this text as 'science' in order to support a narrative of movement from magic, or religion, to rational knowledge. Yet, while the front of the papyrus gives a sequence of chapters on wounds starting at the head, the back has spells against demons: and 'Both sides of the *Edwin Smith Papyrus* belong together.'[47] We want our medicine to make sense, in current terms, but we find it hard to cope with a medicine that mixes science and magic.

There is a further, important, reason for the resurgence of Imhotep as Father of Medicine; the modern priority dispute between him and Hippocrates seeks to reverse a valorization of West over East which has been common in histories of medicine into the twentieth century. For example, in 1931, ending their chapter on Hippocrates, Stubbs and Bligh invited their reader to

> contrast these medical and hygienic achievements of the fifth century B.C. with those of Assyria and Egypt of the seventh century B.C. and realize how utterly impossible it is to conceive that in those two centuries, or ten times those two centuries, the Eastern peoples should have advanced from their dimly lit superstitions and conservatisms to the blazing daylight of the West.[48]

In such histories, even where Egyptian medicine is praised for its content, it is usually seen as non-Western, and attacked for what Withington called 'its non-progressive character'; Greeks speculate and investigate, but Egyptians lack 'love of knowledge for its own sake'.[49] This repeats stereotypes used by Garrison in his much-reprinted 1913 history of medicine, a source for the Wikipedia Hippocrates page: while 'the Father of Medicine was indebted to Egypt for much of his knowledge', the difference between Egyptian and Greek medicine was that Greek medicine was 'entirely free from priestly domination'.[50]

Overturning the traditional priority of the West in favour of a 'stolen legacy' theory,[51] attempting to trace ancient Greek medicine to Egypt, and trying to replace Hippocrates as Father of Medicine with Imhotep, are all influenced by the three volumes of Martin Bernal's *Black Athena* project, published between 1987 and 2006. Bernal argued not only that the roots of ancient Greek civilization and language lay in Egypt and the Semitic Near East, but also that 'the Ancient Egyptian civilization can usefully be seen as African'.[52] These proved controversial claims, but an internet search for 'Who was the true father of medicine?' will now find assertions about Hippocrates such as '... some are of the opinion that the title bestowed upon this man is very misleading. Records show that a man by the name of Imhotep was treating ill patients with modern techniques many generations before Hippocrates [sic] appearance in history.' Imhotep becomes Hippocrates' 'mentor': Hippocrates his 'devotee'.[53] Cited here, and on many other sites, is Sir William Osler, who identified Imhotep as 'the first figure of a physician to stand out clearly from the mists of antiquity'.[54] Yet Osler still regarded Hippocrates as the 'Father of Medicine', so that writers such as James H. Brien are wrong to say that 'in 1928, William Osler proposed that Imhotep was the "real father of medicine" – not Hippocrates'.[55]

Imhotep is also being credited as the author of the *Oath*. The Afrikan Center of Well Being, Inc., which markets a range of holistic medicines, states that 'The Oath is a universal doctrine utilized by traditional Afrikan healers from Imhotep forward along with The Law of Ma'at, centuries before the advent of Hippocrates. Today, the Hippocratic oath is an abridged, allegorical and meaningless document not adhered to by allopaths plus other health professionals!' and, as I mentioned in the Introduction, this site exhorts readers to 'Download a copy prior to your next doctor or dental appointment and conduct a performance evaluation!' A note explains that 'An Aescalapian [sic] is a follower of the God of Medicine, IMHOTEP, the PRINCE OF PEACE!'[56] A new version of the *Oath*, the 'Oath of Imhotep', was composed by Anthony Pickett in 1992 'in recognition of African contributions to Western medicine';

he repeated the Osler claim about Imhotep and the 'mists of antiquity' although he made this 'the midst'.[57]

The name of Imhotep sells news stories about ancient Egyptian medicine. A multi-disciplinary group at the University of Manchester was funded from 2005 by the Leverhulme Trust to study the plants used in ancient Egyptian medicine.[58] At that point, it included Dr Jackie Campbell and Dr Ryan Metcalfe from the KNH Centre for Biomedical Egyptology, and worked with Judith Seath who performed chemical analyses on the plants named in medical papyri, as well as with their partner, the Egyptian Medicinal Plant Conservation Project in St Catherine's, Sinai.[59] On 9 May 2007, the university issued a press release from this project, headlined 'Egyptians, not Greeks, were true fathers of medicine'.[60] They made it clear that the papyri the team had examined were not newly-discovered – they had been known from the mid-nineteenth century – and that the new claims simply 'concerned the efficacy' of the drug substances named in those papyri.[61] This sort of research is part of a recent trend towards making strong claims for the antimicrobial effects of materials used in the past, which may also reflect the 'impact agenda' of universities today.[62]

Imhotep was not mentioned in this press release but, when the *Daily Telegraph* ran the story, it was headlined 'How Imhotep gave us medicine' with the headline of the press release then repeated in the main story: 'The Egyptians – not the ancient Greeks – were the true fathers of medicine'.[63] The story went on to claim that 'The medical history books will have to be revised' because 'a credible form of pharmacy and medicine' had been found in papyri dating to '1,500BC – some 1,000 years before Hippocrates was born'.[64] The reference to Hippocrates is interesting; this did not feature in the 2009 Leverhulme report.[65] The context is the research group pointing out that ingredients in ancient Egyptian remedies would have had physical effects; for example, castor oil as a laxative, cumin for flatulence, substances to redden the skin to treat muscular pain.[66] In framing the story around Imhotep, the *Telegraph* journalist went beyond using his name in the title, claiming that medicine began with 'the likes of Imhotep (2667BC–2648BC), who designed the pyramids at Saqqara and was elevated to become the god of healing' and ending by quoting the lead investigator on the funded project, Rosalie David:

And of all the ancient Egyptians, it is Imhotep who was regarded as being the father of medicine. 'He should have the credit,' said Prof David.[67]

This proved to be a very saleable line. The story was subsequently taken up by Colourful, an African-Caribbean radio station and wider network of sites and groups.[68] *Rasta Livewire* ran a story by Jide Uwechia under the headline 'Imhotep and medical science: Africa's gift to the world,' quoting from Jackie Campbell and opposing 'previously peddled lies which identify Greece as the origin of medicine' while presenting Hippocrates as the 'devotee' of Imhotep.[69] Journalist Deborah Gabriel interviewed Rosalie David for *Black Britain* and reported that

> Imhotep was a man we know from the Egyptian records as the architect of the first pyramid in Egypt – the step pyramid at Saqqara that goes back to the very beginnings of their history to about 2600 BC. In Egyptology we've always thought of Imhotep as an architect, the people later in Egyptian history and indeed the Greeks, regarded him as the father of medical science ... He probably was the founder of medical science in Egypt right back at the time when they were building the earliest pyramids.[70]

The headline now was a variant on the original press release which further increased the authority of the story by putting 'scientists' into the picture: 'Scientists find evidence proving ancient Egyptians were fathers of modern medicine', although the 'new evidence' mentioned in the subheading may raise hopes of rather more than the observation that castor oil is a laxative. The factual statement in a further subheading, 'Ancient Egyptian medical papyri were written before the birth of Hippocrates', is even less 'news'. Gabriel wrote:

> African scholars have long identified Imhotep, the Prime Minister of Pharaoh Djoser, the 2nd King of the 3rd Egyptian Dynasty, as the founding father of medicine, including Dr Molefi Kete Asante, John Henrik Clarke and Cheik Anta Diop.[71]

The reference to 'African scholars' shows how this small story was now moving into a larger narrative: the 'stolen legacy' one.

Once the claims of a press release or published academic journal article are translated into simpler language as they fight for a place in a news site alongside celebrity news, it is perhaps inevitable that they become sensationalist, and that the headline focuses on the sensational element. Contested as it is between an Afrocentric history and historians of ancient Egypt and Greece, the priority war between Imhotep and Hippocrates is unlikely to go away.

Poop proof: Hippocrates' parasites

At the end of 2017, the *Journal of Archaeological Science: Reports* published online a piece by an international team of archaeologists and an anatomical scientist presenting archaeological support for the identification of intestinal parasitic worms mentioned in the Hippocratic Corpus.[72] Presented as a significant discovery demonstrating the benefits of archaeologists working with historians, to the non-specialist this may have looked rather less impressive. The study used finds of worm eggs from four of a total of twenty-five previously-excavated burials on the Greek island of Kea (Ceos), dated to the Neolithic period, the late Bronze Age, and the Roman period, representing a total time range of 4,000 years. Two burials showed roundworm on the pelvis, the location taken as indicating that it came from the faecal contents of the individuals buried, while another two had evidence of whipworm; while these figures may seem very low, the researchers suggest that the fragility of the eggs means those from other species may have been washed away.[73]

This story could have been framed in many ways, but even in a specialized archaeological journal the decision was taken to make it into one about proving that 'Hippocrates was right': indeed, the first word of the article was 'Hippocrates'. This may have been why it had such traction in the media, as otherwise the point that past populations had various types of intestinal worms would hardly be news. The Corpus, the authors assumed, was the work of Hippocrates and his students and showed 'which conditions Hippocrates and his students encountered', although later in the article the students disappear in favour of the 'it's all by Hippocrates' approach, with the article stating that we can become 'much more confident as to the species described by Hippocrates 2500 years ago'.[74] The significance of Hippocratic medicine is that 'they described humoural theory to explain the cause of disease for the first time' (here, 'they' rather than 'he') and this 'theory became the accepted explanation for ill health and influenced medicine for the next two thousand years in Europe and the Mediterranean region'.[75] All of this shows little knowledge of the Hippocratic

Corpus itself, where the humours are only one explanation offered, and the references given to support the comment just quoted include one which never even mentions the humours.[76] The explicitly Hippocratic framing of the story strikes me as very odd, not just because none of the burials was from the period of the Hippocratic Corpus (a period which, for some reason, the article sets a century later than usual, namely in 'the 4th and 3rd centuries BC'), but also because Kea, described in the article as 'not far from Kos', is in fact many miles away: Kea is one of the Cyclades Islands in the western Aegean, Cos one of the Dodecanese Islands in the south-eastern Aegean.[77]

What was the source for the historical comments in this 2017 article? As evidence for their claim that the Hippocratic treatises which say most about intestinal helminths are *Epidemics*, *Prognostics* and *Coan Prognoses*, the authors cite a 2007 article arguing that 'the Hippocratic Corpus provides the first scientific observations about the clinical perception and treatment of helminthic diseases. These observations follow the scientific principles of Hippocrates, the father of modern medicine, who relied on knowledge and observation.'[78] Once again, the image of Hippocrates as the great observer is used. The 2007 article claims to be based on a 'systematic study' of Emile Littré's nineteenth-century translation of the Corpus, but it does not explain what 'systematic' means here – for example, what finding aids were used? what words were selected as significant? – while the extracts it gives are limited. The authors of the 2007 article use the sort of phrasing which implies clear and undisputed authorship of these treatises: 'Hippocrates believes that', 'Hippocrates observed that', 'Hippocrates contributed significantly to the progress of medicine'.[79]

As is now standard academic practice, the 2017 story was, of course, sent to the media via a Cambridge University press release.[80] This too stressed that the finds were able to 'confirm' what Hippocrates said in 'the most influential works of classical medicine'. Although here the dates for Hippocrates were the fifth and fourth, rather than fourth and third, centuries BCE, the press release followed the article in playing up four-humour theory. The story was taken up on Twitter, with Greek History Podcast linking to the bioarchaeologist Kristina Killgrove's story for *Forbes* magazine, headlined 'Archaeologists find intestinal worms in burials from the time of Hippocrates'; although, of course, as the story itself later clarified, it was the eggs rather than worms which were discovered.[81] Microbes&Infection also spread the story, again in terms of 'the parasitic worms that Hippocrates described', although a Twitter feed from the Instituto de Enseñanzas a Distancia de Andalucía more cautiously offered '*may* confirm Hippocrates' textual mention of parasitic worms' [my italics].[82]

David Crystal points out that 'Headlines which are idiosyncratic and ludic attract the reader, and make it more likely that their accompanying articles will be read.'[83] Leaving aside the predictable alliterative headlines ('Poop proof'[84]) here and the general excitement about being able to write 'poo', it is instructive to see how the press presented the story, not only in the headlines but also in the supporting text boxes. *Newsweek* stated that the worms were what 'Hippocrates, the ancient Greek physician widely considered the father of modern medicine, described in his famous medical texts'.[85] The journalist here went on to claim that Hippocrates produced various texts including the Hippocratic *Oath*, 'the pledge all physicians take to do no harm'; 'all physicians'? *Science Alert* headlined 'Ancient poo is the first-ever confirmation Hippocrates was right about parasites.'[86] Hippocrates ('the famous physician and "Father of Western Medicine" who lived from around 460 to 370 BCE') was right ... but about what, precisely? The article opened by addressing its reader: 'You've probably been wondering about this for a while: did the Ancient Greeks ever get intestinal worms like we do today? The answer, we can now tell you, is an unequivocal yes'. But why would we need the confirmation of four skeletons from different periods on Kea to affirm this, when the Hippocratic Corpus and other medical texts from the ancient Greek and Roman worlds already tell us so much about worms? The story goes on to repeat the article's point that three different types of worm are named in the Corpus 'but researchers [formerly] had to guess which worms he meant, since they had found no archaeological evidence'.

The *Daily Mail* of course went further, its headline message being one that emphasized the otherness of the ancient world, in this case that 'Ancient Greece was infested with human parasites'.[87] An accompanying textbox repeated the alleged connection with the *Oath*. The main story stated that the Corpus is 'a collection of 60 texts written by Hippocrates' even though this contradicts the textbox reading 'About 60 medical writings have survived that bear his name – although most of these were not written by him.' The Hippocrates theme was underlined by the inclusion of images of 'Hippocrates' in the *Daily Mail* and *Forbes* stories.[88] For *Forbes*, Kristina Killgrove provided a much more accurate version of the Hippocrates angle – he 'lent his name centuries later' to (rather than wrote) the *Oath* – before summarising the story. Elsewhere, however, the worms were even called 'Hippocrates' parasites'.[89]

The Hippocratic link reached its peak in the *Mental Floss* article opening, 'The long-held mystery of Hippocrates and the parasitic worms has finally been solved.'[90] This piece followed the original article to the extent of having the 'between the 4th and 3rd centuries BCE' dating. Another article, in *LiveScience*, presented the story as one that serves to 'bolster historians' theory about Hippocrates' diagnostic prowess'; nothing new, then, only confirmation of what we already knew, not least that Hippocrates was right.[91] The rest of the story includes confirmation that 'Hippocrates was probably talking about roundworms in his 2,500-year-old medical texts' and that he 'may have conflated' pinworm and whipworm under the name *askaris*. So there is a mystery: we have solved it: and it confirms a hypothesis we already had.

In the final section of their argument, the authors of the original article looked at texts in the Hippocratic Corpus mentioning intestinal helminths, but omitting possibly the most interesting discussion in *Diseases* 4, which distinguishes between flatworms and roundworms as types of 'helminth':

> Now roundworms reproduce, whereas a flatworm does not, although admittedly some people say it does: for a person with a flatworm passes things that look like cucumber seeds from time to time with his stool, which some people identify as the worm's offspring. But, in my opinion, people who say this are wrong, because so many little offspring could not be engendered by a single adult, nor is there enough empty space in the intestine properly to nourish such offspring.[92]

They also miss out many other Hippocratic references to intestinal worms, such as *Prorrhetic* 2.28 on women who vomit up helminths, or *Prognostics* 11 where it is a good sign if helminths are passed in the stools.[93]

I remain unconvinced that trying to match ancient medical descriptions with parasitology really contributes anything here. There is already ancient literary evidence of variation between Greek populations in their experience of intestinal worms – Theophrastus claims that the Athenians did not have tapeworms (except for athletes, who ate pork) although their Boeotian neighbours did – while Pliny the Elder wrote that people in Thrace and Phrygia did not have tapeworm, and nor did Athenians. So there are discussions of differences between ancient populations, which could be relevant, but these are not mentioned here, in favour of creating a false picture of continuity over many centuries and very different parts of the Greek world. In Chapter 2, I mentioned Benjamin Rush's 1806 remark that when Hippocrates is quoted, it is 'to support a fact or an opinion that was discovered or suggested without the aid of his works'.[94] The reverse seems to have happened with the intestinal worms theory: the archaeological evidence is used to tell us something which we already knew from the Hippocratic Corpus.

Julius please her: Hippocratic hysteria

A further example of what Hippocrates is supposed to have done is to name 'hysteria'; for example, in a medical journal article by Cecilia Tasca, 'Hippocrates (5th century BC) is the first to use the term *hysteria*' or, in a fantasy author's blog based on a student essay found online, Nadine Ducca's 'The very father of medicine Hippocrates was the first to coin "hysteria"' or, tying it less firmly to the man himself, 'the name, hysteria, has been in use since the time of Hippocrates'.[95] None of these statements is true, not just because – as we saw in Chapter 2 – we cannot tie any treatise of the Hippocratic Corpus to the historical Hippocrates, but because the word 'hysteria' does not exist in ancient Greek medicine, nor in any other classical Greek text.[96] While it derives from one of the ancient Greek words for womb – *hystera* – this is not the same as saying that 'hysteria' itself is an ancient Greek word. *Hystera* literally means something lower (in spatial terms) or later (in temporal terms). In the first sense, it describes the location of the organ at the lower end of the torso, and perhaps also suggests that it is behind other organs: in the second sense, it echoes the belief that the first woman – Pandora – was a 'late arrival', created after men were made.[97] The adjective rather than the noun, as in *hysterikê pnix* ('suffocation from the womb'), is indeed found in the Hippocratic Corpus and in other medical texts, but it describes a symptom and its supposed origin, rather than 'a disease'. This sensation of suffocation was thought to be caused by the womb physically shifting within the body to put pressure on the organs in whichever place it ended up. The alliterative 'wandering womb' has a strong appeal in our complex reimaginings of the medicine of the past, in which ancient Greek medicine is our ancestor, and 'Hippocrates was right', but also the ancients did 'weird things', as in such clickbait as '10 Truly Disgusting Facts About Ancient Greek Life'.[98]

Within the history of medicine, as Sabine Arnaud has demonstrated, claims for a Hippocratic origin are here intended to create continuity: 'By reading hysteric affection as Hippocrates's discovery, physicians of the sixteenth, seventeenth, and eighteenth centuries became invested in a highly specific genealogy of texts'.[99] Whether or not we believe that there are cases to which the label 'hysteria' can now usefully be applied – and current medicine is divided on this question – it is however misleading to assume the equivalence of the ancient Greek 'suffocation from the womb' and what a later doctor meant by 'hysteria'; for example, a nineteenth-century doctor could mean the four-stage 'hysterical crisis' featuring the body of the sufferer forming an arc shape (the 'arc de cercle' or opisthotonos) as described by Charcot.[100] In the seventeenth century, Jeffrey Boss identified a shift in the scope of various disease labels, changing 'the limits of hysteria, as it united with hypochondria and annexed parts of melancholy's crumbling empire'.[101] Arnaud shows that it was only at the end of the eighteenth century that 'a host of previously known pathologies: uterine furors, suffocation of the womb, fits of the mother, vapors, and hysterical and hypochondriac passions' were 'assimilated into the single category of hysteria', with the label only beginning 'to operate in earnest' in the nineteenth century.[102] The label applied to essentially similar symptoms would depend on the social class of the patient: poor women had 'fits of the mother' (another word for uterus) while elite women had 'the vapours'.[103]

So hysteria is not a Hippocratic word, or a Hippocratic diagnosis, but a very modern one, as well as 'an epithet with which men have stigmatized women across the ages'.[104] The abstract to a 2017 medical article linked that too with Hippocrates, as 'Hippocrates attributed women's high emotionality – hysteria – to a "wandering womb",' before going on to state that Hippocrates 'grouped these heterogeneous symptoms under *hysteria*'.[105] In 1995, Mark Micale argued that the nineteenth-century diagnosis of hysteria '"disappeared" in the early twentieth century due in part to extreme clinical overextension. During the same period, hysteria in the arts and in the social and political arenas also exhausted its metaphorical potential and, as a result, receded rapidly from the scene.'[106] Yet in popular media 'hysteria' remains newsworthy, not least because anything that presents women as less emotionally stable than men continues to play out well, whether this is about using Hippocrates and hysteria to control women now, or about contrasting 'them' and 'us'. In particular, contemporary news stories pick up current media obsessions with sexual frustration. This again misrepresents the ancient world, where 'suffocation from the womb' could indeed be caused by insufficient sex, but where there were many other reasons why the womb was thought to move within the body, and pregnant women were not immune.[107]

In addition, current hysteria stories also pick up the way in which the vibrator has become an icon for female sexual pleasure. In the last twenty years, the myth of Hippocratic hysteria has been promoted through the claim that therapeutic masturbation to compensate for the absence of sex has been a staple of the Western medical tradition since classical Greece. Originally put forward by Rachel Maines in *The Technology of Orgasm* (1999), this has taken on a life of its own, for example in the 2008 movie *Hysteria*, in which a doctor finds he can masturbate more patients per day by automating the process, and where the actress playing the main character is on record as saying that she liked the 'idea that hysteria was this catch-all term to describe any sort of psychological condition in a woman'.[108] Something similar happened in a 1995 book by Laurinda Dixon, *Perilous Chastity*: Dixon merged many different disease categories (including hysteria) applied to women in early modern medicine to make one 'mysterious universal ailment of many names that has afflicted women throughout history': she then used the word 'hysteria' for this merged 'ailment'.[109]

Casual disregard of ancient history and attempts to create a historical pedigree for modern ideas have not helped the plausibility of Maines' claims, which she has subsequently insisted were only a hypothesis even though her book said nothing of the kind.[110] Her case for the nineteenth century was first challenged by Lesley Hall, who noted the extreme care taken by most Victorian medical practitioners to avoid any suggestion of sexual impropriety with patients plus the fear of female orgasm as bad for the health.[111] It has recently been thoroughly debunked by Hallie Lieberman and Eric Schatzberg, two of Maines' fellow historians of technology.[112] For the ancient world, Maines' case rested on highly selective use of primary sources, either read in poor translations or taken out of context.¹¹³ Her version of a story from Galen about a widow who became well again after consulting a midwife and evacuating some thick 'seed' – Galen believed both men and women produced seed, women's normally being thinner and weaker – has not the widow, nor the midwife, but Galen himself performing therapeutic masturbation on the patient.

This myth is the result of a complex line of selective reading; Charles Daremberg's 1856 translation of Galen, Henri Cesbron's 1906 version which took out the reference to the midwife applying the remedy, and then Ilza Veith's 1965 mention of 'digital manipulation'.¹¹⁴ A still more recent retelling by Vern Bullough even adds in a reference to Galen using 'his fingers to masturbate the client'!¹¹⁵ Maines and her users play into a male fantasy of passive women waiting for men to give them pleasure, and assume historical continuity in women's sexual expectations and practices.¹¹⁶ Furthermore, all this overlooks the key point that Galen introduced the widow not even as a case history from his own personal experience but as a story he had encountered.¹¹⁷

In July 2018, the news media picked up a press release from the University of Basle concerning one of the papyri in their collection, due to be published in 2019. It includes what has only now been identified as a description of *hysterikê pnix*, and one which does not correspond to any previously-known medical text. Perhaps because the story broke in the 'silly season' or perhaps simply because sex sells, the UK press embraced this with enthusiasm, *The Sun* newspaper using the headline 'Julius Please Her' and the summary that 'Mysterious 2,000-year-old scroll reveals crazy Roman medical theory that women became HYSTERICAL when they didn't have sex'.¹¹⁸ All the usual clichés of reporting on ancient medicine are here: the 'mysterious scroll' being 'deciphered' after 'decades were spent trying to crack the text' – as if it were in code rather than in ancient Greek – and the previously 'bewildered experts and scholars'. A textbox then attempted to explain 'hysterical suffocation', including the claim that 'Hippocrates, "The Father of Medicine" . . . was the first to coin the term "hysteria"'. The *Daily Mail* headlined with 'it's all about how sex-starved women became hysterical' and, while not making the 'coin the term' connection, claimed that 'Hippocrates, widely-credited as the founder of western medicine, also believed in the diagnosis during the 5th century BC.'¹¹⁹ *Metro*, which repeated the story, called it a 'bonkers Roman theory', the message apparently being that we are far too advanced now to believe this sort of 'very strange theory' about 'single women who did not enjoy regular romps'.[120] Arstechnica.com mentioned the 'surreal sexism of ancient medicine'.[121] As ever, alliteration proved irresistible.

The Smithsonian published its own version of the story, by Meilan Solly, on 13 July, under the headline 'Researchers unlock secrets of Basel papyrus'.[122] While the background to the papyrus was treated well here, Hippocrates was still named as 'the first to coin the term "hysteria"', and this information was referenced as coming from the 2012 paper of Tasca and her co-writers; no ancient sources were mentioned, but of course they do not exist.[123] Solly also quoted 'feminist scholar and neurophysiologist Ruth Beier' whose published lecture includes 'Hippocrates, like Aristotle recognized as a brilliant observer and medical thinker, could not think straight, could not see properly or logically when it came to women.'[124] The other source used was the third volume of Plinio Prioreschi's history of medicine: Prioreschi elides '"hysteric symptoms," that is, "hysteria"'.[125] Clearly some research had been done here, beyond the press release.

The Times was the last major paper to run the story, on 24 July, opening with 'A papyrus that mystified academics for 500 years has been revealed as a lost ancient Roman treatise on the "suffocating hysteria" of sex-starved women', thus managing to combine the themes of mystery and 'lost' with a reinstatement of the label 'hysteria'.[126] Like the version on arstechnica.com (on which it is very dependent), where 'a UV lamp solves the mystery', *The Times*'s story takes the 'science enables us to solve the mysteries of history' approach.[127] Like the Smithsonian, it quoted from Sabine Huebner: '"We therefore assume that it is either a text from the Roman physician Galen or an unknown commentary on his work," Sabine Huebner, of the University of Basle, said', although the Smithsonian had preferred to call Galen 'Greek', making Hippocrates Galen's 'fellow Grecian'. The story went on to emphasize continuity in views of hysteria:

> Galen, a Greek doctor practising in Rome in the 2nd and 3rd centuries AD, followed his predecessor Hippocrates in believing that hysteria caused by abstinence could cause symptoms including anxiety, stupor and a sense of suffocation. Hippocrates argued in the 5th and 4th centuries BC that hysteria was caused by a uterus that was dry due to a lack of coitus. The concept endured into the Victorian period.

Again, the journalist has clearly gone beyond the University of Basle press release, which merely mentioned that 'After Hippocrates, Galen is regarded as the most important physician of antiquity.'[128]

As with the *Smithsonian* story, here too it is possible to see how the various journalists found their material. They rely, of course, as we all do, on what is online, using keyword searching which, 'defined by an individual term, cannot trace a concept as well as a cataloguer who assigns subject headings based on an understanding of the material involved'.[129] And then the material has to be evaluated; research on the search patterns of university students is instructive here. A 1999 study of students using the internet found that 29 per cent 'accepted Internet information regardless, with only 34% considering additional verification important'.[130] In my own conversations with students more recently, I would say that far more than 34 per cent want additional evidence, but it is disturbing – bearing in mind how Chapter 3 showed that print media simply repeat internet material – how many still think a 'real book' is likely to be more reliable.

In addition to students' general approach to what they find online, Leah Graham and Takis Metaxas commented in 2003 on what they described as 'the extraordinary confidence students have in search engines'.[131] Search engines, as Susan Gerhart has shown, do not cover a great portion of the web, despite a 'widely held misconception of search engines behaving somewhat like objective and well-informed librarians'. Not only do they privilege 'organizational', rather than 'analytic' sites, meaning that larger descriptive web pages get more traffic than those analysing data, but also their coverage is partial: in 1999, Steve Lawrence and Lee Giles estimated that 'no search engine indexes more than about 16% of the web', while all search engines combined only reached 42 per cent.[132] Far more pessimistic statistics exist; for example in 2014, *The Tennessean* reported the estimate that Google has only indexed '4 percent of the information that exists on the Internet'.[133] Internet users can take what they like and repeat what they like, but the freedom of information on the Internet cannot mean the user has access only to *good* information. What journalists find is subject to the same caveats as what students locate for their essays; it is likely to be based on what is easily accessible online rather than on any more rigorous assessment, and is subject to the algorithms used by the search engine chosen.

At least one journalist covering the Basle papyrus story – the *Metro* journalist (possibly also the *Daily Mail* writer) – had discovered a primary source, probably online. This is the passage of the Hippocratic *Diseases of Women* (2.126) included in the translated sources of *Women's Lives in Greece and Rome* on the Diotima website; *Metro* even included a link to it.[134] This passage does not, however, mention 'hysteria'; it was only in the mid-nineteenth century, when Emile Littré translated the text and added his own subheadings, that 'hysteria' entered the picture. Unlike the editors of WLGR, he labelled this passage as 'Another description of hysteria attributed to the womb attaching itself to the hypochondria', the location translated in WLGR as 'the upper abdomen'.[135] WLGR also includes another section, *Diseases of Women* 2.123, where the womb moves towards her head, and this causes very different symptoms.

A long history? Meanwhile in Babylon

News stories clearly grapple with the problem of whether hysteria is a historical constant or something originating from a particular context. To some extent, the insistence by historians of medicine that there is no one thing that has always been called 'hysteria' (let alone a thing named by Hippocrates) versus the popular desire for continuity over time represents one skirmish in a wider battle between essentialist and constructivist approaches to the body. Is the body something fixed or something open to interpretation? Back in 1987, the medical anthropologists Nancy Scheper-Hughes and Margaret Lock summarized their response to this in the following way: the body is 'simultaneously a physical and symbolic artefact ... both naturally and culturally produced'.[136]

It is not only in popular responses to 'hysteria' that we can see the essentialist view today. Differences of opinion on this surfaced again when a particularly ambitious claim for historical continuity in 'hysteria' was made in early 2018, in a medical article written by the neurologist Edward Reynolds on 'Hysteria in ancient civilisations': he wrote

> The word 'hysteria' originated in the Corpus Hippocraticum, a collection of about 60 separate works from the Greek classical period of about 420 BCE to

the Hellenistic period and perhaps beyond, as a natural explanation for a variety of diseases in women linked in the Greco-Roman mind to an animate or inanimate womb [2, 3].[137]

He repeated the familiar claim that 'The great achievement of Greco-Roman medicine was in introducing natural causation, including causation linked to the womb, rather than gods or evil spirits': this is the usual view of Hippocrates as separating the natural from the supernatural.[138] Reynolds believes that 'the study of hysteria may be one of the keys to a greater understanding of the relationship between brain and mind'.[139]

Reynolds' aim of showing continuity, tracing what he presents as a single cause for diseases over two millennia, is not the only position that has been taken by medical professionals. In the 1960s, in a famous dispute between Eliot Slater and Francis Walshe, the former argued that 'The diagnosis of "hysteria" is a disguise for ignorance and a fertile source of clinical error', and the 'justification for accepting "hysteria" as a syndrome ... [is] based entirely on tradition and lack[ing] evidential support'.[140] In response, Walshe defended 'the concept of hysteria as a nosological entity in its own right'; note the absence of scare quotes for the disease name here.[141] In 2005, a group consisting of two neurologists, a neuropsychiatrist and a psychologist challenged what had by then become the post-Slater orthodoxy, arguing that it was 'not the quality of the science' shown in the paper which had led to its influence; the paper's impact owed more to 'the memorable eloquence of the conclusion'.[142]

Reynolds has been writing about the ancient world since at least 1990, when in the first output of his long collaboration with James Kinnier Wilson (a retired lecturer in Assyriology and son of a neurologist) he co-wrote a piece for the 'Texts and documents' section of the journal *Medical History* on epilepsy in Babylonia.[143] Here, Reynolds' contributions lie in the commentary which aims 'to interpret the foregoing text in a simple and direct way from the standpoint of modern neurology and modern concepts of epilepsy'.[144] What this means in practice is that some parts of the text are linked to modern views – for example, '"It is he again!" implies an aura' – while others which do not fit so well are downplayed as 'a strange observation by modern standards ... of doubtful medical significance'. Where a common modern symptom such as urinary incontinence is not mentioned in the ancient text, this is noted as 'surprising'.[145] Where a symptom is identified with a modern one, but in modern understanding it only features on one side of the body yet the Babylonian text has the plural 'limbs', then 'the word "limbs" in the translation would require restriction accordingly'.[146] In short, while the authors comment with some caution that 'It is seldom without risk that one interprets former times by the present' it is clear that their method is to do precisely this, downplaying or adjusting anything which does not fit.[147] This contrasts with the approach of another scholar of the Ancient Near East, JoAnn Scurlock, who notes on witchcraft that 'We need to get over the notion that something allegedly caused by something in which we do not believe could not possibly be a real illness.'[148] Kinnier Wilson and Reynolds credit Marten Stol, the great scholar of ancient Near Eastern medicine, for help with translation. Yet, while quoting from their 1990 article in his 1993 book on epilepsy in Babylonia, Stol politely distanced himself from their quest 'to diagnose those symptoms by modern means', making it clear that his own intention was instead to look at how the Babylonians viewed epilepsy within the broader context of medicine in their culture and in the rest of the ancient Mediterranean.[149]

In 2014, Reynolds and Kinnier Wilson wrote a further short article.[150] The abstract stated that 'The Babylonians were remarkably acute and objective observers of medical disorders and human behaviour. Their detailed descriptions are surprisingly similar to modern 19th and 20th century textbook accounts, with the exception of subjective thoughts and feelings which are more modern fields of enquiry.' Again, continuity is emphasized. The article seems to accept the distinction between two types of healer, the asû and the ašipu, as 'physician' versus 'priest or exorcist', something criticized by Scurlock. She argued that, rather than these categories of healer being interested respectively in natural and supernatural causes, and using different procedures for healing as well as different materia medica, the texts 'reflect the same understanding of the nature of disease' and were intended for the ašipu; she concludes, 'we are looking for binary opposites where there are not any'.[151] Furthermore, if anything, the ašipu is 'the closest equivalent to our "physician"' with the asû more like a pharmacist.[152] Reynolds and Kinnier Wilson do not engage with this scholarship. Their approach to ancient Greek medicine comes out in the comment that 'Babylonian medicine was a science formulated before the coming of pathology, the latter undoubtedly being a major contribution of Greek and Roman medicine.'[153]

I have a personal issue with Reynolds' 2018 article; he cites my work as evidence that 'The word "hysteria" originated in the Corpus Hippocraticum', when this is the exact opposite of what I argued in the 1993 chapter he cites. Specifically, I showed at some length that this was wrong: I commented that, as in the example of the long-lived belief that the earth is flat, 'What "everyone knows" is, however, not necessarily true.'[154] After this misguided nod in the direction of my chapter, for the section later in his article when he returns to the ancient Greek material, like Maines, Reynolds relied on the work of Ilza Veith; it is clear there that he has not read my 1993 chapter, as unlike Veith I looked at the original Greek in some detail, and explained how Veith was reliant on poor secondary sources. Reynolds states his 'method': it is to search for key words in PubMed and Medline.[155] As I noted in the Introduction, this appears to be the way that medical authors work, and it means that they miss recent work by historians, and move further and further away from engaging with primary sources.

To write a 'history of hysteria' that goes from Babylonian medicine to the present makes even less sense than taking cemetery evidence from a period of 4,000 years to compare with the Hippocratic Corpus. These claims are part of an attempt to create consistency in the history of the body and of medicine; an attempt which here is seriously misplaced. Instead of seeing different disease categories over time, there becomes just one single condition which has always been associated with women. This glosses over all the interesting detail of the Hippocratic Corpus and of women's medicine in later history, failing to acknowledge the different patterns of symptoms and the different views of their causation.

The Hippocrates detox diet

My final example, like the Imhotep story, originates in a partnership with the monastery of St Catherine in Sinai. While the Imhotep story came from their relationship with the Egyptian Medicinal Plant Conservation Project, this one is from the Early Manuscripts Electronic Library (EMEL).[156] In 2017, news outlets ran a story about a fifth/sixth century CE manuscript of a 'missing' Hippocratic remedy found in the monastery library; 'missing' or even 'lost in a famous Egyptian monastery' are odd ways of describing something which was not previously known to exist, and 'unknown' would be a better choice here.¹⁵⁷ This was a palimpsest, in which the original medical text had been scraped or washed so that the surface – in this case, leather – could be reused for a Bible text. The discovery was made due to the use of spectral imaging to read the underlying text, thus conforming to the pattern by which science uncovers something hidden.¹⁵⁸ Neither the reasons for attributing this remedy to Hippocrates nor the contents of the remedy have so far been revealed, but again the name of Hippocrates sells the story because, as Sarah Gibbens wrote as the opening sentence for the National Geographic website's version of this story, 'There's perhaps no doctor in history more famous than Hippocrates.' This story had to be corrected due to a historical impossibility, as follows:

> Correction: A previous version of this article stated that the 6th century manuscript belonged to Hippocrates. The medical recipe within the manuscript belonged to Hippocrates, but the text was not copied until the 6th century, after the doctor's death.¹⁵⁹

The various versions of this news piece show a high level of confusion. The first announcement on 7 July was in the newspaper *Asharq al-Awsat* but the English version of this used the word 'Palmesit' for 'palimpsest'; this error was followed by Dattatreya Mandal who took this to be a scroll written on leather with 'two layers for rewriting purposes due to the very high cost of leather at the time', adding that 'the library is believed to have quite a few Palmesit scrolls among its impressive hoard of over 6,000 manuscripts'.¹⁶⁰ One version of the story claimed that 'Hippocrates is the world's most famous doctor, but very little is known about his teachings. This new text could help change that.'¹⁶¹

So what is this text? The original stories described a drawing of a herb with text in both Greek and Arabic.¹⁶² *The Times*, however, had more information than most, and announced that this was 'an ancient detox and purification diet'.¹⁶³ This claim was based on an interview with Agamemnon Tselikas, a palaeographer who is part of the EMEL project and 'who authenticated the manuscripts': other reporters quoted only from Michael Phelps (given as Philips in some of the media accounts), Executive Director of EMEL.¹⁶⁴ Tselikas was one of those who deciphered the Antikythera Mechanism and is also on record for arguing that the letter Morton Smith claimed was an authentic letter of Clement of Alexandria, including extracts from a lost 'secret' gospel of Mark, was in fact an eighteenth-century forgery.[165]

Why Hippocrates and detox? As we shall see in Chapter 7, these two seem to go together in the popular imagination: detox is part of his 'ancient wisdom'.[166] According to Carrie L'Esperance, 'a multi-platform free artisan', in *The Seasonal Detox Diet: Remedies from the Ancient Campfire*,

> Hippocrates is said to have offered the Grecian people wise advise [sic]: A healthy mind in a health body should be the goal of all generations in the world. Hippocrates was a vitalist who taught that good health and purity of environment are dependent upon each other ... He knew that Nature made the cure and that the doctor's role was to assist. He believed that the diseased body needed a period of rest – not only a physical rest, but a chemical rest, which he considered even more important. Chemical rest could be achieved only by withholding food, thus giving the organs of the body an opportunity to discharge accumulated waste products and thereby to cleanse themselves.[167]

These detox references call to mind Brian Clement's Hippocrates Health Institute (HHI) in West Palm Beach, Florida, and I shall return to the use of Hippocrates' name here at the end of this book.[168]

Conclusion

The examples I have discussed in this chapter show how, despite some tension as to whether or not he is the Father of Medicine, Hippocrates' name continues to have power. Priority disputes in which he loses that role as Father are part of wider challenges to the hegemony of the West and to Western medicine, but exist alongside claims that Hippocrates represents all that is best in medical ethics. His ethical role is demonstrated by the ease with which people refer to what they think is in the *Oath*; the example of the longevity of the belief that all doctors take, and always have taken, the *Oath*, repeated in memes, tweets and slogans, at the very least demonstrates how we all think we know something about Hippocrates, whether or not we are medical professionals.[169]

As his use in the 1992 doctors' strike suggests, Hippocrates also sells news stories. Everything needs to find its origins in Hippocrates, even if that origin doesn't exist, and it is very easy for 'Hippocratic texts' to morph into

'Hippocrates'. Assuming the continuity implied by finding Hippocratic origins for everything flattens out the past: Galen thought the same as Hippocrates and this continued until the Victorians; every condition of women becomes 'hysteria'. This supposed continuity enables Hippocrates to speak to us today, because nothing has really changed. The construction of these news stories often calls on the prestige of science to 'solve a puzzle' or 'decode a text', but the prestige of Hippocrates remains intact: he named hysteria, he showed his 'diagnostic prowess' and, even if ancient medicine in general is 'bonkers', Hippocrates is right.

The current Hippocrates, because of the essentialist principle of continuity, goes even further. He can still teach us something: the value of a detox, often understood today in terms of a raw food diet, which is particularly ironic when raw foods are not recommended in ancient medicine. I shall explore this further below, first by examining internet use of the various quotes associated with Hippocrates, which show how the authority gained through repetition can be combined with that of an ancient figure, and then by looking at holistic medicine more generally.

5

Hippocrates in Quotes

So far in this book we have seen that there are common views of what Hippocrates is supposed to be about which form part of many people's tacit knowledge. Some have links to the traditional stories told about his character or to specific texts of the Corpus: others, not. In the previous chapter, we saw how writers of news stories still think it is worth invoking his name and tapping into this knowledge, and how such stories move between praising Hippocrates as one of us and distancing us from the weirdnesses of the ancient world, while suggesting 'science' can solve all history's 'mysteries'. In this chapter, I shall start to investigate a range of claims for Hippocrates as an authority, and for the Hippocratic lifestyle and its virtues, through the medium of some of the many 'quotes' going under the name of the Father of Medicine, shared through websites and social media, often independent of what is happening in the news. The next chapter will focus on the food-related quotes which currently dominate online references to Hippocrates.

Sharing such quotes is often the main way in which people become aware of 'Hippocrates' today. They may simply tweet or post on Instagram the alleged words of Hippocrates, complete with his name; their followers, and their own followers, will then retweet the words, perhaps interpreting them very differently from the original tweeter. They may attach to their message an image which moves the meaning of the words in another direction; for example, if someone tweets 'Let food be thy medicine. Hippocrates' and attaches a picture of raw foods, this will have a different meaning from the same tweet accompanied by a picture of one specific food. Throughout, the theme of 'Hippocrates was right' pervades discussions of the Hippocratic lifestyle; the thing about Hippocrates is almost inevitably that 'He knew his stuff.'[1] Words attributed 'to the historical Hippocrates . . . are intended to carry greater weight precisely because of that association'.[2]

First, an example. 'ChefMD' Dr John La Puma promotes 'healthy eating' as 'Both a board-certified practicing internist and professionally trained chef'. Typically pictured at food markets in a white coat with a stethoscope round his neck, La Puma teaches 'culinary medicine' to medical students, presents on PBS and Lifetime TV, blogs, writes for several newspapers and is a YouTube influencer.[3] A striking image combines his logo with three pictures. In one, food is contained in a medical capsule; in the others, raw foods are shaped to resemble the brain and the heart. The use of the multi-coloured capsule reminds me of a point made by medical anthropologists about the symbolic value of capsules over pills within Western biomedicine; patient perception is that 'Capsules are more powerful than tablets, and multicolored capsules are more powerful than single colored ones'.[4] On a 'functional medicine' site, and in other locations online, the power of these images is increased by the addition of a set of four 'quotes' to the right of the image.[5]

These 'quotes' include Thomas Edison, 'The doctor of the future will give no medicine, but will interest her or his patients in the care of the human frame, in a proper diet, and in the cause and prevention of disease.' Is this authentic? Snopes.com found that – other than the 'her or his', and the insertion of 'a proper' – this was indeed something he said in 1902; the context is important, however, as 'He was speaking at a time when very little effective "medicine" existed.'[6] Another quote is from Mark Hyman, a medical doctor, founder of The UltraWellness Center, and best-selling author of the *Eat Fat, Get Thin Cookbook*: 'The fork is your most powerful tool to change your health and the planet; food is the most powerful medicine to heal chronic illness.' Hyman uses a variant of this statement as his banner online, where it is followed by an endorsement from Bill Clinton for one of his books.[7] *Whole Living* magazine is the source of another quote: 'While you can't shut out illness entirely, you CAN make your body a place where health thrives.'[8] Finally, there are two Hippocrates quotes, presented as two sections of the same unnamed text. One, 'Let your food be your medicine and your medicine be your food' – or, to give it that patina of antiquity, 'Let food be thy medicine' – is probably the most commonly-repeated Hippocrates 'quote' today.[9] The other is 'Leave your drugs in the chemist's pot if you can cure the patient with food.' Neither is authentic. Before examining these and other such quotes, I first want to consider how the culture of quotes works online.

Flitting like a bee: Becoming a quote

What does it mean for Hippocrates to have 'become a quote'? Ann Blair drew attention to Descartes' view that reference books should only be used to refresh one's memory, rather than in isolation from their original sources.[10] Yet books of quotations have always existed. Their roots lie in the early modern commonplace book, in which people copied down anything that took their fancy, arranging the phrases and passages under headings.[11] This way of interacting with what one read was originally personal: Erasmus emphasized that the user should 'draw up a list of virtues and vices to suit himself' and when the headings had been fixed should 'arrange them as you please'.[12] Erasmus commented, on the subject of the reading habits of the daughters of his friend Thomas More,

> As they flit like so many little bees between Greek and Latin authors of every species, here noting down something to imitate, here culling some notable saying to put into practice in their behaviour, there getting by heart some witty anecdote to relate among their friends, you would swear you were watching the Muses at graceful play in the lovely pastures of Mount Helicon, gathering flowers and marjoram to make well-woven garlands.[13]

The imagery of the garland recalls the ancient origins of this way of reading: the 'florilegium'. The text could be presented 'as a garden whose elements could be collected, displayed and used'.[14] While its origins were personal, the commonplace book could also enter print, where it told the reader how to think by 'extracting wisdom from classical texts'; the text became a source of such wisdom rather than the reader focusing on the context in which the author had used the extracted phrase, and the phrases then became cultural capital.[15] Collections of *sententiae*, wise sayings of figures of authority, also existed from an early date.

Quotations give the impression of knowledge without the hard work of reading the rest of the text from which they are taken. Early printed books of quotations do not necessarily include anything attributed to Hippocrates; medical texts were far less likely than works of literature to be sampled and shared in this way. John Bartlett's *A Collection of Familiar Quotations* (revised edition, 1856) included just one (abbreviated) Hippocratic quotation, 'Life is short, and the art long', and that only as a footnote to Longfellow's 'Art is long, and Time is fleeting.'[16] As Ann Blair has observed, in its Senecan version of *ars longa, vita brevis*, this has 'proved an especially versatile tag, invoked by both optimists and pessimists about the accumulation of knowledge'.[17]

Quotes can also act simply as decoration. They may be intended to be 'inspirational', as in the title of M. Prefontaine's *The Big Book of Quotes: Funny, inspirational and motivational quotes on life, love and much else*, a book arranged by categories under the subsections of power, relationships, spiritual, fact and fiction, intelligence, the arts, sport, pets, countries, occupations – including 'doctors and medicine' – and the human condition.[18] This extensive collection is described in its marketing material as 'Ideal for pepping up speeches, letters or just for empowering you to live life.'[19] The section on 'Doctors and medicine' includes such gems as 'Never go to a doctor whose office plants have died', attributed to Erma Bombeck (1927–96). Some books of quotes are aimed at an even narrower clientele; there are books for writers, lawyers, and veterinary caregivers, and those aimed at people preparing a speech.[20] This process of using and perhaps transforming the words of others is part of the creation of a sense of self, but also of making a book of 'identity-soothing words' for a particular community.[21]

How has the internet changed the culture of quotation? It is perhaps significant that recent scholarly interest in commonplace books, as a way of organizing and then interacting with knowledge, grew at the same time as the internet became the main source for modern knowledge. Kate Eichhorn linked the commonplace book and the blog as what she called 'archival genres'.[22] Concerns about the difficulty not only of accessing but also remembering all the information available are not new; as discussed by Ann Blair, certainly since the Renaissance there has been too much knowledge for any one person to manage.[23] However, the internet provides the illusion of access to all this knowledge through search engines. What is different is not only that, as we saw in Chapter 3, 'Like a verbal virus, any error committed on one website is quickly replicated on hundreds,'[24] but also that information exists in a state of continual flux, enabled by its interactive nature. As David Crystal has argued, 'People have more power to influence the language of the Web than in any other medium, because they operate on both sides of the communication divide, reception and production. They not only read a text, they can add to it. The distinction between creator and receiver thus becomes blurred.'[25] This clearly has important ramifications for the reception of Hippocrates, as quotes are taken out of context, altered or even created by their receivers.

The difference between a quote and a quotation is no longer the dictionary one in which the first is a verb and the second a noun. An internet quote has various features, some of which are more or less specific to the electronic medium; the quote is usually presented as something someone 'said' rather than 'wrote', it is noteworthy and repeatable, and it has an implicit meaning that is largely taken for granted, so it needs no explanation or commentary. Rather than being the product of a deliberate 'contextomy', in which the snippet is severed from its original text in order to alter its meaning,[26] it requires no context, as the very concept of there being a greater text is absent; Hippocrates quotes commonly give no date and no title of the text from which they are supposed to originate. As an example of how quotes lose context, Garber cites Shakespeare's Polonius saying 'to thine own self be true': a book of quotations would give you this adage, but would lose entirely the significance of the contextual point that it was 'the least self-aware of men' who was originally presented as saying it.[27] Some sites make more effort than others to trace the name of the Hippocratic text from which their Hippocratic quotes originate.[28] The Wikiquote site gives a range of quotes from him, organized by their claimed text of origin, but these are sometimes listed 'as quoted in' another text rather than giving the name or edition of an actual Hippocratic text.[29]

Quotes are repeated and traded between bloggers, tweeters, and participants in chat rooms, used to advertise businesses, and are collected on sites created solely for the purpose of supplying choice phrases, an extension of the tradition of printed collections of sayings.[30] Often, words are left out to make a quote pithier, a process known as 'bumper-stickering'.[31] Quotes hover in cyberspace, offering wisdom in a form that takes only seconds to read, understand, and repeat, and in the case of those I am exploring here often come with a backdrop of an image of Hippocrates or of an inspiring landscape. They can be used in a ritualized fashion to create and maintain relations between social and political groups, to express common interests, enthusiasms, heartbreaks or annoyances.[32] As Clark and Gerrig noted of quotations generally, an online adage can be seen as 'a demonstration of what a person did in saying something,' and the act of quotation paradoxically both separates the quoter from the sentiment and connects them to it.[33]

Ascribing the quote to a historical figure is both a measure of its reliability, and a demonstration of that figure's importance, wisdom and relevance. In a Hippocrates quote, his name as alleged creator becomes part of the quote, while users of the quote somehow incorporate into themselves his authority: Marjorie Garber, who used the term 'cultural ventriloquism' here, noted that the quote 'imparts that authority, temporarily, to the speaker or the writer'. This, she pointed out, contrasts with the use of 'quote-unquote' around words from we wish to distance ourselves or which we want to challenge.[34] Ruth Finnegan quoted David Comins' comment, 'People will accept your ideas much more readily if you tell them Benjamin Franklin said it first.'[35]

It is well-established that many of the most famous quotes are not accurate. In Prefontaine's *The Big Book of Quotes*, Hippocrates (his dates given as '460–370 BC') features with just one quote, the same one as in Bartlett's *A Collection of Familiar Quotations*: 'The life so short, the craft so long to learn.'[36] That is a truncated version of the original, 'Life is short, the art long, the moment fleeting', and Prefontaine's version is correctly identified on Wikiquote not specifically as Hippocratic but as the first line of Chaucer's *The Assembly of Fowles*.[37] Examples of quotes which are not just inaccurate, but imaginary, include Edmund Burke, 'All that is necessary for the triumph of evil is that good men do nothing.'[38] Another example would be '"The more I study science the more I believe in God," Albert Einstein once remarked.'[39] Only he didn't. In 2012, Quentin Schultze and Randall Bytwerk demonstrated that a quote attributed to Joseph Goebbels, beginning 'If you tell a lie big enough and keep repeating it, people will eventually come to believe it', then found on over half a million pages of the internet, was never said by him. They used the term 'referential credibility' for when a quotation is believed by the community using it to have been correctly attributed to a person important to that community.[40]

Gary Saul Morson has analysed the movement 'from quotations to culture'. He describes the process by which words become a quote by using the example of Isaac Newton's 'If I have seen further than others, it is by standing upon the shoulders of giants.' While he was not the first to say something very much like this and, at the time of writing, even Wikipedia is now very clear indeed that the wording existed before his time, on quotes sites the quote is attributed solely to him.[41] Morson writes, 'the quotation is now Newton's because the fact that the words are his has long been part of their meaning. The same words said by anyone but Newton, regarded for centuries as the greatest scientist who ever lived, would not be the same.'[42] Morson compares quotation to the use of found art, in which the object is not made by the artist, but the artist presents it in a different form.[43]

What happens when 'Hippocrates' is quoted online is a more extreme version of what happens when he is quoted in printed sources. A quotation may be an attempt to show that one has mastered the text from which it is taken, in 'a process thought to resemble separating wheat from chaff or selecting gems from stones'.[44] In addition to possible bumper-stickering, the quotation does not have to reproduce the original precisely; quotations, like oral poetry, 'pass from mouth to mouth as well as from text to text. They are frequently spoken, altered, written, and quoted aloud again. Cherished as texts, they also live in their oral use.'[45] The phenomenon of the 'Hippocrates quote' differs from citing proverbs, in which anonymity as well as the absence of a firm date contribute to the sense of 'great age' and to the impression of 'timeless essence and wisdom'.[46] To me, Hippocrates quotes seem to rest somewhere between the quotation and the proverb; what is stated both gains authority from its connection to Hippocrates and presents something which is supposed to be true for all time. I shall now examine some of the most popular Hippocrates quotes today.

First do no harm

In Chapter 4, I explored how, as well as being used by the public as an ideal of how doctors should behave, the *Oath* has been used to create a sense of continuity and an identity for those practising medicine, and I stressed that this is an emotional process as well as a historical one. In the USA, ObamaCare led to a new range of claims for the content and meaning of the *Oath*; for example, from the *Washington Times*, 'When I became a doctor almost 40 years ago, I swore to uphold the Hippocratic Oath — "do no harm." Never has this solemn promise been more difficult to keep.'[47]

This is one of many examples in which one of the most-repeated Hippocrates quotes, 'First, do no harm', is wrongly attributed to the *Oath*, or even regarded as a summary of it: 'The Oath is commonly cited in brief as "first do no harm", but it is actually more involved than that.'[48] Answers.com asks 'What did the Hippocrates [sic] do?' The first answer is 'Nothing!' and the second, 'Rather than nothing, he did say "first do no harm" (primum non nocere, in Latin). This enabled physicians to observe conditions first, rather than prescribe potions, which could be potentially toxic, and even life-threatening.'[49] Once more, the focus is on 'saying' rather than 'writing'. 'Potions', with its hints of magic and poison, is a significant choice of word here, and again the theme is that treatment carries risk.

While the original Hippocratic *Oath* includes 'I will use those dietary regimens which will benefit my patients according to my greatest ability and judgement, and I will do no harm or injustice to them,' this is not quite 'First do no harm.'[50] The nearest wording in the Corpus comes not from the *Oath* but from *Epidemics* 1.11, which includes the injunction 'As to diseases, make a habit of two things – to help, or at least to do no harm.'[51] Like answers.com, many websites telling you that Hippocrates wrote 'First, do no harm' will elaborate that 'originally' this was *primum non nocere*, without necessarily noticing that this is Latin while Hippocrates was a Greek. In Kelly Parsons' thriller *Doing Harm*, the central character Steven first hears this in his first year of medical school from 'one of my older professors who had a proclivity for bowties and Grecian Formula.'[52] Steven 'wondered if Latin really would have been [Hippocrates'] idiom of choice for solemn ethical declarations' but concluded that 'Doctors like to say stuff in Latin because it makes us sound smart.'[53] Elizabeth Vandiver has argued that the classics can lend gravity even to banal sentiments; translated into Latin tags, everyday sentiments about valour and patriotism in the Great War could attain a grandeur they otherwise lacked amongst both those who could read Latin and those who could not.[54] In terms of the familiarity of this phrase to a wider public, a two-part episode of the UK hospital drama *Holby City* broadcast in June 2018 used the Latin as its title and, as I have already mentioned, a few months later the *Assassin's Creed* game section set in ancient Greece included a quest called 'First do no harm', featuring Hippocrates.[55]

Within the medical profession, and for a wider audience, there is now far more awareness that this phrase does not feature in its supposed source, the

Oath, 'just as nobody says "Play it again, Sam" in "Casablanca".'[56] In 2005, the *Journal of Clinical Pharmacology* published a piece in which Cedric Smith tried to trace the origins of the Latin version.[57] As a pharmacologist, Smith was keen to consider the phrase in terms of its relevance to potential adverse drug interactions. One of his key findings was 'Who was the author? Not Hippocrates.'[58] He surveyed earlier literature, trying to pin the phrase on Galen, Ambroise Paré, Thomas Sydenham, Oliver Wendell Holmes or William Osler, but was unable to locate it in any of their writings; the earliest date he found it in use was 1860. He noted that 'like a proverb ... it is a crystallized bit of wisdom ... this maxim has several levels of meaning and can be applied to a wide range of situations'.[59] Importantly, 'It also *sounds* true, especially with its combination with the Latin.'[60] Smith was not the first to observe this: in 1997, the blogger Susan Richards published a piece noting that the words do not come from the *Oath* (and 'nor was [the Oath] actually written by Hippocrates, according to many sources').[61] But Smith's findings were significant because they have been shared widely, for example in an online piece by N.S. Gill on thoughtco.com (a site offering 'expert-created education content') in which she offered a balanced reading of the history of the phrase; however, she did not go far enough, suggesting with regard to the *Epidemics* origin that 'Hippocrates was never proven to be the author of any of these works, but the theories do follow closely with Hippocrates' teachings.'[62] This wording suggests that there is firm independent evidence of 'Hippocrates' teachings' which, as we have seen, there is not. In 2013, Daniel Sokol located 393 articles in the online PubMed database with 'do no harm' in their title and followed Smith in dating the first use in print to 1860; his conclusion was that it is an unhelpful axiom for today, when 'Clinicians inflict harm all the time, whether it is by inserting a cannula, administering chemotherapy, performing a tracheotomy ...'[63]

I suspect that it is precisely because of the invasive nature of much of medicine today that 'First do no harm' plays out so well with the public. The quote is sometimes abbreviated to 'Do No Harm', as in the title of a 2014 memoir by a neurosurgeon, Henry Marsh; a reviewer commented 'But many medical treatments do cause harm: learning how to navigate the risks of drug therapies, as well as the catastrophic consequences of botched or inadvised surgical operations, is a big part of why training doctors takes so long. Even the simplest of therapies carries the risk of making things worse.'[64] A common comment on conventional medicine today is that 'All therapies entail risks' (something nobody has yet, to my knowledge, attributed to Hippocrates!); another example, from the Harvard Health Blog, is 'But if physicians took "first, do no harm" literally, no one would have surgery, even if it was lifesaving.'[65] Steven Miles concluded that the full line of *Epidemics*, with its sense of a calculation of the likelihood of benefits against the risk of damage, was 'worthier of Hippocratic medicine than "Do no harm".'[66]

The 'harm' envisaged by users of this quote can however extend beyond being a side-effect of attempts to heal. As well as the *Holby City* episodes, a film using the phrase as its title was made for American television in 1997.[67] This told the story of a family using the ketogenic diet on their severely epileptic son; this high-fat diet has been used for some epileptic conditions for the past fifty years or so, and came back into prominence in the mid-1990s. In the film, the diet was contrasted with the invasive procedures carried out to diagnose the boy's condition and the various treatments used, which included the rectal administration of a drug seen to melt a plastic cup.[68] Discussion of the film on IMDb included the comment that the title 'comes from the Hippocratic oath which doctors take as part of their vocation', the reviewer adding that the film 'presents a blistering attack on the rigidity and insensitivity of the medical establishment'.[69]

Again, the claimed connection with the *Oath* was important here. The film opens with what are presumably students repeating a very short version of the *Oath* word for word after an older man reads it out: this version, taking lines from various medical oaths, is 'I do solemnly swear that I will be loyal to the profession of medicine and just and generous to its members, that I will prescribe regimen for the good of my patients according to my ability and my judgment and above all else first do no harm.' It thus begins with a line which could be read as doctors looking after their own, and ends with 'first do no harm'. Certainly, the original *Oath* contained clauses which would increase the solidarity of the medical community, teaching each other's children and caring for their own teachers; however, the wording of 'loyal to the profession' here prepares the viewer for a story in which the medical establishment is the enemy, closing ranks to protect its members.[70] While these words are spoken, we see on the screen a well-known image of Hippocrates – the Rubens bust discussed in the Introduction – which is then expanded to show it is taken from an encyclopaedia entry on the *Oath*, thus giving the words even more authority.[71] This recalls the 1937 film *Green Light*, in which one scene sees the entire screen filled with the *Oath*, as a surgeon who made an error in the operating theatre lets a younger colleague take the blame for the death of a patient, finally focusing on the injunction in the *Oath* to keep silent about what one hears both in the context of treating a patient, and beyond.[72]

'Do no harm' also keeps company with 'Let food be thy medicine,' to which I shall turn in the next chapter. As the author of a recent article on how orthodox medicine disadvantages women as patients puts it: 'Hippocrates would be turning over in his grave. A man who admonished caregivers to do no harm, and to use food as our medicine as well to exercise regularly, has to be rather displeased with modern medicine.'[73] It also appeared recently in a setting based around food, in an article promoting Giles Coren's *Truth, Love & Clean Cutlery* – a manifesto for restaurants which produce ethical food. Coren asks that those selling food and drink should give 'an assurance that every possible effort has been made to – in the words of the Hippocratic Oath – "do no harm".[74] Here, the words are used to suggest a meaning that goes beyond medical practice into an approach to the planet.

Walking is the best medicine

'First do no harm' is not in the *Oath*, but does at least have a Hippocratic text behind it. This is not always true of the Hippocratic quotes popular today. According to many sites on the internet, Hippocrates is supposed to have written – although more often to have 'said' – that 'Walking is the best medicine', 'Walking is [a] man's best medicine' or even the excited 'Walking is man's best medicine!', used as the title of a 2012 article in the journal *Occupational Medicine*.[75] This quote has been taken up as the slogan for schemes in orthodox medicine aimed at improving cardiovascular health, such as 'Walk Nebraska' and MacEwan University's Sport and Wellness site, and as a marketing slogan for gyms such as Geneva Fit in Geneva, Illinois.[76] It also features in memes, often accompanied by spectacular scenery of oceans and mountains, or happy couples on the beach.[77] Its users present it as 'a timeless non-pharmacological prescription for well-being and longevity' and as yet more evidence that

'Hippocrates was right', here not least in suggesting something realistic rather than setting an unachievable goal; the article in which these comments feature also recommends parking the car and then walking into the takeaway rather than ordering your food at the drive-up window, or chopping your own vegetables rather than buying them pre-sliced.[78]

Where does this claim about walking originate? In 2017, user Brownturkey wrote on the talk page for the Wikipedia Hippocrates page, 'I can't find any evidence that Hippocrates actually said this (and the citation is not persuasive). Can anyone help?'[79] Before looking at the problems of this particular quote, we can set it within some of the wider claims for Hippocrates and exercise being made today. For example, one of the many Hippocrates exercise memes includes the words: 'Even when all is known, the care of a man is not yet complete… Because *eating alone will not keep a man well*; he must also take exercise. For *food and exercise*, while possessing opposite qualities, yet *work together to produce health* [italics in original].' In this meme, the words are attributed to the Loeb translation of *Regimen* 'Vol.4, 229'.[80] This is not the treatise *Regimen* 4 (also known as *On Dreams*); the passage is found in *Regimen* 1, and the 'Vol.' is a Loeb volume rather than a section of the Hippocratic treatise (*Regimen* 1.2; Loeb, *Hippocrates* IV, 227–9). In the Roman Empire, Galen considered that those who attributed the first book of *Regimen* to Hippocrates were probably wrong, although the second book 'might perhaps with good reason be thought worthy of Hippocrates'.[81] The balance between food and exercise is the cornerstone of the *Regimen* books, as expressed in *Regimen* 3.69 (Loeb, *Hippocrates* IV, 383): 'whether food overpowers exercise, whether exercise overpowers food, or whether the two are duly proportioned. For it is from the overpowering of one or the other that diseases arise, while from their being evenly balanced comes good health.' The concept of balance translates all too easily to modern culture, but the immediate sense of recognition and the superficial similarity cover over many important differences in what is being 'balanced'.

While it features on general health sites and in alternative medicine, the idea that health is a balance between food and exercise also plays a key role in sports medicine. It has been used as part of the attempt to create a history of the EIM (Exercise Is Medicine) movement – a health initiative launched by the American College of Sports Medicine in 2007 and which has since spread across the world. One example of this creation is Charles Tipton's 2014 article, 'The history of "Exercise Is Medicine" in ancient civilizations'.[82] Tipton was not the first to try to provide a history for EIM; in 2010 Jack Berryman wrote 'Exercise is Medicine: A Historical Perspective' for *Current Sports Medicine Reports*.[83]

Tipton's piece in particular provides yet another example of the impulse to find a history for a new initiative, and he ranges widely across ancient civilizations seeking to identify their 'contributions ... to the emergence and acceptance of EIM'. He credits the Indian Susruta with being 'the first "recorded" physician to prescribe moderate daily exercise' although Hippocrates was the first 'recorded' 'to provide a written exercise prescription for a patient'; I will examine this claim shortly.[84] Tipton considers that Hippocrates deserves recognition for providing the centrality of exercise in EIM from the following statement in *Regimen in Acute Diseases* (25, p. 62):

> I say then, that this question [regimen] is a most excellent one and allied to many others, some of the most vital importance in the art [medicine], for that it can contribute much to the recovery of the sick, and to the preservation of health in case of those gymnastic [athletic] exercises, and is useful to whatever one wish to apply it.[85]

'25' here is not a Loeb volume, which is what Tipton used elsewhere for his Hippocratic quotations, but the Francis Adams translation. Nor is that translation quoted accurately: the final phrase as given here makes no sense, and part of the passage is missed out. Adams gives '... and to the preservation of health in the case of those who are well; and that it promotes the strength of those who use gymnastic exercises, and is useful to whatever one may wish to apply it'.[86] The Loeb translates instead:

> But I am confident that this inquiry is wholly profitable, being bound up with most, and the most important, of the things embraced by the art. In fact, it has great power to bring health in all cases of sickness, preservation of health to those who are well, good condition to athletes in training, and in fact realization of each man's particular desire.[87]

As to whether the Loeb's 'inquiry' is the same as Adams' 'question', glossed by Tipton here as 'regimen', the context of the opening section of the treatise is indeed that previous physicians have not given regimen the attention it deserves. The section immediately before this one focuses on how ordinary people find it difficult to take the medical art seriously, because different practitioners treat acute diseases with such different remedies.

Tipton, then, has missed out the full range of benefits described in the passage, presumably to focus on its relevance to his audience. He suggests that Hippocrates has even more to contribute to modern society, commenting that 'it is surprising that the current crusade against obesity has not invoked Hippocratic views in its efforts', bearing in mind that *Regimen* 1 talks about how food can overpower exercise. As for his plea for Hippocrates to be recognized as having provided 'a written exercise prescription for a patient with a disease (consumption)', while this is supposed to be a reference to *Diseases* 3 (using Potter's translation, Loeb VI), I have not been able to identify it there. There are certainly references to exercise as a remedy for what is usually translated into English as 'consumption' (in Greek, variations of *phthisis*), but there is no idea of a single disease entity behind this label; instead, there are descriptions of various severe lung conditions. So, in *Diseases* 2, a 'consumption' patient 'takes walks out of the wind and sun', and in another variant of consumption the advice includes 'have him do a few exercises, take walks'.[88] In *Internal Affections*, in a variant of *phthisis*, the advice is 'Have the patient take walks in conjunction with his meals ... If walks are beneficial to the patient, let him take them; if they are not, he must keep his body as quiet as possible'; here, then, walking is not a blanket recommendation.[89] For another type of *phthisis*, the patient is given a pattern of diet and exercise lasting for a year. In the first month, for example, 'On arising from his sleep, have him walk at least twenty stades that day; on the days that follow, let him walk an additional five stades each day until he reaches one hundred stades.'[90] Nothing here matches Tipton's 'written prescription', which anachronistically suggests an individual patient being given words on papyrus.

Food and exercise thus appear as the two features of a healthy life which balance each other. But this is still not as specific as 'Walking is the *best* medicine'. At the end of 2016, a Greek team led by Nikitas Nomikos and consisting of two members of a faculty of Physical Education and Sports Science, a medical historian working in a Faculty of Medicine, and an orthopaedic specialist, published 'The Role of Exercise in Hippocratic Medicine' in the peer-reviewed *American Journal of Sports Science and Medicine*.[91] They identified *Regimen* in

Health as the source of Hippocratic exercise theory, although their quotations come from *Regimen* 1, 2 and 3 as well.[92] For all of these, they use the 1931 Loeb translation by W.H.S. Jones, although – for reasons I do not understand – they attribute it throughout to 'E.J. James'. For them, Hippocrates is 'the great physician of antiquity', 'the founder of Greek and global medicine' and 'the father of modern Medicine'.[93] Their method is to summarize the text (there is no doubt in their minds that all these treatises are by Hippocrates) and to intersperse some references to modern medical studies with comments on what Hippocrates 'means' in modern terms. Thus he is presented as understanding the importance of a warm-up, the dangers of overtraining syndrome and the value of post-exercise recovery. His observations are invariably 'confirmed' by modern research; for example, the advice that running in a cloak heats the body and so is good for weight loss leads the authors to reflect on the benefits of exercise kit designed to increase sweating.[94]

Hippocrates, once again, was right: of course. However, the insistence in modern sports medicine that Hippocrates is the origin of exercise in medicine (or even Exercise Is Medicine) is misplaced. As Lesley Dean-Jones has shown, athletics trainers and medical experts in classical Greece had very different aims.[95] The treatise *On Places in Man* (35) presents gymnastics and medicine as opposites, and *Regimen* (1.24, Loeb IV, 261–3) is hardly flattering about the exercise trainer, whose art is 'how to transgress the law according to law, to be unjust justly, to deceive, to trick, to rob, to do the foulest violence most fairly'.[96]

Nomikos and his co-writers correctly quote the Loeb as saying that 'Walking is a natural exercise, much more so than the other exercises', so it is possible that this passage should be seen as the best match for this particular Hippocratic quote.[97] However, that is not the whole of this *Regimen* sentence; on walking, it continues '...but there is something violent about it'. In *Regimen* 2, not only does the author go on to distinguish different types of walking – its effects depend on the time of day – but also the statement needs to be read alongside the previous chapter which distinguishes between 'natural' (*kata physin*) and 'violent' (*dia biês*) exercises.[98] The natural exercises here are not walking, but sight, hearing, voice and thought, all of which 'move the soul'. This is clearly not the world of sports medicine or of any other simple statements today that 'Walking is the best exercise'.

In the next chapter, I shall turn to the food-related Hippocrates quotes which dominate the internet today. Many of these come from a range of different alternative forms of medicine; for example, Jensen's *Foods That Heal* opens with the epigraph 'Let food be thy medicine', attributing it to 'Hippocrates circa 431 B.C.' and he claims to 'use many of Hippocrates' practices and principles in my own work' because 'he believed in foods and natural cure' and 'the power of positive thinking'.[99] He claims that 'Curiously, however, Hippocrates' writings on foods have been all but ignored by the American medical mainstream.'[100] As we shall see, this is not the case: mainstream medical writing, too, repeats this quote. What, however, does it mean? Where are the boundaries drawn between food, and medicine? Sometimes it refers to a general principle of rejecting drugs – playing into the opposition to Big Pharma – but in other cases, as we shall see, it is used to support using specific foods to cure specific conditions.

6

Let Food Be Thy Medicine

By far the most popular Hippocrates quote today is the one for which this chapter is named, often presented as the most Hippocratic sentiment of all. 'HIPPOCRATES said, "Let food be thy medicine and medicine be thy food." Just about every nutrition related professional I know has that quote displayed somewhere in their office, probably to convince reluctant patients that a really smart guy a really long time ago predicted that food could actually heal the body.'[1] It features on T-shirts, key rings, clocks, mugs and aprons, and is widely quoted in complementary and alternative medicine.[2] It is also found beyond the world of healing. Advertising a Canadian meal-delivery service, 'The Greek Physician Hippocrates, said in his scriptures, "*let food be thy medicine, and medicine be thy food*" and to a large extent, this is a good and true statement.'[3] A questioner on WikiAnswers asks: 'Did Hippocrates say let food by [sic] thy medicine and medicine by [sic] thy food?' The question is short, misspelled, but thoroughly to the point, and the sole answer comes as a single word: 'Yes.'[4] Its use online repeats themes already discussed in this book, such as the priority dispute with Imhotep, to whom 'Let food be your medicine, let medicine be your food' is also ascribed.[5] A blogger writes: '"Let Food be they [sic] medicine, medicine be thy Food". Words first spoken by the true father of medicine: Imhotep; who inspired the Greeks; Hippocrates the father of "Western Medicine".'[6] Occasional attacks on this quote can be found; for example, a discussion on agnostic.com in September 2018 in which a typical comment was 'As a species, we've learnt a lot in the last two-and-a-half thousand years. If you want to turn your back on all that, it's up to you.'[7] However, this scepticism is the exception to the rule.

Why is this quote so popular and how is it being used? A recent special issue of the *Journal of the History of Medicine and Allied Sciences* celebrating the movement of the history of food into the historical mainstream was introduced in a piece entitled 'Introduction: Food as medicine, medicine as food'.[8] Correctly noting that 'Let food be thy medicine' is a misquotation and not the words of Hippocrates, the authors noted that its popularity today 'illustrates the desire to view recent nutritional science as a confirmation of past wisdom, and past dietetic practices as intuitive anticipations of modern knowledge'.[9] The quote may also benefit from the fact that, as mentioned in the previous chapter, there is just so much on diet in the Hippocratic Corpus. Following the enthusiasm aroused by the excavations at the temple of Asclepius at Cos from 1902 onwards, Richard Caton even speculated in the *British Medical Journal* that one room was 'the culinary department, where the special diet to which the Coan School gave so much attention was prepared'.[10] However, although sometimes it is restricted to our category of 'nourishment', both food and drink, the ancient Greek word *diaita* can cover far more than just 'food': it means the entire regimen or way of life.[11]

The writer of *On Ancient Medicine* 3, for example, was clear that those who are sick require a different regimen from those who are healthy, 'regimen' here covering not just food but also exercise, as it does in *Airs Waters Places* 1.[12] In ancient medicine generally, *diaita*, drugs and surgery were used, although that order of preference was not fully established until the first century CE.[13] *On the Nature of Man* 9 states that diet is not the cause of disease, because those 'who drink wine and those who drink water, those who eat barley bread and those who eat wheat bread, those who do a lot of exercise and those who do little' are all affected by disease. This seems to refer to a situation in which everyone is affected by the same disease, which is not the usual scenario in the Corpus, where more commonly an individual becomes ill because of a situation that is specific to him or her.[14] While the *Anonymus Londinensis* papyrus comments on diet as something Hippocrates regarded as important for healing, this may just be further evidence that the writer of this late Hellenistic papyrus is making Hippocrates into what he wants him to be, and in the ancient world it was usually Herodicus of Cnidos, not Hippocrates, who was seen as the first discoverer of dietetics.[15] Modern scholarship on ancient Greek medicine has now come to the conclusion that the use of diet not just to prevent, but to cure, diseases was a 'relatively late development' in the late fifth century BCE.[16]

Food, then, plays a large part in the concerns of ancient medicine, but does that make food 'medicine' or medicine 'food'? In an important article, Laurence

Totelin has shown that Hippocratic writers were fully aware of the difference between medicines (*pharmaka*) and food (*sition*) and regarded both as having the power to cause change in the body. However, they deliberately blurred the boundary because many materials were used in both ways; for example, garlic was part of the normal diet, but also recommended for patients as part of their treatment. It was only later, in the Aristotelian tradition, that medicines were seen as the opposite of foods.[17] In a very loose sense, then, we could argue that food and medicine were not entirely distinguished in Hippocratic medicine.

However, the quote itself is another matter. Several variations on the basic 'Let food be thy medicine' currently circulate. These include 'food should be our medicine and our medicine should be our food' (in which an egalitarian 'we' are all working together rather than experts telling patients what to do); 'if you don't eat food as medicine, medicine becomes your food' (warnings against the negative effects of a poor diet, or perhaps of comfort-eating); and various examples of non-standard English, such as 'Allow food be thy medicine as well as medicine be thy food.'[18] Sometimes it is rephrased to use 'your' rather than 'thy' (thus losing the otherwise appealingly archaic feel) and it is interesting that, in introducing the quote, the verb 'say' is usually preferred over 'write'; as we have seen already, there is something in the immediacy of speech which seems to appeal to users of Hippocrates.

Mainstream medicine uses the line without references although sometimes with an acknowledgement that this is not a genuine quote. A feature in the journal *BMJ Global Health*, by public health experts, used it in the title: 'Let food be thy medicine: linking local food and health systems to address the full spectrum of malnutrition in low-income and middle-income countries'.[19] Without citing any primary sources, the authors stated that Hippocrates 'was among the first to recognize the centrality of diet in disease prevention and treatment' and then observed that, in the *Oath*, 'I will apply dietetic measures for the benefit of the sick according to my ability and judgement' preceded the comments on drugs and surgery. After this almost ritual nod to Hippocrates, the rest of the article was about improving diet in poorer parts of the world by modelling good behaviour through hospital food, developing gardens attached to hospitals and clinics, and holding farmers' markets at healthcare institutions; an unusually broad interpretation of the quote.

Outside the mainstream, 'Let food be thy medicine' appears alongside a very wide range of claims, and apparently without any awareness that it is not in the Hippocratic Corpus. Some are more cautious than others; for example, an organic wholefood cooking school site saying, 'When I say "Let food by [sic] thy medicine", under no circumstances am I suggesting that food alone can help to prevent or heal every illness there is.'[20] Others are more militant. Many focus on just one food for one condition; for example, using it to introduce their prescription of curry soup for glaucoma, or celery for nerve function.[21] I shall examine some specific claims of this type later in this chapter.

So why is this quote so widespread? Modern Western cultures have a complex relationship with food. The range of foods available, all year round, seems to overwhelm us, making us easy prey for anyone who proposes that we should simplify our diet in some way. David Gorski wrote, 'I like to view the fetishization of "food as medicine," to cite Hippocrates, as one of the best examples out there of the logical fallacy known as the appeal to antiquity; in other words, the claim that if something is ancient and still around it must be correct (or at least there must be something to it worth considering).'[22] The aphorism is repeated not least because it appears to be 'centuries-old wisdom . . . as true and important today as more information becomes available about the limitations and drawbacks of drugs', as claimed in an advertisement for 'Medicinal Foods' in *Vegetarian Times* for January 1988.[23] But our current obsession with food is not new; in 1888, in his Preface to *Eating for Strength, or, Food and Diet in Their Relation to Health and Work*, Martin Luther Holbrook commented 'In no period of the world's history has there ever been so deep an interest in the subject of foods as at the present' and observed that it is 'a subject now attracting more attention than at any former time'.[24]

In particular, as I noted in Chapter 3, Alan Levinovitz has argued that diet culture uses the language of religion: purity versus sin.[25] The religious status of diet and the fetishization of 'food as medicine' are significant at a time when we know far more about the science of diet than anyone in the past: deficiency diseases and the components of a healthy diet could only be described when developments in chemistry made it possible to isolate the various substances involved, and the vitamins were only identified in the early twentieth century.[26] In news stories, as I demonstrated in Chapter 4, 'science' is often presented as the way in which a 'mystery' of the past has finally been 'solved', but the science of diet is rarely brought into the discussion of 'Let food be thy medicine.' As is often the case, however, Hippocrates is presented as having got there first: 'Hippocrates was ahead of his time when, around the year 400 BC, he advised people to prevent and treat diseases first and foremost by eating a nutrient-dense diet'.[27] This is from the website of Dr Josh Axe, doctor of natural medicine, doctor of chiropractic and clinical nutritionist, who runs a clinic in Nashville where 'vegetable juice and Paleo donuts' are available for office breakfasts, but this view of Hippocrates is hardly unique to him.[28] While there are certainly plenty of Hippocratic treatises that discuss diet, in the wider sense of the entire regimen or way of life of the person, at no point in the Hippocratic Corpus is anything comparable to 'a nutrient-dense diet' advised; there is instead awareness that the normal diet differs from city to city.[29]

Back to the source?

But where is this particular quote supposed to have originated? On answers.com someone asks, 'Hippocrate [sic] said Let food be your medicine but where or when or in which book?' and receives the distinctly unhelpful answer 'It may be in The Hippocratic Corpus which was written either by Hippocrates or his students.'[30] Like 'First do no harm,' 'Let food be thy medicine' can also be linked into the narrative of the *Oath*. I have already mentioned the reference to 'dietetic measures' in the *Oath* but as with 'First do no harm' some locate the source of this quote *itself* in the *Oath*. One of Gwyneth Paltrow's supporters, Steven Gundry, wrote that

> fifteen years ago I resigned my position as Professor and Chairman of Cardiothoracic Surgery at a major medical school to devote myself to reversing disease with food and nutraceutical supplementation, instead of bypasses, stents, or medications, just like Hippocrates asked you and me to do when we took our oath: 'Let food be thy medicine.' He also instructed that all disease begins in the gut. And finally, he taught that a physician's job was to search out and remove the obstacles that are keeping the patient from healing themselves.[31]

I shall be exploring the quote 'All disease begins in the gut' in the final section of this chapter.

In 2013, Rob Kutch wrote a blog post on the importance of good bacteria to diet. He stated, 'Hippocrates, a famous Greek physician, in the year 440 BC said, "Let food be thy medicine and let thy medicine be food". We have finally come to fruition with that fact, 2,383 years after his death.'[32] In 2014, Kutch returned to Hippocrates and did the sums rather differently, writing: 'The amazing thing about Hippocrates is that twenty-five centuries ago he was teaching that quality food is powerful medicine to prevent diseases.'[33] Kutch imagines his blog, 'Renovating Your Mind', in a dream dialogue with Hippocrates (who here prefers to be addressed as 'Crates' rather than 'Hip').[34] A section reads as follows:

> RYM: 'Then what do you think is the healthiest foods available to us today?'
> Hippocrates: 'Anything that comes from the Mother Earth without man's intervention like fruits, vegetables, nuts and seeds.'
>   Don't know if history ever corrected itself when it said one of my quotes was 'let food be thy medicine and medicine be thy food.' I actually said, 'your nutrition is your medicine!'
> RYM: 'Really Crates, I am shocked! I never read that in Greek history.'
> Hippocrates: 'Hey, I am just busting your togas! I am so damn old I don't remember what the hell I said. Sorry kid.'
> RYM: 'You really had me going there Doc.'[35]

What, however, does the quote mean for Kutch? Later in the discussion, Hippocrates says that he is not opposed to the prescription of 'a "safe" and effective drug'. While food is preventative, drugs also have a place, although the hope is that they will not become necessary. Kutch's Hippocrates says, 'I had a stone worker with an inflammatory condition which I would prescribe anti-inflammatory foods twice daily. Listing out the food choices and appropriate recipes.' No reference is given; this could derive from *Epidemics* 4.20c, 'scaliness and blisters, as with the mason Acanthius', but no treatment was suggested there for this condition. While discussions of Hippocratic awareness of inflammatory conditions are widespread online – for example, 'Hippocrates didn't know about the biochemistry of immunity and inflammation in 400 BCE, but he did figure out that some system in the human body was responsible for healing and recovery – what we now know as the immune system. Inflammation is one of its jobs ...' – I have not found any discussions of this 'stone worker'.[36] Kutch's imaginary dialogue with 'Crates' shows some awareness of the fact that 'Let food be thy medicine' is not found in the Hippocratic Corpus, even though the net result is merely a restatement of the concept.

There is in fact a Hippocratic source behind this particular quote, but it requires some work to reach it. The phrase comes from an adapted translation of *On Nutriment* 19: *en trophê pharmaeiê ariston, en trophê pharmakeiê phlauron, phlauron kai ariston pros ti*.[37] Jones put the date of composition of this treatise at around 400 BCE, based on style and on comments recalling the philosopher Heraclitus, such as matter being 'in a state of continuous change' with any element affecting the body being good or bad depending on the circumstances.[38] More recent scholars, however, have dated *On Nutriment* to the second or first century BCE, with von Staden characterizing it as 'self-consciously archaizing' in its 'unsuccessful attempt at "Hippocratic" authenticity'.[39] This places *On Nutriment* in Hellenistic Greece under the Ptolemaic kings, roughly contemporary with the original collation of the diverse medical texts into the Corpus, and post-dating by several centuries the historical Hippocrates.

What did the phrase originally mean? In a rough and very literal translation, it would be 'In food [and] medicine the best, in food [and] medicine the least, least and the best according to which[ever is appropriate?]'. In his Loeb translation, W.H.S. Jones offers something rather more specific: 'In nutriment purging excellent, in nutriment purging bad; bad or excellent according to circumstances.' This uses a narrower interpretation of *pharmakeia* not as 'medicine' in general but rather as those substances used to expel material from the body, a widespread practice throughout the Hippocratic Corpus; and the term can have this sense.[40] Jones seems to suggest that this enigmatic fragment expresses the variability of what is required medically; purging can benefit the nutrition of the human body, or it can be harmful, depending on the circumstances. This reflects the fact that the Hippocratic texts frequently stress variation in people's physical and mental constitutions, different regimens being needed for these variables. Jones notes that the author of *On Nutriment* uses 'the aphoristic style and manner', and suggests that he has written in this opaque way in order that 'more than one interpretation might legitimately be put upon his words'. This difficulty of translation and interpretation presents a dilemma for the translator, so 'In my paraphrase,' Jones tells us, 'I have tried to give the most obvious meaning, although I have often felt that other meanings are almost equally possible.'[41] For this particular passage, however, he offers no alternatives, leaving the contradictions in the awkward phrase to speak for themselves.

I know of no translation of the Corpus giving 'Let food be thy medicine' here. Francis Adams regarded *On Nutriment* as spurious, arguing that it 'must be the production of some metaphysician, rather than a medical practitioner, such as we know Hippocrates to have been'.[42] John Chadwick and William Mann's 1950 *The Medical Works of Hippocrates*, the basis of the easily-available Penguin Hippocrates, also omits *On Nutriment*; while they did not think we can work out which texts of the Corpus were written by Hippocrates, 'it is at least possible to sift the wheat from the chaff by the test of medical accuracy and worth,' so *On Nutriment* counted as 'chaff'.[43] Menahem Luz, who regards this as a fifth-century text with 'later explanatory insertions', argued that the phrase was a later gloss on the previous section, and translates it 'In nutrition, purging is best, in nutrition purging is bad – both bad and best are relative.'[44] It seems that, although Jones's version is far from 'Let food be thy medicine', it is still as near as we are going to get. But this still does not explain where the common wording of the quote originates.

One possible suspect, as ever with interpretations of Hippocrates, is Galen, who saw himself as the true heir of Hippocrates who had understood the master's words while others had not.[45] While correct, Hippocrates 'needed interpretation, like a proverb or a religious text, whereon, from a brief, pregnant statement, one can construct lengthy sermons and whole philosophies of life or of medicine'.[46] Galen's views were not identical to those of the Hippocratic texts on regimen; he considered that a drug acted on the body, while the body acted on foods.[47] His interpretation of *On Nutriment* 19, translated here by Mark Grant, is however strikingly similar to the internet's 'let food be thy medicine':

> Some substances relax the stomach as they have medicinal powers mixed in them ... This appears to be what Hippocrates meant when he said 'In food medicine'. Thus it is good not only to lend an ear to these ideas, but also the argument can be explained from those foods that possess no nutritive or purgative quality. For they say that these things not only serve frequently as foods, but also as medicines by heating, moistening, cooling and clearly drying us.[48]

Galen seems to be saying that 'medicine' is to be found in food, because it has qualities that extend beyond simply supplying nutrition to the human body.

Certain foods can dry, moisten, warm or cool the body, and thus regulate the person's condition. These are understood as medicinal attributes which physicians can use to alter the bodies of their patients as seems necessary. Galen presents the Hippocratic sense as focusing on purgation ('relaxing'), although he thinks we should go further. He proposed that 'everything of average temperament . . . is only a food, not a medicine' as it does not alter the body's heat or functions 'but in every way maintains the body nourished in the same state that it was encountered'.[49] Food nourishes and allows the body to continue working; medicine encourages the body to react differently (for example, sweating, promoting or stopping excretion). Some foods acted as medicines when applied correctly.[50] Galen does not reference the full phrase recorded in *On Nutriment*, but instead quotes only the first three words: ἐν τροφῇ φαρμακείη.

In a short but important article from 2013, which has reached at least some medical professionals, Diana Cardenas surveyed the use of this aphorism in medical journals from 1979 to 2012. She showed that the allegedly Hippocratic phrase is a 'misquotation' and a 'literary creation' 'lying at the root of an entire misconception about the ancient concepts of food and medicine'.[51] Following Robert Joly's 1967 French translation, she translated *On Nutriment* 19 as 'In food excellent medication, in food bad medication, bad and good relatively'.[52] None of this suggests – as does the version widespread today – that food should be one's sole 'medicine'. Her work suggests that it is the recent rise in interest in nutrition in medicine which has led to the repetition of the aphorism.

Cardenas' article went live on 1 December 2013. How did this affect the popular tradition? On 31 December 2013, on the Wikipedia Hippocrates page, an editor added something to the end of the section 'Direct contributions to medicine': 'Hippocrates often used lifestyle modifications such as diet and exercise to treat diseases such as diabetes, what is today called lifestyle medicine. He is often quoted with "Let food be your medicine, and medicine be your food" and "Walking is man's best medicine"'. The reference cited is 'Chishti, Hakim (1988). *The Traditional Healer's Handbook*. Vermont: Healing Arts Press. p. 11'; this is Ghulam Chishti, *The Traditional Healer's Handbook: A Classic Guide to the Medicine of Avicenna*, which will be discussed in Chapter 7. It was not until 25 August 2014 that a further phrase was added to this statement, with a reference to Cardenas' article, by user 'Pineali': 'however the quote "Let food be your medicine" appears to be a misquotation and its exact origin remains unknown'. Despite taking nearly a year from Cardenas' publication for it to be added to the 'Hippocrates' entry, this remains at the time of writing (20 February 2019), still with the comment that 'Let food be your medicine' (here, 'your' rather than 'thy') '*appears to be* a misquotation' [my italics]; at one point this was 'is an apparent misquotation'.

What Cardenas could not do, however, was to identify the source for modern writers in English of the exact wording we know so well, 'Let food be thy medicine'. One other person has tried to push this wording back before the start date of the research for her article; Matthew Dalby, in a blog post published on 31 October 2017.[53] Using Google Books Ngram Viewer, he traced trends in the popularity of various versions of the quote, noting that the archaic 'thy' version was first used in the 1920s and increased in usage in the 1960s. Using Google Books, his first hit was in a 1921 issue of the periodical *Public Opinion*, although this did not include the name of Hippocrates.[54] Joanna Brown has, however, found that we can go back much further than this, if we include the phrase without the attribution and if we loosen up the search terms.[55] An early use in a slightly different form is found in an 1850 popular medical journal, where an editor admonishes an unhealthy correspondent, one Frederick Mansel of Kenilworth: 'Were you to swallow pills by the gross, mixtures by the gallon, and powders by the pound, you would never be well. Why be so enamoured of physic? Make food your medicine, not medicine your food.'[56] The phrase is here used to discourage the use of 'physic' in favour of eating healthily, and thus approximates its modern usage. However, it is not ascribed to Hippocrates, or to anyone else; perhaps it was already so well known that the name was not needed, or it existed before it took on his name, or the similarity is a coincidence.

Dalby also cited Otto Carqué's *The Key to Rational Dietetics* (1926), which opened with this as an epigraph, again without the name of Hippocrates. Brown located another early naturopathic example of the use of 'Let food be your medicine' in the same year, in Gustave Haas, *Health Through Sunshine and Diet*; this has now also been identified by Barry Popik, an etymologist, in a blog post in 2013.[57] Discussions of Haas within naturopathic literature are hard to find, but he is cited by the National Institute of Chiropractic Research on their 'Chronology of Naturopathy' as the author of a piece on 'chiropractic orthopaedics'.[58] Haas uses 'let food be your medicine' here both to lend authority to his own thesis, and also to advertise a product explicitly promoted by him. He works from the understanding that all life on earth requires the rays of the sun in order to survive, and suggests that people in the modern era have failed to remember this truth. The human diet should consist of 'fresh-sun-ripened fruits and vegetables' which are 'Nature's natural foods' through the consumption of which 'we can reap the product of the sun's rays'.[59] Applying this understanding, he produces a list of peoples whom he claims understood the use of diet to treat illness, including Native Americans, 'Kaffirs, Aborigines and Mexicans'. The mention of peoples with an ancient lineage and non-Western medical traditions is intended to lend authority to his claims. However, his first appeal to authority is made instead to the father of Western medicine: 'Like Hippocrates of old I firmly believe that food is the best medicine, but it is not my desire to start a food reform … but rather to advise in each bodily ailment a modified diet which … will do much to bring about a speedy recovery.'[60] This is clearly a version of *On Nutriment* 19. 'Food is the best medicine' suggests that food is different from medicine, and far superior to it; true medicine is nutritional, and what is commonly referred to as 'medicine' is in fact not medicinal at all. Here it is the antiquity of Hippocrates that renders him authoritative: he is 'of old', rather than 'of Cos'.

Haas announced his appreciation of 'the assistance rendered by Frank W. Bower, food chemist and dietitian … [who] has presented to the world the incomparable food remedies, NORMALETTES', and directed the reader to Bower's advert at the end of his own volume.[61] The advert describes 'a line of concentrated food preparations which … contain in concentrated form the Organic Salts, the Vitamins, the Chlorophyll and other life-giving elements … so often lacking in the customary daily meal'.[62] At the head of the column of text stands the adage 'LET FOOD BE YOUR MEDICINE', this time uncredited. Here, the phrase is expounded upon in the rest of the text; the sentiment refers to Frank Bower's tireless work researching the nutritional value of plants, and disseminating this research to the malnourished public in the form of pills. Because they contain 'Vital Elements from Food Plants' these items are marketed as belonging to 'food' rather than 'medicine', despite what we may see as the highly artificial state of their manufacture; 'Drugless Physicians … can prescribe them since they are a food'. Bower's advert also advertises 'The Dr Haas book, "Health Through Sunshine and Diet"' even though the piece itself is published within the very book it promotes.[63] Thus, the book promoting sunshine (something free to all) and a largely vegetable diet (something inexpensive) advertises a product that claims naturalness while existing in pill-form, which itself then feeds back by advertising the book. All this is bound together by the authority of 'Hippocrates of old', who said 'food is the best medicine' or 'LET FOOD BE YOUR MEDICINE'. Hippocrates himself, it seems, would have prescribed Bower's Normalettes.

Other uses of the Hippocratic injunction can be found in texts expounding drugless treatments in the years before the extensive popularization of alternative health movements in the 1970s. For example, Gayelord Hauser's *Dictionary of Foods*, first published in 1932, consists of a list of various foods and their individual properties, followed by recommendations to the 'housewife' on how to keep her family healthy. Hauser's introduction begins with Hippocrates, who is cited not only as the father of medicine, but also as the 'father of food science; for it is he who first said, "Your food shall be your medicine."'[64] Hippocrates' injunction is contrasted with the money-making dictates of the 'mechanical age, in which we are now living [which has caused] a decline in natural health'.[65] In contrast, Max Gerson, famous for his creation of a special diet for the treatment of cancer, stated that 'The majority of nutrients are regarded as 'pharmakon' according to the doctrine of Hippocrates; this means a medication prescribed for a special purpose in a special dosage. The dietary regime, therefore, does not attempt to compose nutritional principles of general value.'[66] This passage seems to refer back, however vaguely, to *On Nutriment* 19, in its conflation of nutrient and *pharmaka*. Gerson's dietary plan included the 'Hippocrates Soup', based on leeks, celery and parsley, which as the name suggests is supposed to come from a (never specified) Hippocratic treatise. The soup is 'miraculous' or even 'magical', and is promoted as cleansing the kidneys, repairing damaged cells and aiding the digestion of an otherwise raw diet.[67] 'Hippocrates, the father of ancient greek [sic] medicine conceived this magical soup to treat his chronically ill patients. He used it to detoxify their bodies and stimulate healing.'[68]

Another comparable use of 'let food be your medicine' comes from adverts published in the *Vegetarian Times* from the early 1980s onwards. 'Alive Polarity Programs' from California opened its advert with 'Hippocrates said, "Let food be thy medicine"' and announced that through the use of its regimen, 'you'll learn how your diet & your body work together. We'll show you how to use your body as a laboratory to find which foods are best for you.'[69] Unlike later naturopathic literature with its aggressive opposition to the methods of conventional science, Alive Polarity introduces the body as scientific testing ground, encapsulated in the word 'laboratory'. Through trial and error, the patient will learn which foods he or she requires to maintain health, the reference to the laboratory supplying scientific validation on top of Hippocrates' moral or antique validation. Here, the use of 'let food be thy medicine' has shifted from simply providing authority to individuals' claims for the efficacy of a particular food, and advertises a specific programme, run by one particular company. This dual approach, using Hippocrates' supposed words both to advertise a company's particular regimen and to supply authority to the practitioner, becomes a feature of the self-promotion of various suppliers and theorists in the internet age.

Which foods? Liver, garlic and watercress

Like Gerson's 'Hippocrates soup', many recipes bearing the name of Hippocrates make no attempt whatsoever to find a source in the Hippocratic Corpus. The Hippocrates Health Institute, discussed further in Chapter 7, also promotes 'Hippocrates' Famous Green Juice', 'an alkaline nutritional powerhouse'.[70] Such recipes are invariably based on fruit and vegetables. Yet, when it comes to identifying 'good' foods, we often have very different views from those of the writers of ancient medical texts.[71] For us, 'an apple a day keeps the doctor away,' and there is even a claim on answers.com that Hippocrates 'was first to suggest that people eat more fruits and vegetables and exercise more for a healthy diet'.[72] This is far too modern a reading. *Regimen* 2.55 lists the properties of all fruits, which are 'rather relaxing'; this is in the sense of being laxative. Of these fruits, 'Sweet apples are indigestible, but acid apples when ripe are less so.'[73] In Galen, too, all fruit should be regarded with extreme caution, with a similar view of apples; they are 'difficult to concoct, slow to pass and unwholesome' until they are thoroughly ripe, when they could be baked in pastry and given 'to strengthen the stomach'.[74]

'Let food be thy medicine' is not restricted to advice on achieving a healthy diet, fruit- and vegetable-based or otherwise; it can also be attached to specific foods acting as 'medicine' for specific conditions. Take, for example, night blindness (*nyctalopia*, although in ancient Greek the word was used for both day- and night-blindness).[75] One website on vitamins claims that 'It is recorded in the history that Hippocrates (about 500 BC) cured night blindness. He prescribed to the patients ox liver (in honey), which is now known to contain high quantity of vitamin A.'[76] A cardiologist, Hajar Al Binali, set this remedy in the context of how his own father was cured of nyctalopia within a week, using fish liver oil rubbed on the eyes; the oil was produced by cooking the liver on charcoal. Al Binali ingeniously suggests that this works because, as well as juices from the cooked liver being put in the eye, the patient cannot resist eating the liver itself – and this provides the patient with the vitamin A in which he or she was deficient.[77]

What is the Hippocratic origin of this treatment? Here is the relevant passage:

> As a medication for nyctalopia let the patient drink squirting-cucumber juice, have his head cleaned, and reduce his neck as much as possible, compressing it for a very long time. When remission occurs give him raw bull's liver dipped in honey, and have him drink down as much as he can, one or two.
>
> *Sight* 7, Loeb IX, 385[78]

What is clear here from this is that, in contrast with discussions of liver today, in Hippocratic medicine the liver is raw, not cooked. Glancing back to ancient Egyptian medicine does not help here; in the Ebers papyrus roasted ox liver is pressed on the eye, while in the Kahun papyrus a patient with an eye problem is given what may be raw ass liver.[79] Furthermore, in the Hippocratic *Sight* the liver is 'drunk down' (Elizabeth Craik prefers 'gulped down') rather than even being put on the eyes; this suggests that what is used is fluid, so perhaps the liver is simply placed in the honey and the resulting liquid taken by the patient. Craik suggests another route out: to emend the Hippocratic text so that the liver is not raw.[80]

Taking a different approach, in a discussion of the various post-Hippocratic medical writers who recommend a different animal liver, that of the goat, for day- or night-blindness, von Staden notes that this particular animal could be used because goats were believed to have excellent night vision.[81] The specific action described in the Hippocratic *Sight* also contrasts with discussions of night blindness in those later authors; for example, Dioscorides (*On Simples*, 3) where (fluid from?) boiled goat's liver is 'injected into the eye' or vapour from the cooking process allowed into the eye, but it is 'also to be eaten'. In Celsus, *On Medicine* 6.6.38, those with night blindness are advised to put on to their eyes 'the stuff dripping from a liver whilst roasting ... and as well they should eat some of the liver itself'. This is far closer to Hajar Al Binali's suggestions. There cannot, of course, be any connection with vitamin A in these texts, because it was as-yet undiscovered.

'Let food be your medicine' is very strongly present in the modern naturopathic and dietetic literature of the 1970s and beyond. An anonymously-edited booklet entitled *Garlic, Compiled by Health Research*, published in 1983, collected comments and brief articles on the use of garlic, ranging from excerpts from Culpeper's seventeenth-century herbal, to modern anecdotes: 'If you are ill, you may take garlic judiciously, along with the sagacious advice of Hippocrates who long ago said, "Let food be your medicine."'[82] He 'gave garlic first place in his herb codex' – which is of course an entirely imaginary text.[83] Writing in the same year, Gary Hullquist claimed that Hippocrates 'classified garlic as an effective laxative and diuretic. No doubt he was thinking of garlic when he advised his fellow physicians: "Let food be your medicine."'[84] Unusually, here Hippocrates is speaking to other physicians rather than to his patients, or by extension to us, and had just one particular plant in mind, which is of course the plant promoted by the author.

Other foods recommended in current literature are seen more generally as 'superfoods' rather than as remedies for specific conditions. For example, Channel 4's "Food Unwrapped" 'travels the world to uncover the truth about the food we eat'. A 2014 episode included a feature on the health benefits of watercress. Dr Steve Rothwell, owner of 'Vitacress', was asked by the presenter about why he thinks watercress is so good. He responded:

> People have known about it for a long time. Hippocrates, the father of modern medicine, when he built the world's first hospital, he built it by a fast-flowing stream because he wanted to grow watercress which he deemed essential to the care of his patients. And it's really the last sort of hundred years, that we've valued the taste and texture of eating watercress.[85]

There are several points worth noting here in addition to the alleged Hippocratic endorsement. Hippocrates is not just 'father of medicine' but father of *modern* medicine. Not only did be build the world's first hospital (another entirely false claim), but its location is described. The myth of this hospital next to a watercress bed is surprisingly ubiquitous, as websites copy other websites. For example, from a 2009 piece on watercress:

> Fortified with more than 15 essential vitamins and minerals, even since ancient times its health giving properties have been highly valued. In fact Hippocrates – the Father of modern medicine – is said to have deliberately located his first hospital beside a stream so that he could grow a plentiful and convenient supply of watercress with which to help treat his patients.[86]

The place where it was grown is sometimes a river, sometimes a stream, or even in 'natural springs'.[87] Some widely-repeated versions of the Hippocrates and watercress story include a special title for watercress: the 'cure of cures'. For example, 'Hippocrates was particularly convinced of the health benefits of watercress, a plant he often referred to as the "cure of cures". Hippocrates is known to have built his first hospital in Kos, Greece, near a river where he could grow watercress to help treat his patients.'[88] Tammi Hoerner's Mompositive blog ('Vibrant living starts here') instead ties watercress to a specific group of conditions: 'My favorite fact about watercress is that Hippocrates (the father of modern medicine) built the first hospital along side a river where he'd plant watercress so that he'd have access to this powerful green to treat blood disorders. Isn't that cool? "Let food be thy medicine and medicine be thy food".—Hippocrates.'[89] Other claims made for ancient watercress include its use as 'a brain food, a hair tonic and aphrodisiac by the Romans'.[90] Sometimes the myth includes a date – Hippocrates did this 'in 400 BC', an attempt, perhaps, to anchor the myth in an accessible chronology, to a date with a clear round number.[91]

European watercress is *Nasturtium officinale*; it is native to Europe and to Asia. In Greek, this is *sisymbon* (σίσυμβρον). Some websites will tell you that the Greek for watercress is *kardamon* (κάρδαμον): 'Hippocrates, the father of medicine, is thought to have decided on the location for his first hospital because of its proximity to a stream so he could use only the freshest watercress to treat his patients. The ancient Greeks called watercress kardamon; they believed it could brighten their intellect, hence their proverb "Eat watercress and get wit."'[92] However, *kardamon* is not watercress, but garden cress, the

Latin *Lepidium sativum*. Within the texts associated with the name of Hippocrates, garden cress seeds feature almost exclusively in the Hippocratic gynaecological treatises, cleansing both the milk and the womb.[93] In a list of foods recommended for a woman undergoing a long and complicated process of healing for the movement of her womb to the hip, both watercress and cress feature alongside leeks, radishes, garlic and seafood; the purpose of the diet and the other forms of treatment – fomentations and suppositories – is to soften the mouth of the uterus.[94] Cress seeds are also used to soften the mouth of the uterus in the treatise *Superfetation*.[95] In one of the rare uses outside gynaecology, in the treatise *On Ulcers* the leaves of 'narrow-leaved *kardamon*' are used to fill an ulcer. There is still nothing here that matches the internet myths.

Another story circulating on the internet is that 'The ancient Greek general, and the Persian king Xerxes ordered their soldiers to eat Watercress to keep them healthy'.[96] A variation is that 'the Persians did observe that soldiers were healthier when watercress was part of their daily diet' or that 'Persian King Xerxes fed watercress to his soldiers, to keep up strength and stamina'.[97] 'The ancient Greek general' here is named on other sites as Xenophon, and the reference (which none of these sites gives) is actually to Xenophon's *Education of Cyrus*, 1.2.8. However, this story has nothing to do with soldiers; instead, it is about Persian ways of bringing up children so that they will learn self-restraint. The passage reads: 'Furthermore, they bring from home bread for their food, cress for a relish, and for drinking, if any one is thirsty, a cup to draw water from the river.' Further on, at 1.2.11, cress is described as food for failures: 'Those of this age have for relish the game that they kill; if they fail to kill any, then cresses.' Common to all these internet references seems to be one assumption: that if an ancient precedent can be found for the use of a plant, this is proof of the plant's efficacy in medicine. This does not mean that the users of the references have been anywhere near an ancient text.

Death begins in the gut: Constipation and Hippocrates

The other side of food consumption is, of course, its excretion. In his history of constipation, James Whorton reported the comment of the American humourist Dave Barry that the 'international symbol for the middle class' should be 'a stick drawing of a little person trying to read the fiber content on a cereal box'.[98] Whorton has argued that this contemporary concern originated in the nineteenth century with the rise of industrial society and was reflected in a growing interest in the model of the body as a factory, complete with 'waste products' that must be evacuated before they can cause disease; the theory of 'autointoxication', in which fears about constipation merged with knowledge of germs, proved merely the most extreme example of this.[99] From at least the nineteenth century, constipation was presented as 'civilization's curse', a curse then addressed in the twentieth century with claims for the health benefits of colonic irrigation and of fibre in the diet. The interest in fibre began within unorthodox medicine but by the 1970s, following the work of Hugh Trowell and Denis Burkitt in particular, it was increasingly accepted in the mainstream too.[100] The role of fibre is no longer considered so simple; in 1990 the *British Medical Journal* published a review article by K.W. Heaton – a Reader in medicine at the University of Bristol – with the tag-line, 'After 21 years of study the verdict remains one of fruition and frustration.'[101]

Hippocrates has been enlisted to support a high-fibre diet, with a range of quotes about both disease and death originating in the gut, because – as we know now – 'Hippocrates was right.' 'All disease begins in the gut' is commonly attributed to Hippocrates, and often linked now to the modern idea of the mind-gut connection.[102] It can also be connected to claims that Hippocrates recommended apple cider vinegar, something which – as we have already seen – needs to be challenged.[103] Other sites with slightly different agendas state that he performed colonic irrigation: 'Death begins in the colon and an unhealthy colon is the root cause behind many health problems. Colon cleanse is one of the methods to take care of your colon. This was believed to be the case by Hippocrates of Cos, a famous ancient Greek physician (*ca.* 460 BC–*ca.* 370 BC). Modern science has shown that he was correct.'[104] Here, 'All disease begins in the gut' has morphed into 'Death begins in the colon.' Hippocrates is not the only person associated with this second version of the quote: there are also claims that Bernard Jensen (the 'Father of Colonics') came up with the phrase from his own research, to describe 'self-poisoning', and 'Death begins in the gut' is also widely attributed to Elie Metchnikoff to describe his research on intestinal flora, for which he received the 1908 Nobel Prize for medicine.[105]

Medical journals are not exempt from making these statements. The editor of *Gastroenterology & Hepatology*, Gary Lichtenstein, introduced a special issue on gut microbiota with the unreferenced statement that 'The importance of the gut in human health has long been a point of emphasis in medicine, warranting comment from such luminaries as Hippocrates, who flourished during the 4th century BCE and warned that "bad digestion is the root of all evil" and that "death sits in the bowels."'[106] Elsewhere, however, 'Death sits in the bowels' is given as an 'old German proverb'.[107] The etymologist Barry Popik has tried to find sources for either Hippocrates or Metchnikoff ever writing this; he traces 'Death begins in the colon' to at least 1944, with a peak of usage after 1976.[108]

Even without a convenient Hippocratic quote, Hippocrates was enlisted as a supporter in the earliest days of the fibre fashion; at the beginning of the twentieth century, this was particularly associated with John Harvey Kellogg, the inventor and promoter of flaked cereals who, as Whorton notes, 'was effectively born a health reformer' with his combination of a Seventh Day Adventist background, hydrotherapy training and a medical degree.[109] Kellogg promoted vegetarianism and fresh air, but had a particular interest in 'autointoxication'; in 1928 he stated that 'Hippocrates was also a believer in bran'.[110] This 'bran Hippocrates' became widespread among unorthodox healers who supported raw food diets. Here is Sylvester Graham, founder of the Grahamite movement and promoter of the Graham cracker, on Hippocrates: 'styled the father of medicine', he 'depended far more on a correct diet and general regimen, both for the prevention and removal of disease, than he did on medicine, [and] particularly commended the unbolted wheat meal bread "for its salutary effects on the bowels"'. Graham added that 'the ancients' knew such bread led to good health, being 'better adapted to nourish and sustain them than that made of the fine flour'.[111]

So what is the Hippocratic origin for such claims? Graham gave no source for his quotation on the 'salutary effects' and I have not been able to identify it.[112] The wording appears to suggest a laxative effect, and that knowledge is what is commonly attributed to Hippocrates even in modern literature; for example, Hugh Trowell, from the 1974 issue of the *American Journal of Clinical Nutrition*: 'Since the time of Hippocrates it has been observed that wheat bran is laxative.'[113] A chapter on the history of dietary fibre states that 'the concept that coarse foods of plant origin help to combat constipation goes back to Hippocrates ... in the 4th century BC who commented on the laxative action of the outer layers of cereal grains', while another chapter in the same handbook summarizes and then quotes Graham: 'The link between the ingestion of unprocessed foods and good health is chronicled as far back as Hippocrates (4th century BC) who recommended the eating of wholemeal bread for its "salutary effects upon the bowels".'[114]

In addition to observing the laxative effects of fibre, Hippocrates is also quoted by nutritionists as stating that 'whole meal bread makes larger feces than refined bread'.[115] In his book *Food Intolerance*, Dr Maurice Lessof attributes the following words to Hippocrates: 'Wholemeal bread cleans out the gut and passes through as excrement. White bread is more nutritious as it makes less faeces.'[116] In this version, unlike in the unorthodox medicine version, Hippocrates believed that white bread was nutritious because it did not contain any material that the body was unable to absorb. The source for Lessof's Hippocratic quote appears to be *Regimen* 2.40: 'The meal together with the bran has less nourishment, but passes better by stool. That which is cleaned from the bran is more nourishing, but does not pass so well by stool.'[117] However, there is one important point here: this passage is discussing not wheat flour, but barley flour, yet the modern references assume that it concerns wheat.

The Greek term for wholemeal or wholewheat bread is *autopurites artos* or, in Latin, *panis artopuros*; the majority of the few references to it are 'remedial'.[118] Outside the medical texts, it features in Petronius' *Satyricon*, where we are told that such bread is strengthening, and 'when I do my business, I don't grumble'; that is, it eases bowel motions, echoing what is implied in the Hippocratic source text.[119] Wholemeal bread has just one mention in Athenaeus, *Sophists at Dinner* – that repository of ancient food references – without any indication of whether it is an enjoyable or useful food.[120] Celsus describes bread using 'the meal from which nothing is extracted' as being of middling strength.[121] In the second book of *Method of Medicine to Glaucon*, Galen describes how to make a cataplasm – a sort of bread poultice – to disperse a swelling. He compares barley and wheat breads and mentions *autopuros* bread made with the whole flour, noting that people prefer to eat bread made with more refined flour, but for cataplasms he recommends bread made from the finest wheat flour.[122]

In the Hippocratic treatises, too, there is more interest in using whole wheat bread in treating diseases rather than as part of the normal diet, although here it is ingested rather than being used in a cataplasm. There are three references to *autopurites* in *Internal Affections*. In chapter 20, to treat excess phlegm, the use of wholewheat bread is recommended; wheat bread in general 'draws the phlegm very well', while wholewheat bread features after a period of rest following vomiting.[123] In chapter 22, excess phlegm has turned to dropsy, and the aim is explicitly to 'dry out the patient's cavity': as part of this, 'fresh warm dark whole-wheat bread' is given.[124] In chapter 30, where the issue is bile in the spleen, the use of wholewheat bread in conjunction with acid, salty and sour foods could be read in terms of encouraging the bowels to work: 'At the beginning, the patient accepts his food, but does not pass it through very well; as the disease progresses, his colour becomes pale-yellow, violent pain besets him, his collarbones become lean, he no longer accepts his food as he did at the beginning, but now becomes full on a little.'[125]

Conclusion

The quotes I have examined in detail in this and the previous chapter are, of course, only the tip of a very large iceberg. Perhaps the most convenient of all is the claim that Hippocrates said, 'Foolish the doctor who despises knowledge acquired by the ancients,' a sentiment which gives support to all the other quotes around. It appears, for example, on a site 'sourcing and importing select herbs and superfoods of the highest purity from mountainous regions of Greece. We believe that a healthy diet paired with Loose Leaf herbal teas can greatly improve one's quality of life.'[126] I have not found any attempt to locate it in a Hippocratic text, but nor have I found any challenges to its authenticity.[127]

Nevertheless, 'Let food be thy medicine' remains the most popular at the moment, even more so if we add in the other quotes which offer the same message. In October 2011, 'Flourella' posted in the online forum historicum. com, asking if anyone had a source for 'the (allegedly) Hippocratic quote' 'Leave your drugs in the chemist's pot if you can heal the patient with food'. Flourella expressed doubts about the authenticity of the axiom, having 'only managed to find it quoted on assorted dubious websites (most of which are attempting to sell me equally dubious forms of alternative medicine for various ailments I don't have)'.[128] There were two responses: one suggesting looking at *On Nutriment*, and the other from someone who carried out further searches and failed to find any evidence that it was from a Hippocratic treatise. The quote is often found on sites promoting locally-grown, organic food, often in conjunction with 'Let food be your medicine and your medicine be your food.'[129]

SHINE (Self-Help in Natural Enrichment) included it in its list of 'Hippocrates Quotes', a list distinguished from most in two ways; first, there are dates by some quotes, with the 'chemist's pot' one having 420 BCE while 'To do nothing is sometimes a good remedy' is dated to 400 BCE, and second, because some quotes have the name of a treatise beside them.[130] This quote, however, does not, which is not surprising because it is not Hippocratic. The version given in this list also changes the verb from 'heal' to 'cure': 'Leave your drugs in the chemist's pot if you can cure the patient with food.' The 'chemist's pot' aphorism features in printed sources as well, used as evidence that 'the paradigm of a preventive approach' goes back to Hippocrates.[131] It can be found in the work of Seventh Day Adventist Gunther B. Paulien; his *The Divine Prescription and Science of Health and Healing* uses it twice, once in the standard form but again with the unique archaizing variant, 'Leave thy drugs in the chemist's pot if thou canst heal the patient with food.'[132] The phrase 'chemist's pot' is an odd one, as another use of it is in a poem by Edward Hopper, *The Dutch Pilgrim Fathers*, first published in 1626 and reprinted in 1865; here, the 'chemist's pot' is where all the different nations forming America are mixed together and 'the scum thrown out'.[133]

Quoting Hippocrates, as discussed in this and in the previous chapter, works by presenting an allegedly Hippocratic 'truth' in isolation from any of the texts of the Hippocratic Corpus or any idea about what Hippocrates is supposed to have represented. In Chapter 7, I shall move from these separate elements and turn to the case of 'holistic' medicine today in order to discuss further what people think Hippocrates' contribution to medicine now covers. This offers another slant on the dietary Hippocrates, but in the context of an entire approach to the body and its healing.

7

The Holistic Hippocrates: 'Treating the Patient, Not Just the Disease'

In this final chapter I want to look at the Hippocrates of today not through specific uses in news stories or in quotes, but through the invocation of his name in holistic (or, as we shall see, 'wholistic') medicine. Holism today presents itself as a return to a superior past, and brings Hippocrates in as part of this strategy. The model of the history of medicine implicit – or sometimes explicit – in holistic users of Hippocrates is one in which there was a golden age until 'the turn away from holism in medicine allowed diseases to be located in specific organs, tissues or cells'.[1] While there is something in this where ancient medicine is concerned, with its basis in fluids rather than organs, this is of course also a tried and tested strategy for convincing an audience of the value of a 'new' thing: you claim it is 'old', or ancient, or just traditional. Tracing the lineage of a treatment or approach back to Hippocrates is, as ever, a winning move in a power game. New is bad: traditional, having a history, is good and, if that goes back to the Father of Medicine, it is even better.

After discussing what can be meant by 'holism', I shall start by considering various approaches which operate under the umbrella of 'holistic medicine' today, and outline their reception of Hippocratic medicine. I shall also locate some of the claims made, in relation to the texts of the ancient Mediterranean world and to the earlier history of holism. I find useful here the model of 'projection', described in Chapter 2.[2] How does the holistic Hippocrates fit into this practice of projecting our utopias or nightmares? What versions of holism are currently being projected back on to the classical past, what does this tell us about current views of what medicine should be, and how are the classical texts then used to reinforce what their new users mean by holism? Returning to questions raised throughout this book, whose Hippocrates is he anyway – does he belong to orthodox medicine or to alternatives to this – and is he the founder of a system, or the rebel trying to overthrow it?

The self-healing body

James Whorton has shown in general terms how and why alternative practitioners often consider Hippocrates to be 'their doctrinal father'. In orthodox medicine, Hippocrates was designated the Father of Medicine because he had rejected supernatural phenomena as the causes of illness: the 'alternative' Hippocrates was valued for his 'natural' methods of healing and his belief in an 'inborn ability of the human body to respond to the insult of illness or injury and restore itself to health'.[3] In both cases Hippocrates is a champion of the natural, but the end result can be very different, depending on whether his opposition is to the supernatural or to the artificial.

This alleged ability of the body to heal itself is often linked to the phrase *vis medicatrix naturae*, 'the healing power of nature', a tag which features heavily in alternative medicine and which is sometimes traced back to Hippocrates, sometimes in the mistaken variant *vis mediatrix naturae*; as we have already seen for *primum non nocere*, Latin looks good, even if it is not correct.[4] Some scholars have attributed the origin of the phrase in its Latin form to the eighteenth-century William Cullen.[5] One article I have found by naturopaths, citing as one of their sources the entry for *vis medicatrix naturae* in 'Wikipedia 2010', comments on the Hippocratic origins of the phrase, 'some writers maintain there is little evidence that he used the term vis medicatrix naturae' and states instead that he 'used the term *physis*, the ability to heal oneself, or nature in Greek'.[6] The Wikipedia page on 'Vis medicatrix naturae' presents the phrase as being the Latin form of the Greek 'Νόσων φύσεις ιητροί ("Nature is the physician(s) of diseases")'.[7] While it has recently been seen as something entirely un-Hippocratic,[8] it does in fact translate the three opening words of the fifth section of the Hippocratic *Epidemics* 6, which begins 'The body's nature (*physis*) is the physician in disease. Nature finds the way for herself, not from thought ... without instruction, Nature does what is needed'. As Wesley Smith pointed out, however, 'the text of the manuscripts shows signs of commentators' interference' and *physis* here seems to mean both the nature of the body, and *physis* in a philosophical sense, as opposed to *logos*.⁹ In the nineteenth century, perhaps in a reaction against the excessive interventions of 'heroic medicine', the Latin phrase was reclaimed by some orthodox practitioners but, at least from the 1830s to the 1860s, 'art' was still believed to trump 'nature'.¹⁰

Another naturopath, Pauline Nelega, whose approach to holism will be discussed in more detail later in this chapter, wrote: 'Hippocrates, who is considered the father of modern medicine, was a physician in ancient Greece in around 400 BC. He emphasized a holistic approach to medicine, *warning doctors not to interfere with the body's ability to heal itself*.'¹¹ This last phrase seems to bring *vis medicatrix naturae* towards 'First do no harm.' Holism, Hippocrates and the self-healing body reinforce each other: presenting Hippocrates as the person who first understood that the body can heal itself also links him to nature and suggests the safety of his healing methods, while providing an antique seal of approval for later methods concerned with maintaining a balance with an external 'nature'. The ideology of alternative medicine often uses 'nature' as 'a symbol redolent with beliefs and meanings about health, the body, and the ideal state of the human being'.¹² The body has an original healthful state which is one with nature, and it desires to return to that state. Rosalind Coward has pointed out that 'nature' and 'old' or 'traditional' shade into one another; if it has been used for thousands of years, it must be safe, and if it is 'traditional', it must be natural.¹³ Holistic systems suggest that the alternative to orthodox medicine and its drugs lies in a return to 'natural' approaches to health, concentrating on diet, exercise, herbal medicines and positive thought patterns.

Both holism and 'let food be thy medicine' are manifestations of what Norman Gevitz has called the 'drugless systems', important in US medicine from the nineteenth century onwards.¹⁴ The use of Hippocrates as a forefather by the modern alternative health movement can be traced in its popular literature throughout the first half of the twentieth century and, as we saw in the previous chapter, the dietary Hippocrates was often invoked. Today, 'Let food be thy medicine' is commonly appropriated by practitioners and advocates of vegan raw food diets. In this set of beliefs, even life-threatening conditions such as terminal cancers can be cured through the strict application of a diet using only raw 'living' foods. The critique of orthodox medicine implicit, or often explicit, here asserts that orthodox physicians do not see their patients as individuals and are blind to their emotional needs, while conventional medicine destroys the body whether or not it destroys the disease (that is, it 'does harm').[15] Coward argues that alternative medicine's antipathy towards artificial products is grounded in 'hostility to the destruction of an original wholeness'.[16] This image of a primeval but recoverable wholeness can be particularly attractive to those experiencing the bodily fragmentation of chronic illness; Jessica Hughes has shown that the experience of fragmentation was also present for patients in the ancient world.[17] Alternative methods focus upon non-invasive, 'natural', dietetic treatments which promise endless energy, 'optimal health', and self-healing, so long as the patient maintains the regimen constructed for them. At the end of this chapter, I shall glance briefly at one of the most powerful uses of the name of Hippocrates in this context today, one which continues to have considerable press coverage: Brian Clement's Hippocrates Health Institute (HHI), which has brought Hippocrates' name into the public domain in the USA and beyond.

How far does any of this have its roots in the Hippocratic Corpus? It would be logical for those claiming Hippocratic roots for holism to discuss the Hippocratic whole/parts claim from Plato's *Phaedrus*, where as I noted in Chapter 2 priority is given to 'the whole'.[18] In modern discussions of holistic medicine, while this is rarely cited explicitly, it often lies in the background. For example, consider Robson and Baek's 'Hippocrates held the belief that *the body must be treated as a whole and not just a series of parts*, which is the underlying concept of the recently emerging *systems biology*'; by omitting any mention of Plato, this supports the impression that the whole/parts point can indeed be traced to a specific Hippocratic text.[19] What is meant by 'the whole' in Plato is in any case far from clear. Is it, as Galen and subsequently Littré thought, the universe, or is it the whole body?[20] Is it 'all external factors that influence health'?[21] And does the passage tell us more about Plato than about what the Hippocratic writers, let alone Hippocrates himself, originally meant? For Wesley Smith, it was 'the nature of the whole man', 'the nature of the cosmos' and perhaps also 'the nature of all body'. Smith argued, 'As always, Plato uses his language precisely and self-consciously, and if he is purposely ambiguous he will take account of all the meanings he has suggested.'[22] So, rather than either/or, perhaps we should see this as both/and: the 'whole' is all of these things.

The specific promotion of raw foods in order to enhance the body's self-healing powers has to ignore the inconvenient Hippocratic treatise *On Ancient Medicine* which offers a history of human diet in which people gained health only by rejecting the raw diet of animals, because this was too 'strong' for them. In the process, some foods were removed entirely from the diet because human nature could not 'overcome' them.[23] Ralph Rosen has further argued that, for the author of *On Ancient Medicine*,

> dietary regimen is not a 'natural' phenomenon. Nature may go to great lengths to heal the diseased body, as Hippocratic treatises are fond of saying, but it does not in fact do such a good job of directing humans towards foods and dietary habits that will keep them healthy or heal them when sick. That requires the intervention of intelligence and agency: the τέχνη of regimen, in other words, addresses a deficiency that needs to be rectified, and this is the polemic on which much Hippocratic medicine seems to have been based; it forms, in fact, the rationale for the very notion of medical intervention. It is not insignificant that Hippocrates was credited in antiquity with saying that medicine was a 'servant of Nature', for servants are brought in to do what masters cannot or will not do themselves.[24]

When it comes to the implications of allowing Nature to heal the body, there is clearly variety among the treatises of the Hippocratic Corpus. Nature, alone, is unlikely to be enough; she needs a helping hand. However, this is also precisely why modern holistic alternatives make money despite their enthusiasm for Nature; they argue that, without their specific interventions, Nature will not be able to carry out her healing work.

Beyond the Hippocratic texts, a range of meanings of 'holism' existed in the ancient Greco-Roman world: it could concern the relationship between mind (or soul) and body, or advocate considering the body as a whole, or focus on the body's unity with the cosmos, this last meaning being the one chosen by Paul Carton, one of the French naturopaths who promoted what he considered Hippocratic holism in the 1920s as part of a return to simplicity as an 'antique virtue'.[25] Modern holistic medical approaches, while rarely constrained by any of these meanings, also tend towards the larger, 'cosmic' interpretations. Often combined with using the name of Hippocrates, they promote better ways not only to treat illness, but also to live. The slogan of hippocrate.net, a French site which sells a range of short courses including the 'Academy of Alchemists', is

'I improve my health and my life'.[26] When we read on a website advertising the Apivita cosmetics range that its founders were inspired by 'the holistic approach of Hippocrates to health, beauty and well-being' and that this approach influences their 'make-up, fragrances, soaps, hair products and sunscreen, all of their unique products are designed to act beneficial [sic] to the body, spirit and soul',[27] the word 'holistic' is being used in a deliberately imprecise way; what is most important is, firstly, that whatever it means it is supposed to be a Good Thing and, secondly, that its credibility is somehow enhanced here by its attribution to Hippocrates.[28]

Fears about Big Pharma also play an important part here. Whorton linked the resurgence of drugless alternatives to the loss of confidence in pharmaceutical treatments following the Thalidomide tragedies of the 1960s. At this point, he argued, it became normal to attack medicines as dangerous, and alternative practitioners were able to exploit popular anxiety.[29] The enthusiasm for 'natural' approaches to health exploded in the late 1970s with the growth of a medical counter-culture. Beginning as a critique of psychiatry, this widened to include other medical issues, claiming that holism saw the patient as a 'whole' being, rather than as a disparate collection of organs and symptoms.[30] Coward adds that the emergence of AIDS in the 1980s disrupted traditional understandings of both treatment and contagion, and further highlighted the limits of conventional medicine. She argues that, for heterodox practitioners, 'Aids [was] the prototypical disease of our age' as it was 'a disease which made visible [a] heralded collapse of immunity', which they insisted had been compromised through the bombardments of a highly artificial mode of life in the West.[31] Following this, admissions from orthodox practitioners that some 'alternative' methods may be effective for some conditions (although not AIDS) only strengthened the revival of naturopathy in America.[32]

Hippocrates in contemporary holistic medicine

In this section I shall examine in more detail how ancient Greek medicine features in holism today, by looking at the claims made and the sources used by some specific examples. The website 'Greek Medicine' is a good place to start, not least because it is so widely used by other online materials, whether or not they credit it as their source; these include a sample essay from a UK-based 'essay mill', worryingly entitled 'A Brief History into Greek Medicine History Essay'.³³ 'Greek Medicine' is run by David K. Osborn, who describes himself as 'Master Herbalist – Astrologer – Holistic Health Consultant and Educator' and who explained its genesis as 'a website about traditional, holistic, Greek Medicine'; the juxtaposition of 'tradition' and 'holism' is significant.³⁴ He is also a trained acupuncture practitioner and certified yoga instructor; current practitioners of holism often use a range of methods, contrasting with specialism, where one person is an expert on a very narrow field. Healers also project their range of healing methods back in time so that the sanctuary of Asklepios in Cos becomes 'a holistic healing centre' which 'contained infirmaries, temples, hot springs, hostels, a school for physicians and much more';³⁵ taken from a Greek tourism website, this wording picks up and gives a 'holistic' spin to an older scholarly view that healing sanctuaries were much like modern health spas frequented by 'health tourists'.³⁶

Osborn's online bio describes how his life changed when he found a book which 'correlated the astrological signs and planets with the four temperaments and humors of Greek Medicine. This gave David the Golden Key to medical astrology; he was then able to relate everything he had learned and studied in holistic healing to astrology. This key to medical astrology also started David's study of Greek Medicine.'³⁷ His basic approach is that 'Truth is one, but the sages of these different traditional medical systems call it by different names.' Holism, then, is broader than anything we have so far encountered: it concerns a single medical truth which connects all forms of medicine. For Osborn, Greek medicine is 'truly a natural healing system for the whole world' as well as being 'the traditional healing system from which modern medicine grew and evolved'.³⁸ One truth: whole world. Here, holism is about more than treating the body as a whole: it concerns treating medicine itself as a whole, with different local models expressing the same truth, and being the ancestors of 'modern medicine'. In his history of naturopathy, Whorton labelled this trend 'world medicine'; we also have met it in Chapter 5 as 'global medicine'.³⁹

While there is no reason why users of the site would necessarily read Osborn's bio, he also writes a blog, where in March 2017 he celebrated ten years of the greekmedicine.net site.⁴⁰ He explained there that the book which gave him that Golden Key was *L'Astrologie Médicale* by Sylvie Chermet-Carroy, an astrologer and graphologist.⁴¹ This is an example of how the greekmedicine.net site adds to its image of authority by Osborn's practice of giving 'acknowledgements' of some of the books he has used, a common internet strategy which plays into a model in which books must surely be (even) better than online materials. However, Osborn does not use the standard printed works we would perhaps expect; those deriving from scholarship on ancient medicine. On Hippocrates and his works, Osborn thinks we can be 'fairly certain' that some of the works of the Corpus can be attributed to him; specifically, *Airs Waters Places*, *Aphorisms* and *On Ancient Medicine*. He writes that Hippocrates led a 'band of renegade physicians' who moved with him from Cnidos to Cos. His source here is acknowledged as another printed work, Ghulam Chishti, *The Traditional Healer's Handbook: A Classic Guide to the Medicine of Avicenna*.⁴²

That 'band of renegade physicians' phrase is repeated widely online; greekmedicine.net was cited in 2009 by a chiropractic blog using it.⁴³ The entire section of greekmedicine.net in which it appears was copied with attribution by Jim Putnam in his blog *The Colton Points Times*, 31 January 2017, as part of a piece on the Hippocratic *Oath*.⁴⁴ The phrase also features extensively without attribution; for example, on a site selling nutritionals, *Tested Nutrients*, which proudly proclaims 'We are people in search of science.'⁴⁵ It also migrated from online materials into supposedly academic publications, including those 'published, print-on-paper sources'.⁴⁶ A 'band of renegade physicians' sounds almost like Robin Hood ('riding through the glen/ … with his band of men'), and immediately identifies Hippocratic medicine with the forces of the Resistance; Hippocrates himself can become 'The medical renegade who came to be called the Father of Medicine.'⁴⁷ The resistance story has other internet variations, and recalls the myth that he was imprisoned for 'opposing the infrastructure' of ancient Greece, discussed in Chapter 3.

In Chishti's and thus Osborn's narrative, holism is used to explain the alleged move from Cnidos to Cos. Both say that Cnidian medicine 'considered the body to be merely a collection of isolated parts, and saw diseases manifesting in a particular organ or body part as affecting that part only, which alone was treated'; not a holistic approach. This part of the Osborn/Chishti model is repeated widely, including on the website of Red House Australia, an independent centre for the treatment of eating disorders majoring on superfoods eaten in a community environment, where it appears on a page on

'Hippocrates' influence on Red House philosophies, principles, and practices.'[48] Red House quotes the Osborn/Chishti idea that 'The Cnidian school considered the body to be merely a collection of isolated parts', alongside what was then the opening of the Biography section of the Hippocrates page on Wikipedia:

> Historians agree that Hippocrates was born around the year 460 BC on the Greek island of Kos. He is renowned as the 'Father of Modern Medicine' – in recognition of his lasting contributions to the field as the founder of the Hippocratic School of Medicine. It was Hippocrates who finally freed medicine from the shackles of magic, superstition, and the supernatural.[49]

Use of the Wikipedia line 'Hippocratic medicine was humble and passive' (discussed in Chapter 3) also betrays the origins of this Red House page. While I have not yet been able to work out the origin of this widely-repeated line – it could simply be the creation of a Wikipedia editor – it proves a particularly useful marker for reliance on what holistic practitioners often wrongly call the 'wonderful Hippocrates wikipedia page'.[50] For Chishti and Osborn, holism thus characterizes Cos and marks its superiority over Cnidos. As it is from Cos, it must also be the approach of Hippocrates.

Chishti himself clearly had Plato's *Phaedrus* in mind, although not naming this as the source, when he wrote that 'He [Hippocrates] viewed the human body as a complete, integrated whole (as opposed to a collection of parts) and his system of treatments was of a general nature, rather than a specific treatment against one set of symptoms.'[51] From this formulation we also learn that, in addition to being opposed to specialisms, holism supports treating the whole person rather than 'specific' treatments. Here is Osborn's development of this: 'As a holistic healing system, Hippocratic medicine treated the patient, and not just the disease.' This is interesting wording. In 2013, in one of his assaults on alternative medicine, Edzard Ernst – formerly Chair in Complementary Medicine at the University of Exeter – noted that when he asks alternative practitioners 'What do you treat effectively?' he was given answers like 'Alternative practitioners, unlike conventional clinicians, do not treat diseases' or 'I treat the whole person, not just the disease.' In response to these answers, Ernst argued that 'any good medicine always has been and always will be holistic. High-jacking [sic] holism as a specific characteristic for alternative medicine is misleading and an insult to all conventional clinicians who do their best to practice good medicine.' Ernst's concern is that, by claiming a monopoly on holism and saying that they treat the whole person, alternative practitioners then receive what Ernst calls 'a "carte blanche" for treating any disease or any condition or any symptom'.[52]

Osborn's statement about Hippocratic medicine and the answers Ernst was given echo, whether consciously or unconsciously, the quotation I have used in the title of this chapter. Found on many holistic medicine internet sites, sometimes as 'It is more important to know what sort of person has a disease than to know what sort of disease a person has', or bumper-stickered into 'treat the (whole) person, not the disease', it is a saying associated with one of the greatest physicians of the modern era, Sir William Osler (1849–1919): 'The good physician treats the disease; the great physician treats the patient who has the disease.'[53] It has however so far proved impossible to source this in Osler's writings; the nearest quotation may be 'Care more particularly for the individual patient than for the special features of the disease.'[54] As we saw in Chapters 5 and 6, Hippocrates does not have a monopoly on 'fake quotes'. As applied to Hippocrates, the axiom also recalls Lasagna's 1964 version of the *Oath*, which includes 'I will remember that I do not treat a fever chart, a cancerous growth, but a sick human being.'[55]

Unlike many other modern users of Hippocrates, practitioners of holistic medicine tend not to give 'quotes' but instead simply invoke the name of Hippocrates in support of their beliefs. For example, Sandra Sigur, a practitioner from Florida of reflexology, yoga, reiki and aromatherapy, and a former doula, author of *Healing Groovy* (2015),[56] was interviewed for the blog 'Windermere Sun' in 2016:

> Natural or holistic medicine has been around for over 5,000 years. Hippocrates, who is considered the Father of Modern Medicine, emphasized a holistic approach to medicine, warning doctors not to interfere with the body's ability to heal itself, as well as to treat the body as a whole – mind, body and spirit. The early Hippocratic Oath was revised to exclude the word 'spirit' because it was thought to mean religion, when in actuality our spirit is what defines us as unique individuals (i.e., how we respond differently to life's circumstances).[57]

Holistic here becomes another word for natural, and the dating suggests that the system had been around for millennia before Hippocrates; it is unclear, therefore, what makes him the 'Father'. That exclusion of 'spirit' is perhaps a reference to those versions, such as the Revised Hippocratic Oath proposed by the British Medical Association in 1997, which have dropped the opening invocation of the Greek gods.[58]

The site *Natural Wellbeing* goes into more detail, featuring a page on 'The History of Holistic Medicine: The Ancient Greeks and Holistic Medicine', by Paulina Nelega.[59] Written in 2009, this is part of a short series, all written by Nelega, on the allegedly-long history of holistic medicine; the ancient Greeks provide 'another forebearer [sic]'. Nelega is a clinical herbalist based in Vancouver who describes how her passion for 'exploring our relationship with nature and the healing properties of plants' developed from growing up surrounded by 'majestic cedars [which] shared their timeless wisdom as I sat beneath them'. She then took a 'conventional path', becoming a medical laboratory technologist, which taught her 'the benefits – and shortcomings – of allopathic medicine' and encouraged her to understand 'our body's innate wisdom and profound intelligence to heal – *vis medicatrix naturae*'.

In holistic circles, as we have already seen, 'Vis medicatrix naturae' may be taken to mean that there is a natural healing force in everybody, or that nature tends towards health and should either be left alone or should be given encouragement to get on with it. There is however a further use: as here, it may be used to suggest that healing depends on actual contact with 'Nature', whether that is growing a plant in a pot or being in a forest. Nelega did not only learn from the cedars, however; she also trained at Coastal Mountain College of Healing Arts in Vancouver. Currently, this no longer seems to be operating, and at one point it was merged with Wild Rose College, a school which offers individual online courses at around $200–300, and a 'Wholistic [sic] Therapist Diploma' at $1,697, payable in monthly instalments.[60] For a mere $97, you can submit a 'Wholistic Therapist Thesis' and 'you have one year from date of approval to complete your thesis'.[61] 'Our emphasis is on the wholism of the individual – the integration of the body, mind, and spirit. We believe wholistic healing is an art to be cultivated through a sound investigation.'[62]

Wider discussions of what Hippocratic medicine involves thus lie behind Nelega's version of Hippocrates. It is significant that she claims Hippocrates as the ancestor of holism, not of biomedicine, when she writes: 'While Hippocrates is considered the father of modern medicine, many of his practices bore more resemblance to what is today considered holistic or alternative medicine. Many of today's holistic practices date back to the understandings of Hippocrates and the ancient Greeks.'[63] Elsewhere on the same page she develops these claims:

> Hippocratic medicine bears more resemblance to today's holistic medicine than it does to allopathic (traditional) medicine. Hippocrates based his methods on 'vis medicatrix naturae' – the healing power of nature. According to Hippocrates, the body contained the ability to *heal itself* through balancing the four humors (blood, black bile, yellow bile and phlegm). When one of the humors was out of balance, the body became ill, and Hippocrates taught that administering certain natural substances would bring about a rebalancing of those humors.

Here the suggestion is that, while you can intervene (using 'natural substances', of course), what you are doing is merely stimulating a natural process of 'rebalancing'.

Wild Rose College's 'wholistic' medicine with a 'W' deserves some attention, as other holistic sites too prefer this spelling. Loma Linda University, a Seventh-Day Adventist school in California, has as its motto 'To make man whole.'[64] Once again, this concerns the body's natural tendency to heal itself. In 2008, Loma Linda announced its Pediatrics Wholistic Medicine Clinic, merging 'modern Western medicine' with 'ancient treatments from the East'.[65] Another 'wholistic' site, 'Wholistic kids and families', offers a different merger under the same label. It presents wholistic medicine as 'neither entirely conventional or ultra-holistic'; they prefer diet and herbs, but they use antibiotics when necessary. Their aim is to 'treat your child as a whole'.[66]

Adventists have a particular affinity with (w)holism. They 'believe the key to wellness lies in a life of balance and temperance' and recommend – although do not insist on – a vegetarian diet.[67] In 1898, Ellen G. White, revered by Adventists as a prophet whose writings are second only to the Bible in their relevance, published *The Desire of Ages*, where she retold stories from the gospels about Jesus as the Great Physician who taught that 'health is the reward of obedience to the laws of God'.[68] She stated that 'For the sick we should use the remedies which God has provided in nature, and we should point them to Him who alone can restore.'[69] In *The Ministry of Healing* she wrote that the holistic principles were 'Pure air, sunlight, abstemiousness [avoiding things that are harmful], rest, exercise, proper diet, the use of water, [and] trust in divine power – these are the true remedies … Those who persevere in obedience to her laws will reap the reward in health of body and health of mind.'[70] These 'Eight Laws of Vibrant Health' sound much like the six Galenic non-naturals – air, exercise/rest, sleep/waking, diet, evacuation/retention and passions/emotions – and there has been much discussion in other contexts of whether or not White was a plagiarist.[71]

By putting the W into holism, Loma Linda University claim to be separating themselves from the 'quacks and false promises' present in the field of holistic health.[72] Across the world, there are now many other medical centres calling themselves 'wholistic'; for example, in Sydney, Melbourne, Atlanta and London. They often combine a range of methods which sound scientific, rather than 'natural'. At one such centre in Marylebone, which says it is attended by patients from all over the world, the mission statement does not use 'the great physician treats the patient who has the disease' but states this in these words: 'Patient individuality is our prime concern. What helps one person may not suit another with the same condition.'[73] The founder, Dr Shamim Daya, and her team offer 'food therapy', which – in another echo of the claims for Hippocrates – they describe as 'Food as Medicine'. This gives 'A greater feeling of being anchored and grounded'.[74] It is practised alongside processes which sound very scientific, such as 'Therapeutic PEMF' to counter 'electrosmog' which 'comes from electric wiring and equipment' including power lines, TVs and mobile phones.[75]

Somewhere in the marketing for its version of wholism, nearly every such centre will invoke Hippocrates' name, although not necessarily where one would expect to find it. At the Marylebone Wholistic Medical Centre, that unreliable Hippocrates quote about disease beginning in the gut is attributed to Daya herself, in the form 'The origins of most disease processes lie in the gut and therefore healing starts with normalizing the function of the gut.'[76] However, Daya does cite Hippocrates in another section of the Centre's website, on digital infrared thermal imaging offered for breast screening: she includes 'In whatever part of the body excess of heat or cold is felt, the disease is there to be discovered. Hippocrates, 400 BC.'[77]

Invoking Hippocrates through history

These examples show how references to Hippocrates support a range of alternative healing practices which operate under the 'holistic' – or 'wholistic'

– umbrella. In their repeated reclaiming of the true Hippocrates from the hands of a mistaken or deliberately-distorting orthodoxy, the imagined moral core of the man remains intact, even though many different versions of 'his' views have been constructed. One of the patterns of engagement with the image of Hippocrates, found throughout the history of medicine and still strong today, is to contrast him with whatever the speaker or writer perceives as most negative in mainstream medicine: 'appeals to Hippocrates were explicitly and most fundamentally appeals to the past which expressed considerable discomfort with contemporary science and, more generally, with the world that science had created'.[78] This clearly happens with contemporary holistic medicine websites.

What is different in the present uses of Hippocrates is partly that none of the standard concern for identifying a 'genuine work' seems to interest those promoting holistic medicine today, and – like the spread of quotes online – their claims about Hippocrates are constructed with very little reference to any texts. This may stem from the period between the World Wars, when the neo-Hippocratic movement developed as 'a revolt against the system, formalism, academics, professionalism, materialism, and analysis of the nineteenth century', favouring instead 'vitalism, humanism, individualism, and synthesis, a return to Hippocratic doctrine'.[79] There were regional variations: in Britain, the neo-Hippocratic movement was about Hippocrates as generalist rather than specialist, while in France it provided support for both homeopathy and naturopathy.[80] Through selective reading, the different treatises of the Hippocratic Corpus could be called upon to support homeopathy's practice of curing like with like as well as allopathy's cure by opposites.[81] Homeopathy has had a particularly strong relationship with Hippocrates as 'an ancestral figure worth of veneration' but also as a practitioner of direct observation of the patient, although this is not always a feature of current holism, as the practitioners discussed in the previous section of this chapter demonstrate.[82] For example, Nelega consults at a distance, inviting readers to ask her any questions and to 'let me know if I can assist you with a health consultation and custom-compounded herbal formula'.[83] Readers fill in a very simple form and send in the money. In the form, you give your details (age, gender, weight, current pattern of smoking, caffeine, alcohol and water consumption, exercise) and your 'primary health concern' and tell her what existing conditions you have, attaching any lab reports and a list of medications and dietary supplements.[84]

Analysing why the name of Hippocrates was so important for the emerging holistic movement in 1920s and 1930s France, George Weisz argued that 'The notion that was most identified historically with Hippocrates was that of "nature" or "natural" healing'; Emile Littré had defined 'hippocratisme' as 'the doctrine which attempts to imitate Hippocrates, giving to this imitation the particular sense of following nature, that is to say of studying the spontaneous effort that it makes and the crises that it produces'.[85] Ideas of the healing power of nature were able to find plenty of support in the Hippocratic Corpus; for example, in the section from *Epidemics* 6 mentioned at the beginning of this chapter: 'The body's nature is the physician in disease. Nature finds the way for herself, not from thought ... without instruction, Nature does what is needed.' Such ideas had also been widely discussed in American medicine of the 1860s. John Harley Warner has argued that this interest in Nature was a reaction to changing therapeutic interventions, as doctors moved from trying to reduce fever and inflammation by attacking with bleeding and purging, to seeing their role as being more about building up the strength of the patient.[86] The conclusion reached was that while 'bloodletting had indeed been carried to absurd excesses greatly impeding nature's work ... this did not mean that bloodletting was necessarily bad in principle'.[87] Nor did believing that diseases were self-limiting mean that the answer was to do nothing, as the role of the doctor could be to support the body in healing itself. Here, too, the current uses of Hippocrates in holism are not new.

Today, however, alleged Hippocratic holism does not even have to be an 'alternative': mainstream medicine wants to claim it too. For example, in 2000, the Royal Society of Medicine held a conference on the topic 'Healthcare for the Whole Person: Is Holistic Medicine More Healthy?'[88] An article by a medical student, Sneha Mantri, in the 2008 edition of the American Medical Association's *Journal of Ethics*' online section, *Virtual Mentor*, argued for the humanistic integration of Hippocratic holism with modern knowledge. Mantri stated that medicine has moved 'from prescientific holistic approaches to modern, scientifically supported explanations of pathology', and contrasted 'the integrative Hippocratic view ... [with] the specialization view'.[89] This, apparently unconsciously, echoes the concerns of inter-war British neo-Hippocratics, who emphasized Hippocrates as generalist rather than specialist and, looking back at the First World War, criticized what they saw as the specialization of German education and the centralization of its institutions, as opposed to the greater focus on the individual and on personal initiative in British society.[90] They saw the unity of the organism as a key principle, and – according to the leading neo-Hippocratic Alexander Cawadias – a focus on the 'whole individual patient' was essential.[91] Mantri ended with a call for fuller integration to take into account 'both the individuality of illness and the universality of disease etiology'.

Mantri's contrast between 'the integrative Hippocratic view' and 'the specialization view' is worth exploring further. The history of medicine has long been interested in the history of specialisms. Vanessa Heggie's 2010 article in *Medical History*, 'Specialization without the Hospital: The Case of British Sports Medicine', summarized the main approach as follows: 'Specialization in medicine acts to normalize categories of health and sickness that, once constructed, can appear to be obvious and rational divisions of the body, of disease, or of populations.'[92] This underlines the point that, while decisions on how we divide the body into organs or systems or other sorts of 'part' are arbitrary, once these categories exist they can then take on a life of their own. As Roger Cooter argued for the emergence of fracture treatment under the control of orthopaedics, a specialism also needs 'professional interests and aspirations' to propel it into existence; its emergence was partly due to the Second World War leading to a greater interest in accidents and trauma, and partly to orthopaedists 'enlarg[ing] their professional space'.[93] Cooter argued that 'accidents and trauma cut across the "organ geography" of medical and surgical specialties' and argues against the claim that orthopaedics can trace its lineage to 'traditional bone-setting [which] appears to legitimate orthopaedic surgeons as the rightful menders of broken bones'; nevertheless, that claim of antiquity was important.[94] Orthopaedics emerged 'as a specialized branch of general surgery … in the early twentieth century in terms of a holistic physiological vision of the structures and functions of the musculoskeletal system—a naturalized division of labor' but later became fragmented into separate smaller branches: 'the surgery of the hand, the foot, the ankle, the spine, and so on'.[95] This increasing fragmentation was at least partly due to the various technical developments in the field, in which 'knowledge appeared to increase year after year';[96] 'There is no mind so comprehensive that it can keep pace with all the requirements of modern surgery', as Robert Jones had said in a lecture delivered in May 1925.[97] So, here we have spurious claims of historical continuity (those traditional bone-setters), then the emergence of specialisms due to social and economic factors and also to new techniques, further division into sub-specialties, and then – perhaps – a return to holism?

While mainstream medicine can now claim to be holistic, hits on search engines suggest that there is still more *popular* interest in holism than *mainstream* medical interest.[98] I have already alluded to the veiled criticism of allopathy: holism is seen as a 'whole life approach' rather than being about 'fragmented (i.e. nonholistic), episodic (i.e. lack of continuum of services), and external symptom-based (as opposed to dealing with the root cause of illness) diagnostics and treatment, mostly depending on the one-fits-all approach and yet on the trial-and-error for treatments'.[99] Here holism comes a little closer to 'personal medicine' – individualized and empowering to the patient[100] – but, once again, holism is defined in opposition to how mainstream medicine is perceived: unlike that medicine, it is not about fragmentation, nor about specialists clinging to their little empire of one organ or system.

Hippocrates branded

Commentators have noted that the draw of alternative methods is greatest amongst those who have chronic or potentially fatal conditions, 'where orthodoxy has least to offer', or who are undergoing traumatic treatments such as chemotherapy.[101] Here, in its darkest formulations, the quote 'let food be thy medicine' in particular can be used to encourage desperate people with life-threatening conditions to reject drugs and instead to undertake, against medical advice and at great expense, drastic and demanding dietary regimes. Big Pharma here is more than the enemy: it is presented as the devil. Brian Clement, who runs HHI, asserts that 'Doctors back 100 years ago and before that were all natural doctors. There was no such thing as the pharmaceutical industry then, no pushing drugs just for the heck of it.'[102] The HHI website also argues that the *Oath*'s 'I will give no deadly medicine to anyone' has been 'disregarded by much of modern medicine as physicians blindly and reflexively embrace the marketing campaign of every new pharmaceutical drug coming off industry assembly lines'.[103] It thus draws on 'Let food be thy medicine' and the *Oath* while embracing the 'drugless medicine' approach; a 2011 TripAdvisor review of HHI from an enthusiastic user, 'islandler', states 'Let food be your medicine and examine what should be your food that is the most nutritious' [sic].[104] Clement's claims have been dismissed in much of the press as 'nothing but pure American pseudoscience' and his claimed degrees are from diploma mills; he is only state-licensed as a nutritionist.[105] While he apparently no longer calls himself 'Dr' he still mentions the PhD, in addition to making much of his own journey to health from being 'unfit and gasping for air' as a young man.[106]

Why is this the 'Hippocrates' Health Institute? Not because it is easy to spell; in a radio interview, Clement spelled it out for his listeners, because it 'is a big, hard name for most of us'.[107] But it is clearly worth using. In 2010, in his book *Supplements Exposed*, Clement presented Hippocrates in holistic terms as 'Perhaps the greatest practitioner of this ancient wisdom tradition' as he 'and other innovators of the complementary healing system examined no part of the human condition in isolation from its other parts'.[108] Clement has also used the very vague quote 'Medicine is woven into the stuff of our mind. Hippocrates', which comes from the Hippocratic *Decorum* 6 and is found widely on the internet.[109] The HHI website underlines that the name was selected because of the holistic aspects of Hippocrates: 'As a fifth-century BC Greek physician, Hippocrates treated the body as a whole, not just a series of parts, and taught a natural healing process centered on a wholesome, natural diet.'[110]

HHI traces the history of its raw vegetable diet to its claimed founder, Ann Wigmore; Clement claims that she used this diet to reverse her own stage four colon cancer, while he himself benefitted by 'eliminating death and dying from my menu'.[111] In an interview in 2012, he said how much he enjoyed his work, because 'Can you imagine watching people come back to life?'[112] Interviewed as an 'entrepreneur' in August 2018, Clement said that 'Our institute is proudly named after its founder, Ann Wigmore, who said that Hippocrates principles of health are the natural rules for obtaining physical wellness, hence establishing an Institute around those principles and practices.'[113] Yet it is not the 'Wigmore Institute'; what has happened is that the title Wigmore gave to her own clinic in 1960s Boston has been taken over by Clement. Hippocrates' name has become a commodity here, and not only for patients; a spokesperson for the Ann Wigmore Foundation commented in 2015 that 'She lost the name Hippocrates and we're not connected.'[114]

The year 2015 was significant for HHI, as Clement was ordered to 'cease and desist' from practising medicine after two children were taken out of conventional cancer therapy to attend HHI, and one of them died.[115] The State of Florida did not pursue this, apparently because HHI has no need for a licence because it does not accept payments from medical insurance.[116] The expense of HHI is mentioned by reviewers: in 2018 one commented, 'There was a constant pressure to buy more goods and services every single day' and added 'I am weak and just as exhausted and fatigued and in pain as before attending Hippocrates.'[117]

Beneath the application of the apparently relaxed 'Let food be thy medicine' quote, there are interesting suggestions of something more sinister at HHI. The language of religion is often applied, including by its users. Frank D described his experience as a 'rebirth' – 'I am opening the door and my heart to a rebirth for me, only me, no one else but me' – and wrote that HHI was 'My Mecca'.[118] As we saw in Chapter 3, when the story about Hippocrates in prison was taken up by the weeksmd.com site it included the idea that Hippocrates competed with the priestly system of medicine in which 'Whether the cure worked or not, depended upon your degree of sin and the priest kept the payment regardless', and this idea of one's personal morality affecting the efficacy of a cure is also used by HHI.[119] Current concerns in holistic medicine with overall well-being and perfectible health present health as something to be attained through dedication and effort, so guilt is generated when, despite the effort (and the financial investment), the patient does not improve or recover.[120] While earlier Western religious discourses of guilt and perfectibility centred around the purification of the soul as separate from the corrupted body, modern alternative health movements in the 1980s locate the body as 'the place where this perfectibility is to be found'.[121]

Clement asserts that 'both health and healing are dependent upon our beliefs'.[122] While this can be viewed (and often is viewed) as a method of self-empowerment for a sick individual, it can also be used (and indeed is used) as a stick with which to beat the noncompliant HHI 'guest'. Reviewer 'tmaddow' (who gave only one star) suggested that 'When MANY of the residents did not achieve the results they were promised the staff turned on them . . . and had the audacity to insinuate that the residents in question were preventing their own healing through lack of faith.'[123] Conversely, a positive reviewer on Tripadvisor suggests that the negative reviewers 'are missing the whole point of the self healing [sic] process' which includes 'tak[ing] responsibility for your own health care' and 'examin[ing] your thinking as it relates to your health, do you deserve good health?'[124] Health thus becomes something that is a reward for the morally responsible or pure, and the body withholds it from the person who is not thinking in the correct manner.

The example of HHI also shows that part of the appeal of holism is that it is not an easy route to health; their programme runs for twenty-one days and, as a user puts it, 'This is a HOLISTIC healing center, not a quick fix, so don't go there expecting that.'[125] Reviewers are clear that they have 'now lost faith in the western medical establishment and realise that the natural way is the best way, as it gets the most results.'[126] Yet amidst the insistence on the 'natural', the trappings of biomedicine are still used, even at HHI: users note that 'Blood samples are taken on arrival and departure' and there are 'scientific references aplenty.'[127] In a 2018 interview, Clement mentioned the technology available as a selling point; he said 'At Hippocrates Health Institute, we have numerous cutting edge electromagnetic, high frequency healing modalities such as QRS, Hwave, Cyberscan and Biowell.'[128]

Another holistic healer who uses the H-word in her brand – and whose approach has been extensively challenged – is Rebecca Carley, who developed what she calls 'the Hippocratic protocol' which she says can cure autoimmune diseases, autism and cancer.[129] After being suspended as an MD in 2003, Carley – who believes she can reverse what she identifies as vaccine-induced diseases – promptly repackaged herself as a 'holistic' healer. As her archived website for 'the Hippocrates Academy Protocol' puts it, 'Note that Dr. Carley does NOT practice medicine, and does NOT give medical advice. Rather, she teaches her students what she would do if she were you after reviewing your individual history of assaults to your immune system.'[130] Holistic healers seeking to avoid prosecution insist that they are not healing the patient: the patient is healing herself, courtesy of the self-healing body with a little help from the healer who offers a way to stimulate the healing process.

Conclusion

Everyone – in biomedicine and in various branches of alternative medicine – wants Hippocrates on their team. Considering the whole, whether that is the whole body rather than an organ or system, or the body in relation to its wider setting, clearly has a long history, and several 'medicinal utopias' are currently held under the umbrella of 'holism'. The term 'holism' is always used in a positive way, but in its alternative medicine uses it often contains a barely-veiled criticism of Western biomedicine. The holistic Hippocrates conjures up nightmares of excessive specialization and 'toxic' drugs alongside more positive dreams of the individual being heard and understood and participating in a worldwide natural healing system.

Contemporary holistic medicine goes well beyond arguing that a knowledge of the whole body is essential to understanding what is wrong with a part of it. Holistic medicine presents Hippocrates as its ancestor, using the strategy of the claim to be returning to the 'original', the 'ancient'. The past is a time of integration, holism and Hippocrates, and the answer to our present problems is to reject fragmentation and return to this holistic Hippocrates. Comparing this with other current uses of Hippocrates as a projection screen on to which we place our ideals of medicine, holism too may not go far beyond using a 'quote' – for example, 'Let food be thy medicine' – which may or may not have its origins in any text of the Hippocratic Corpus. Yet, despite having a rather promising potential source text in Plato's *Phaedrus*, very few holistic medicine sites referencing Hippocrates make any use of this. I wonder if the problem is that it is in Plato, not the Hippocratic Corpus, that the key sentence about the whole and the part is found?

Conclusion: Strange Remedies?

Hippocrates is, indeed, a pretty quotable guy. He has never been the sole preserve of either mainstream or alternative medical systems, and today he remains a trump card to be played in any medical competition. But, in the absence of any reliable knowledge of his own medical views, what that card shows always remains blurred, until someone puts it down. As Vivian Nutton wrote of the *Oath*, 'far from the *Oath* imposing its values on society, it has always been society that has imposed its interpretation and values on what that *Oath* is and means, and it has been constantly changed to accommodate the demands, the concerns, and, at times, the prejudices of society at large'.[1] The malleability of 'Hippocrates' reproduces that of the *Oath*. Ann La Berge drew attention to Louis Peisse, a journalist and a member of the Academy of Medicine, who in 1857 stated that 'each has the right to hippocratise to his delight' and to make Hippocrates – 'the old sage' – into a follower of any of the then-current medical sects; she commented, 'Hippocrates could stand for virtually any position within Paris medicine, and was used in inconsistent and contradictory ways'.[2]

In 1860, the caricaturist Cham (Amédé Charles de Noé) wrote *Cours d'Hygiene*. It is a short illustrated parody of advice literature, noting for example how the movement of bile around your body is improved when you find your servant sitting reading the newspaper for which he has kept you waiting for over two hours.[3] Here is the title page (Figure 4):

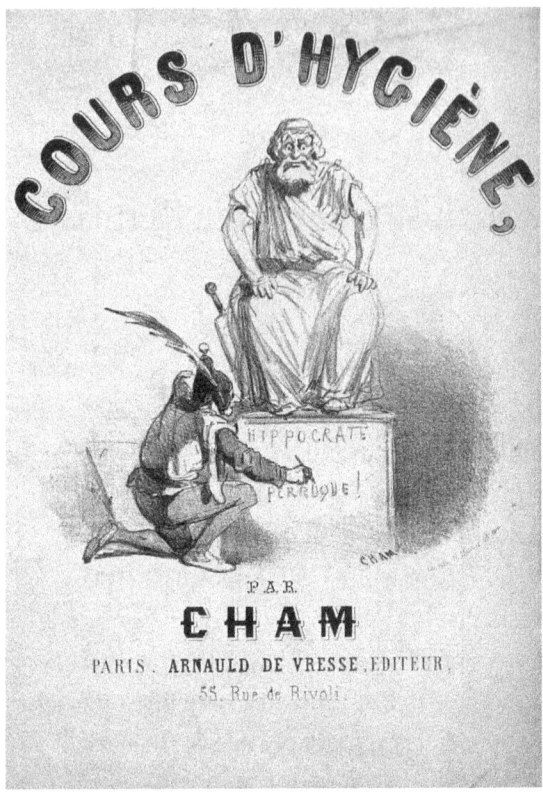

Fig. 4 A fool is writing an insult on the pedestal of a statue of Hippocrates. Lithograph by Cham, *c*. 1850. Wellcome Collection. CC BY.

The fool, in his cap and bells, writes 'Hippocrate perruque!' Hippocrates, meanwhile, looks furious. What does the inscription mean? 'Perruque', 'wig', is used for someone who is too old for his job, or who follows old-fashioned ideas.[4] This would suggest that Hippocrates' ideas on diet are now out of date, and this is consistent with the book's images of the realities of the strains of modern life. However, the one who is writing is a fool: perhaps, therefore, the message is that Hippocrates is not really out of date at all.

In some ways, nothing has changed. Hippocrates can still be used in many different ways. The Hippocrates of the internet age is still blurred, until brought into focus through the lens of whoever is using him for whatever purpose. I am struck by how Hippocrates is often described in religious terms; it is a heresy to say he did not exist, quotes may be produced like Bible verses, his gospel is promoted, and he is claimed as a patron saint. The *Oath* can mark the entry into the priesthood of the orthodox medical profession, or be waved around like a censer. Is he saviour, or scientist? Humane, or detached? Characterized by his empathy, or by his powers of observation and note-taking? He can be any one of these. Recent works proclaim that he is not dead, that he is crying, or that he is turning over in his grave. One point of consistency is that Hippocrates is 'right', or 'ahead of his time'. Just occasionally he lets us down – in particular, he was unable to cure his own baldness – but these exceptions are striking because they are so unusual.

But in other ways, things are different. While once alternative forms of medicine tried to claim him as their founder in order to take on his antiquity and his moral respectability, today he is more likely to be a medical renegade, misunderstood by the Establishment, dedicated to overthrowing the very medical system which used to honour him as Father. While stories have been made up about him for a very long time, four factors strike me as new, or at least exaggerated, today. The first is that we encounter Hippocrates in quotes. Ever since Galen, we have identified as Hippocratic the treatises we like the most, those which most resonate with us in terms of their theory or their practice, but in his popular reception these are now forgotten, and instead isolated quotes – some of them nothing to do with any Hippocratic text – are interpreted, displayed and combined at will. The separation of this Hippocrates in quotes from the traditional debates about which of the treatises he really wrote is part of the fragmentation of knowledge; medicine, in all its forms, has moved away from the discussions that are still going on in the humanities. Quotes can be decorative, or claim knowledge, but they are shared without explanation or commentary, and they may lose all sense that there ever was a larger text. Robert Goldberg, writing about modern fears about medicine, wrote that misleading claims 'becom[e] apparent truth through sheer repetition'.[5] This could also be said of quotes. Phrases such as 'let food be thy medicine' become more loaded with significance with each re-tweet or re-post. The sheer number of these draws authority into the phrase, and cements the idea that Hippocrates 'said' it. Does the quote mean that one food cures one condition, that we should follow a complete dietary and lifestyle plan, or that we should all eat superfoods alleged to prevent many diseases? Does it support a raw food diet or a high fibre diet? That depends on the user of the quote but, by using it, one shares in the authority of Hippocrates.

Secondly, we are more aware than before that we lack anything against which to measure the stories that are told; Hippocrates has always been a construct, but we are now even less confident that we can judge between a use and an abuse of his name. It is not just that it is difficult to find reliable information about him; there is simply no such information. In the modern market of knowledge, Wikipedia holds the key place, and those looking for material will find it or one of its derivatives; however, for many people the first places they will learn about Hippocrates are news stories, answers sites or social media. In news stories, he is usually proved 'right', and he is used to support the idea of continuity; for example, the myth that he 'named hysteria' promotes disease categories fixed across time. The effect of this claimed continuity is to make the words of Hippocrates retain their value now: if diseases are the same, why would a cure not continue to work? In many ways, this makes no sense; Christopher Wanjek asks 'why do we yearn for other ancient cures and customs born of the same logic, from an era when most people died young from diseases we've since licked?'[6] Robert Goldberg speculates about those who refuse to allow their children to receive MMR vaccinations, noting that 'few parents had ever seen the diseases that immunization had rendered rare or extinct, and, as a result, failed to comprehend their danger.'[7] Yet the appeal of the past is a real one, particularly when modern society and its medicine seem so complex and confusing.

The third factor is one which tries to compensate for the absence of any fixed point; in its place, we have the personal connection with Hippocrates which people can feel. 'Hippocratic texts' have always tended to morph into 'Hippocrates' the man – sometimes it is just easier to write 'Hippocrates said' rather than 'in this Hippocratic text we read' – but this process is particularly exaggerated today. While he is eminently quotable, with his quotes acquiring the status of proverbs, it is very important to users that he is also real. 'To antiquity it mattered less whether the ideal was historical than whether it was personified. The ideal physician needed a name, and Hippocrates supplied it.'[8] Pinault's conclusions are still valid, but Hippocrates also seems to have moved beyond the texts which may or may not have been his work, to become a fellow-traveller on whatever path the writer is taking. Today, we find people wanting to believe in him and longing to read his own words. You can chat with him as Dr Hip or as Crates and see what he thinks. You can sit under 'his' tree or one of its descendants. You can look at his face and yearn for his excellent bedside manner. You can use his juice, drink his soup, follow his protocol or attend the Institute named for him; all of these are ways people meet Hippocrates today.

Fourthly, I think something new is the level of creativity which has come into play because of the lack of fixed points; and, while this can be playful, it is often very serious. As any interest in deciding which of the existing treatises he wrote has declined, imaginary treatises have entered the picture: *The Complicated Body*, *Natural Exercise*, the book he would have written from his notes on diseases of the mind, his herb codex. People have always made up their own Hippocrates – from the time of Plato onwards – but the prison story and the enthusiasm with which it is embraced shows a far higher level of imagination. Yet even the prison story is not entirely divorced from the older traditions; it plays into the tradition of his high ethical standards, as he has done nothing wrong, and he goes on treating prisoners in jail. But this story also makes him into a figure driven by a Protestant work ethic, continuing to write the greatest of all his books and making the best of his situation.

The Hippocrates we meet today, with his respect for Nature, is the result of unease about the invasive nature of modern medicine which, by definition, 'does harm'; he reflects the fact that, in the USA in particular, 'mistrust haunts the public's and medical professionals' view of the health-care system'.[9] He has been enlisted by those who believe, in the words of Alan Levinovitz, that 'Modernity is dangerous and unnatural, and the solution to numerous fearsome ailments lies in returning to the lifestyle of paradise past', the myth 'behind every single blockbuster diet of the last decade'.[10] Hippocrates is the enemy of Big Pharma and its commodification of drugs, and the supporter of the pure and the natural; yet, of course, the holistic devotees of Hippocrates themselves have something to sell. There is, not surprisingly, a Hippocratic quote for this too: 'Now laymen do not accurately distinguish those who are excellent in this respect (treating acute diseases) from their fellows, but rather praise or blame strange remedies', from *Regimen in Acute Diseases* 6.[11] The passage continues 'it is in the proper treatment of these illnesses that ordinary folk show their most stupid side, in the fact that through these diseases chiefly quacks get the reputation of being physicians'.

Hippocrates is not dead; in many ways, he is more alive than ever before.

Notes

Introduction

1. http://www.fitnessnetwork.com.au/resources-library/let-food-be-thy-medicine-nutrition-for-inflammation accessed 20 February 2019.
2. E.g. http://www.brainyquote.com/quotes/authors/h/hippocrates.html (no attributions); http://todayinsci.com/H/Hippocrates/Hippocrates-Quotations.htm (attributions) accessed 20 February 2019; certain of these turn up frequently on social media.
3. The Hippocrates Prize for Poetry and Medicine, http://hippocrates-poetry.org/2019-hippocrates-prize-for/index.html accessed 20 February 2019. https://www.hippocraticpost.com is 'The world's first global blogging site specialising in medical issues', accessed 20 February 2019.
4. Julius Rocca, 'Present at the creation: Plato's "Hippocrates" and the making of a medical ideal' in Brita Alroth and Charlotte Scheffer (eds), *Attitudes towards the Past in Antiquity. Creating Identities. Proceedings of an international conference held at Stockholm University, 15–17 May 2009* (Acta Universitatis Stockholmiensis, Stockholm Studies in Classical Archaeology, 14 (Stockholm: Stockholm University, 2014), 285.
5. Emily Wilson, *The Death of Socrates: Profiles in history* (Cambridge, MA: Harvard University Press, 2007).
6. http://www.aspeninstitute.org/seminars/socrates-program-seminars accessed 1 November 2015; https://www.socratesacademy.us/our-school accessed 20 February 2019.
7. See further below. 'Hippocrates' soup', based on leeks, celery root and parsley root, is popularized in the Gerson diet to cure cancer; http://gerson-research.org/hippocrates-soup/ accessed 20 February 2019. On the raw-food programme of the Hippocrates Health Institute, see below, Chapter 7. For the face cream, see https://www.facebook.com/pg/hippocratescream/about/ accessed 20 February 2019; it contains 'Organic Olive Oil, Beeswax, Propolis, Selvia, Chamomile, Rosmarino, Dictamo, Chios Mastic'.
8. Robert Jütte, 'The historiography of nonconventional medicine in Germany: a concise overview', *Medical History*, 43 (1999), 343.
9. James C. Whorton, *Nature Cures: The history of alternative medicine in America* (New York: Oxford University Press, 2002), 299; Bruce Barrett et al., 'Themes of

holism, empowerment, access, and legitimacy define complementary, alternative, and integrative medicine in relation to conventional biomedicine', *Journal of Alternative and Complementary Medicine*, 9.6 (2003), 938.
10 Quoted in Whorton, *Nature Cures*, 300.
11 https://cmda.org/product/hippocratic-oath-framed-silver/ accessed 20 February 2019.
12 http://www.acwbinc.org/icm.html accessed 20 February 2019; a link takes the reader direct to a translation of the Hippocratic *Oath*.
13 http://unhcr.refugeefilm.org/2016/en/the_man_who_mends_women/
14 Cannon's True Towel Tales, 1994, no.4: 'Maybe this Roman bath was built for a conquering Caesar. Well, today it's being used by Joe Doughboy', https://www.magazine-advertisements.com/bathroom-accessories/cannon-mills/ accessed 20 February 2019.
15 Charles Martindale, *Redeeming the Text: Latin poetry and the hermeneutics of reception* (Cambridge: Cambridge University Press, 1993), 89.
16 For a useful guide to current thinking in the reception field, see Ika Willis, *Reception* (Abingdon and New York: Routledge, 2018); on the professional and lay readers, 90–1.
17 Elizabeth M. Craik, *The 'Hippocratic' Corpus: Content and context* (London: Routledge, 2015), 286.
18 David Cantor, 'Introduction: the uses and meanings of Hippocrates' in Cantor (ed.), *Reinventing Hippocrates* (Aldershot: Ashgate, 2002), 1.
19 Ibid.
20 Vivian Nutton, *Ancient Medicine* (London and New York: Routledge, 2004), 53 summarized the 'three converging tendencies' which led to these earlier biographies as a desire to know more about famous people; the tendency of other works to be drawn in to an existing group of texts; and a way of interpreting the texts which prioritizes some over the others and then claims the prioritized ones are by Hippocrates. See further Chapter 2, below.
21 https://www.fanfiction.net/u/133158/StillWaters1, profile updated 26 May 2013, accessed 20 February 2019. On reception and fan fiction, see Willis, *Reception*, 51–4 and 91–2.
22 https://www.fanfiction.net/s/6392078/1/A-Hippocratic-Proof, 12 October 2010, accessed 20 February 2019.
23 An episode of *Deep Space Nine* first broadcast on 16 October 1995 is entitled 'Hippocratic Oath', http://memory-alpha.wikia.com/wiki/Hippocratic_Oath_ (episode) accessed 20 February 2019; see further David Cantor, 'Western medicine since the Renaissance' in Peter Pormann (ed.), *The Cambridge Companion to Hippocrates* (Cambridge: Cambridge University Press, 2018), 382–3.

24 Cantor, 'Western medicine since the Renaissance', 382.
25 Anon., review of M.S. Houdart, *Études historiques et critiques sur la vie et la doctrine d'Hippocrate, et sur l'état de la médecine avant lui*, Edinburgh Medical and Surgical Journal 51 (1839), 495.
26 John Harley Warner, 'Making history in American medical culture: the antebellum competition for Hippocrates' in David Cantor (ed.), *Reinventing Hippocrates* (Aldershot: Ashgate, 2002), 200-1.
27 Robert Jütte, *Geschichte der Alternativen Medizin. Von der Volksmedizin zu den unkonventionellen Therapien von heute* (München: Beck Verlag, 1996).
28 Clemens von Bönninghausen, *Die Homöopathie, ein Lesebuch für das gebildete, nichtärztliche Publikum* (Münster: Coppenrath, 1834), 70, cited by Jütte, 'The historiography of nonconventional medicine, 355; see also 344.
29 Jütte, 'The historiography of nonconventional medicine', 353-4.
30 https://www.healthyhildegard.com/about-hildegard/ and https://www.healthyhildegard.com/hildegard-of-bingen-medicine/ accessed 20 February 2019.
31 Oliver Micke and Jutta Hübner, 'Traditional European Medicine: after all, is Hildegard of Bingen really right?' *European Journal of Integrative Medicine*, 1.4 (2009), 226; https://www.healthyhildegard.com/healing-plants/ accessed 20 February 2019.
32 Warner, 'Making history', 201-2.
33 Ibid., 202-3.
34 Patrick Guinan, *Hippocrates is Not Dead: An anthology of Hippocratic readings* (Bloomington IN: AuthorHouse, 2011).
35 Peter E. Pormann, 'Introduction', *The Cambridge Companion to Hippocrates* (Cambridge: Cambridge University Press, 2018), 1.
36 William F. Petersen, *Hippocratic Wisdom: For him who wishes to pursue properly the science of medicine* (Springfield IL: Charles C. Thomas, 1946), xv.
37 Guinan, *Hippocrates is Not Dead*, back cover.
38 John F. Brehany, 'The indispensability of Hippocrates' in Guinan, *Hippocrates is Not Dead*, 24.
39 Michael A. Taylor, *Hippocrates Cried: The decline of American psychiatry* (Oxford: Oxford University Press, 2013), 49.
40 Maya Dusenbery, *Doing Harm: The truth about how bad medicine and lazy science leave women dismissed, misdiagnosed, and sick* (New York and London: HarperCollins, 2018).
41 Julia E. Hubbel, 'How doctors manage to make us even sicker: the problem with being female and needing healthcare', 31 July 2018, online article, https://medium.com/@jhubbel/how-doctors-manage-to-make-us-even-sicker-a3c83d1d3d96 accessed 20 February 2019.

42 Susan E. Lederer, 'Hippocrates American style: representing professional morality in early twentieth-century America' in David Cantor (ed.), *Reinventing Hippocrates* (Aldershot: Ashgate, 2002), 241.

43 John Fabre, 'Medicine as a profession: Hip, Hip, Hippocrates: extracts from *The Hippocratic Doctor*,' *BMJ*, 315 (7123) (1997), 1669.

44 Lederer, 'Hippocrates American style', 242; Allen Browne, 'The death and resurrection of Hippocrates' plane tree', 3 May 2014, http://allenbrowne.blogspot.com/2014/05/the-death-and-resurrection-of.html accessed 20 February 2019.

45 https://www.nationalgalleries.org/art-and-artists/63270/spirit-collection-hippocrates and http://www.yorku.ca/agyu/archive/archive/e2002_borland.html accessed 20 February 2019.

46 Presented by Dr Thomas Doxiades; https://repository.duke.edu/dc/homartifacts/homst15001 accessed 20 February 2019.

47 J.V. Pai-Dhungat, 'Hippocrates – Father of Medicine', *Journal of the Association of Physicians of India*, 63 (2015), 18, http://www.japi.org/march_2015/004_hippocrates.pdf accessed 20 February 2019; the tombstone, now in the British Museum, is shown on https://www.britishmuseum.org/research/collection_online/collection_object_details.aspx?objectId=399641&partId=1 accessed 4 November 2018.

48 https://www.nationalgallery.org.uk/paintings/peter-paul-rubens-portrait-of-ludovicus-nonnius accessed 20 February 2019.

49 Helen King, *Midwifery, Obstetrics and the Rise of Gynaecology: Users of a sixteenth-century compendium* (Aldershot: Ashgate, 2007), 95.

50 Francis Clifton, *Hippocrates upon Airs, Water and Situation* (London: J. Watts, 1734), frontispiece. On images of Hippocrates, Gisela M.A. Richter, *Portraits of the Greeks* (London: Phaidon Press, 1965), vol.1, 151–4 and figs 855–74.

51 'Plato', 'Hippocrates the father of medicine', 12 March 2013, accessed 20 February 2019 and using the 1638 engraving: https://classicalwisdom.com/hippocrates-the-father-of-medicine/. Compare Charles Picard, 'Sur l'iconographie d'Hippocrate d'après un portrait d'Ostie', *Comptes rendus des séances de l'Académie des Inscriptions et Belles Lettres*, 91–2 (1947), 332: 'cette figure ridée, fatiguée, mais animée encore de son bonhomie bienveillante, où l'intelligence et la curiosité respirent.'

52 James Finlayson, *Hippocrates: A bibliographical demonstration in the library of the Faculty of Physicians and Surgeons of Glasgow, 23rd November 1891* (Glasgow: Alex Macdougall, 1892), 9.

53 In 1940, in the tomb of a first-century CE doctor at Ostia, a damaged stone bust was found which has been identified as a Roman copy of a Greek original of Hippocrates, although there is no name given for the individual it shows, and one

dissenting voice suggested it was in fact Pindar. See Mark V. Barrow, 'Portraits of Hippocrates', *Medical History*, 16.1 (1972), 86. On initial reactions to this find, Picard, 'Sur l'iconographie d'Hippocrate'.

54 Johannes Antonides van der Linden, *Magni Hippocratis Coi opera omnia* (Lugduni Batavorum [Leiden]: Gaasbeeck, 1665), frontispiece.

55 Barrow, 'Portraits of Hippocrates', 86 and fig. 1; he notes how many busts initially identified as Hippocrates because of their resemblance to this coin have subsequently been re-identified as the philosophers Chrysippos or Carneades.

56 Jody Rubin Pinault, *Hippocratic Lives and Legends*, Studies in Ancient Medicine 4 (Leiden and New York: E. J. Brill, 1992), 17.

57 Benjamin Rush, 'Lecture 12, On the opinions and modes of practice of Hippocrates', Nov 1806, in *Sixteen introductory lectures, to courses of lectures upon the institutes and practice of medicine, with a syllabus of the latter. To which are added, Two lectures upon the pleasures of the senses and of the mind, with an inquiry into their proximate cause* (Philadelphia: Bradford and Innskeep, 1811), 272.

58 Barrow, 'Portraits of Hippocrates', 87; fig. 11, a version from 1809, is almost entirely bald.

59 https://guides.gamepressure.com/assassins-creed-odyssey/guide.asp?ID=46686 accessed 20 February 2019: for more on the game see https://www.rockpapershotgun.com/2018/10/22/assassins-creed-odyssey-hippokrates-how-to-complete-the-side-quests/ accessed 20 February 2019. This possibly alludes to Julius Caesar's insecurity about his own baldness, which 'troubled him greatly'; Suetonius, *Life of Julius Caesar*, 45.2.

60 Aristotle, *Politics*, 1326a15–17; the Brussels 'Life' (see Pinault, *Hippocratic Lives and Legends*, 13 and 25: *Traditur autem ceteris corporibus Yppocratem fuisse minorem, capite tamen delicate*.

61 Daniel Le Clerc, *The History of Physick, or, an account of the rise and progress of the art* (London: D Brown et al., 1699), 359; Pinault, *Hippocratic Lives*, 12 on the other ideas of his appearance in the 'Life' by Soranus, ch. 8 and 17.

62 https://healthywildandfree.com/hippocrates-kidney-cleansing-healing-soup-recipe/ accessed 20 February 2019.

63 http://www.answers.com/Q/FAQ/8893 and http://www.answers.com/Q/Did_Hippocrates_get_put_in_prison accessed 20 February 2019.

64 https://fuehairdoctor.co.uk/hair-loss-prevention/l0014825-portrait-of-hippocrates-from-linden-magni-hippocratis/ and https://fuehairdoctor.co.uk/hair-loss-prevention accessed 20 February 2019.

65 https://en.wikipedia.org/w/index.php?title=Hippocrates&diff=prev&oldid=453325065 added 1 October 2011.

66 https://en.wikipedia.org/w/index.php?title=Hippocrates&diff=next&oldid=453325065.
67 https://en.wikipedia.org/w/index.php?title=Hippocrates&diff=next&oldid=484226091.
68 http://www.alopeciaworld.com/profiles/blogs/men-s-baldness-in-history accessed 20 February 2019.
69 http://www.history.com/news/history-lists/9-bizarre-baldness-cures posted on 25 September 2012, https://www.wimpoleclinic.com/blog/weird-and-wonderful-historical-hair-loss-treatments/, posted 1 March 2015, accessed 20 February 2019.
70 https://www.history.com/news/9-bizarre-baldness-cures 25 September 2012, accessed 20 February 2019.
71 https://www.wimpoleclinic.com/blog/weird-and-wonderful-historical-hair-loss-treatments/ posted 1 March 2015, accessed 20 February 2019.
72 E.g. http://www.newsbf.com/moyieboy/170504bald.html, 'pigeon droppings to inspire the domes of his patients to sprout', 4 May 2017, accessed 20 February 2019. On their wider use in ancient medicine, see Caroline Petit, 'The torture of therapeutics in Rome: Galen on pigeon dung,' which describes Galen applying this substance to the shaved head of a woman who was spitting blood, as a heating and drying remedy, https://recipes.hypotheses.org/12783 accessed 20 February 2019.
73 'Eunuchs do not go bald', 29 June 2005, https://www.hairlosstalk.com/interact/threads/eunuchs-do-not-go-bald.13868/ based on http://www.independent.co.uk/life-style/health-and-families/health-news/how-to-keep-your-hair-on-5544434.html posted 28 June 2005, accessed 20 February 2019.
74 https://www.thetimes.co.uk/article/breakthrough-in-search-for-baldness-cure-b90ppl8hssc 16 May 2007; https://www.thetimes.co.uk/article/then-and-now-baldness-sk7txpnl58m 8 November 2003; accessed 20 February 2019.
75 http://articles.baltimoresun.com/1997-01-22/news/1997022090_1_baldness-hair-growth-hair-follicles 22 January 1997, accessed 5 November 2018; this link is no longer live in Europe but repeats Charles P. Vallis, *Hair Transplantation for Male Pattern Baldness* (Springfield IL: Charles C. Thomas, 1982), 40.
76 http://recipes.hypotheses.org/2057.
77 Laurence Totelin, *Hippocratic Recipes: Oral and written transmission of pharmacological knowledge in fifth- and fourth-century Greece*, Studies in Ancient Medicine 34 (Leiden and Boston: E.J. Brill, 2009), 262, using the chapter numbering of the Littré edition; in the most recent translation, by Paul Potter (Loeb, *Hippocrates XI*, 409) this is renumbered as chapter 80 and translated 'If all the hair falls out, apply a plaster with cumin, pigeon excrement, ground radish, onion, beet or stinging nettle.'

78 https://archive.org/about/ currently has 15,000,000 books in full-text as well as another 550,000 more recent works which can be borrowed using a free account. The Europeana Collections are also very useful, for images as well as texts; https://www.europeana.eu/portal/en and https://ec.europa.eu/digital-single-market/en/europeana-european-digital-library-all accessed 20 February 2019.

79 Helen King and Monica Green, 'On the misuses of medical history', *The Lancet*, 7 April (2018); https://www.thelancet.com/journals/lancet/article/PIIS0140-6736(18)30490-2/fulltext.

80 Helen King, *The One-Sex Body on Trial: The classical and early modern evidence* (Aldershot: Ashgate, 2013), 100.

81 Kelly Parsons, *Doing Harm* (New York: St Martin's Press, 2014).

82 http://www.wbur.org/npr/597159133/how-bad-medicine-dismisses-and-misdiagnoses-womens-symptoms accessed 20 February 2019.

83 https://slate.com/technology/2015/10/research-suggests-google-books-isnt-as-helpful-as-some-believed.html 13 October 2015, accessed 20 February 2019.

84 Cantor, 'Western medicine since the Renaissance', 383; Willis, *Reception*, 92 on de Certeau.

Chapter 2

1 On the blank page, see Jack Winkler, 'Gardens of nymphs: Public and private in Sappho's lyrics' in Helene P. Foley (ed.), *Reflections of Women in Antiquity* (New York: Gordon and Breach, 1981), 63, citing Monique Wittig and Sande Zeig, *Lesbian Peoples: Material for a dictionary* (London: Virago, 1979), 136.

2 'A good practical physician in relying more on general measures than on drugs', in the words of Ronald Campbell Macfie, *The Romance of Medicine* (London: Cassell and Co., 1907). Macfie was a medical doctor and poet who believed in the 'imaginative aspect' of medical discovery. A review in *Athenaeum* (19 October 1907), 485 regarded Macfie's ancient sections as 'brief but accurate' but *The Spectator* (11 January 1908) commented 'About earlier times he does not seem to know very much.'

3 John Precope, *Hippocrates on Diet and Hygiene* (London: Williams, Lea and Co., 1952), 13; Herbert Ratner, 'Hippocrates has vital meaning for physicians' (originally published in 1953), in Guinan, *Hippocrates is Not Dead*, 17; how Hippocrates could be the perfect Christian physician is explored fully by Owsei Temkin, *Hippocrates in a World of Pagans and Christians* (Baltimore MD: Johns Hopkins University Press, 1991).

4 Richard Armour, *It All Started with Hippocrates: A mercifully brief history of medicine* (New York: McGraw Hill, 1966), 27.
5 I. Mazzini and G. Flammini, *De conceptu: Estratti di un'antica traduzione latina del Περὶ γυναικείων pseudoippocratico l* (Bologna: Pàtron, 1983), 53 quoted by Laurence Totelin, 'Old recipes, new practices? The Latin adaptations of the Hippocratic *Gynaecological Treatises*', *Social History of Medicine*, 24.1 (2011), 86.
6 David H. Newman, *Hippocrates' Shadow: Secrets from the house of medicine* (New York: Simon & Schuster, 2008), xvi; https://well.blogs.nytimes.com/2008/09/23/what-would-hippocrates-do/ accessed 20 February 2019.
7 Paul Hoedeman, *Hitler or Hippocrates? Medical experiments in euthanasia in the Third Reich* (tr. Ralph de Rijke, Sussex: Book Guild, 1991). As Robert Jay Lifton, *The Nazi Doctors: Medical killing and the psychology of genocide* (New York: Basic Books, 1986), 32 notes, 'Heinrich Himmler himself embraced Hippocrates as a model for SS physicians' https://phdn.org/archives/holocaust-history.org/lifton/contents.shtml.
8 David H. Newman, *Hippocrates' Shadow*, xvi–xvii.
9 Wesley D. Smith, *Hippocrates: Pseudepigraphic writings letters-embassy-speech from the altar-decree*, Studies in Ancient Medicine, 2 (Leiden: Brill, 1990), 51.
10 On the 'authentic "firstness"' of Hippocrates, see John Harley Warner, 'Making history in American medical culture: the antebellum competition for Hippocrates' in Cantor (ed.), *Reinventing Hippocrates*, 200.
11 Denying his existence 'was done in an inaugural dissertation published some years since at Paris, to the no small annoyance of the medical dignitaries of the day, who were outraged by so great a heresy': Anon., 'Review of Houdart'. In Houdart's book (Paris: Baillière, 1836), 3 this is 'une espèce de sacrilege'. In 1930, Edith Bruce Paterson, 'Hippocrates', *Medical Life*, 37.6 (1930), 304 and 306 also referred to 'those who deny that Hippocrates wrote anything'.
12 He was, apparently, 'spot-on' because 'Let food be thy medicine' – which will be discussed in Chapter 5 – is 'One of the most powerful quotes ever, and still accurate to this day', according to a site promoting the home-based business 'American-Dream-Nutrition', http://www.ibosocial.com/philschaefer/pressrelease.aspx?prid=613377 5 October 2018, accessed 20 October 2018 (no longer available). On the 'smart' Hippocrates, https://asthma.net/living/how-did-hippocrates-diagnose-asthma/ accessed 20 February 2019.
13 https://www.psychologytoday.com/blog/the-athletes-way/201506/hippocrates-was-right-walking-is-the-best-medicine accessed 20 February 2019; https://www.omicsonline.org/proceedings/hippocrates-was-right-all-disease-begins-in-the-gut-new-insights-at-the-forefront-of-gastroenterology-71904.html accessed 20 February 2019.

14 Ludwig Edelstein, 'The genuine works of Hippocrates', *BHM*, 7 (1939); reprinted in Owsei and C. Lilian Temkin (eds), *Ancient Medicine: Selected papers of Ludwig Edelstein* (Baltimore, MD and London: Johns Hopkins University Press, 1967), 133–44.
15 Edelstein, 'Genuine works', 143.
16 Jaap Mansfeld, 'Plato and the method of Hippocrates', *Greek, Roman and Byzantine Studies*, 21 (1980), 342.
17 W.H.S. Jones, 'General introduction' in Loeb, *Hippocrates I* (Cambridge, MA: Harvard University Press and London: Heinemann, 1923), xxxv.
18 Jacques Jouanna, *Hippocrates* (Baltimore, MD and London: Johns Hopkins University Press, 1999; Fr. original *Hippocrate*, Librairie Arthème Fayard, 1992), xii.
19 Charles Reginald Schiller Harris, *The Heart and the Vascular System in Ancient Greek Medicine from Alcmaeon to Galen* (Oxford: Clarendon Press, 1973), 267; see also Wesley D. Smith, *The Hippocratic Tradition* (Ithaca and London: Cornell University Press, 1979); 2002 revised edition at http://www.biusante.parisdescartes.fr/ressources/pdf/medicina-hippo2.pdf, 106: 'At different times Galen has seduced people into crediting him whole, as Hippocrates' direct heir, or half, taking Hippocrates as the source of true science perversely misunderstood by those after him. Galen's rhetorical posture would seem to gain credence because in a sense it reflects his real situation: to a great extent he was a unique genius and the unique prophet of his version of medicine and of intellectual history.'
20 Rocca, 'Present at the creation', 285.
21 Paul Potter, 'Why we go back to Hippocrates', Thirteenth John P. McGovern Award Lecture, 6 May 1998 (Wellcome Collection), 9–10.
22 Smith, *Pseudepigraphic Writings*, 8.
23 Ann E. Hanson, 'Hippocrates: the "Greek miracle" in medicine', https://www.ucl.ac.uk/~ucgajpd/medicina%20antiqua/sa_hippint.html accessed 20 February 2019. I shall return to the contributions of Plato and Aristotle below.
24 G.E.R. Lloyd, *Methods and Problems in Greek Science: Selected papers* (Cambridge: Cambridge University Press, 1991), 194.
25 G.E.R. Lloyd, *In the Grip of Disease. Studies in the Greek imagination* (Oxford: Oxford University Press, 2003), 41.
26 See now Aileen R. Das, 'New material from Galen's *On the Authentic and Spurious Works of Hippocrates*,' *Classical Philology*, 113.3 (2018).
27 Jacques Jouanna, 'Galen's reading of the Hippocratic treatise *The Nature of Man*: The foundations of Hippocratism in Galen' in Philip van der Eijk (ed.), *Greek Medicine from Hippocrates to Galen: Selected papers* (Leiden and Boston: Brill, 2012), 321 discusses in detail Galen's changing views on this treatise.

28 Lloyd, *In the Grip of Disease*, 42; Jouanna, *Hippocrates*, 62; on the ancient views on the authorship of this Hippocratic treatise, see Volker Langholf, 'Structure and genesis of some Hippocratic texts' in Manfred Horstmanshoff and Marten Stol (eds), *Magic and Rationality in Ancient Near Eastern and Graeco-Roman Medicine* (Leiden: Brill, 2004), 244–7. Mansfeld, 'Plato and the method of Hippocrates', 344 notes that this section is now 'safely attributed' to Polybus.

29 Eric Nelson, 'Tracking the Hippocratic Woozle: Pseudepigrapha and the formation of the Corpus' in Lesley Dean-Jones and Ralph Rosen (eds), *Ancient Concepts of the Hippocratic. Papers Presented at the XIIIth International Hippocrates Colloquium, Austin, Texas, August 2008*, Studies in Ancient Medicine 46 (Leiden and Boston: Brill, 2016), 117. This important collection will hereafter be referred to as DJR.

30 Véronique Boudon-Millot, 'Ce qu' "hippocratique" (ἱπποκράτειος) veut dire: la réponse de Galien' in DJR, 378–98.

31 In particular, see Smith, *Hippocratic Tradition*.

32 Plato, *Phaedrus* 270c1–5; Lloyd, *Methods and Problems*, 195, summarizing Smith, *Hippocratic Tradition*, 47–8; Boudon-Millot, 'Ce qu' "hippocratique" (ἱπποκράτειος) veut dire'; Jordi C. Saumell, 'New lights on the *Anonymus Londiniensis* papyrus,' *Journal of Ancient Philosophy*, 11.2 (2017), 130–1 and n.57.

33 Ann E. Hanson, 'Hippocrates: the "Greek miracle" in medicine'; Jouanna, *Hippocrates*, 62.

34 Rebecca Flemming, 'The pathology of pregnancy in Galen's commentaries on the *Epidemics*' in Vivian Nutton (ed.), *The Unknown Galen*, Bulletin of the Institute of Classical Studies, 45 (2002), 101.

35 Jouanna, 'Galen's reading of the Hippocratic treatise *The Nature of Man*', 331.

36 Ibid., 336.

37 *Assassin's Creed: Odyssey*, episode 'First Do No Harm': extract on http://www.ign.com/videos/2018/08/08/assassins-creed-odyssey-12-minutes-of-exclusive-mission-gameplay accessed 20 February 2019. See also http://assassinscreed.wikia.com/wiki/Hippokrates accessed 20 February 2019; at present this suggests that some areas were so 'conservative' that Hippocrates needed to treat patients there in secret.

38 Owsei Temkin, *Galenism. Rise and decline of a medical philosophy* (Ithaca and London: Cornell University Press, 1973).

39 R.J. Hankinson, 'Galen on Hippocratic Physics' in DJR, 432.

40 Smith, *Pseudepigraphic Writings*, 11.

41 Boudon-Millot, 'Ce qu' "hippocratique" veut dire', 397: 'dans quelle mesure Galien croyait-il lui-même à l'Hippocrate qu'il avait ainsi forgé?'; Hankinson, 'Galen on Hippocratic Physics', 441.

42 Smith, *Pseudepigraphic Writings*, 11.
43 Pinault, *Hippocratic Lives and Legends*, 29–30.
44 Smith, *Pseudepigraphic Writings*, 8, on Dioscorides and Capiton; Jouanna, 'Galen's reading of the Hippocratic treatise *The Nature of Man*', 320.
45 Craik, *'Hippocratic' Corpus*, xxiv; Ernst Nachmanson, *Erotiani vocum Hippocraticarum collectio cum fragmentis* (Upsala, 1918), online at https://archive.org/stream/erotianivocumhip00erotuoft#page/n5/mode/2up (accessed 20 February 2019); Renate Wittern, 'Zum Hippokratesglossar des Erotian κατάπηροι im Corpus Hippocraticum', *Sudhoffs Archiv*, 55.1 (1971).
46 Pilar Pérez Cañizares, 'The treatise *Affections* in the context of the Hippocratic Corpus' in DJR.
47 Iain M. Lonie, 'The "Paris Hippocratics": teaching and research in Paris in the second half of the sixteenth century' in Andrew Wear, Roger K. French and Iain M. Lonie (eds), *The Medical Renaissance of the Sixteenth Century* (Cambridge and New York: Cambridge University Press, 1985), 162.
48 Jole Shackelford, 'The chemical Hippocrates: Paracelsian and Hippocratic theory in Petrus Severinus' medical philosophy' in Cantor (ed.), *Reinventing Hippocrates*, 63 and 69.
49 Andrew Cunningham, 'The transformation of Hippocrates in seventeenth-century Britain' in Cantor (ed.), *Reinventing Hippocrates*, 103.
50 Houdart, *Etudes historiques et critiques sur la vie et la doctrine d'Hippocrate*, 183, quoted in Finlayson, 'Hippocrates: A bibliographical demonstration', 11–12; Craik, *The 'Hippocratic' Corpus*, 50–1 summarizes the scholarship on the relationship between these three treatises, with *Coan Prognoses* now being seen as based on *Prognostic* rather than the other way around.
51 Mansfeld, 'Plato and the method of Hippocrates', 356–8; Smith, *Hippocratic Tradition*.
52 On the earliest computer analyses based on sentence length and vocabulary, see William C. Wake, 'Who was Hippocrates?', *The Listener*, 29 December 1966, 966–7. His conclusion (based on his 1951 PhD) was that *Prognostics*, *Regimen in Acute Diseases*, *Fractures* and *Joints* 'could all have been written by one author' but that *Epidemics 1* and *3* (traditionally seen as by Hippocrates) could not be by that one author.
53 Mansfeld, 'Plato and the method of Hippocrates', 344.
54 The first quotation is from Jouanna, *Hippocrates*, 59–61; the second from Smith, *Hippocratic Tradition*, 56; the third from Mansfeld, 'Plato and the method of Hippocrates', 344. On the papyrus, see now the Teubner edition by Daniela Manetti, *Anonymus Londiniensis. De medicina* (Berlin: de Gruyter, 2011).

55 David Wootton, *Bad Medicine: Doctors doing harm since Hippocrates* (Oxford: Oxford University Press, 2007 edition with postscript), 29, 7–8. Criticisms from reviewers focused on Wootton's use of hindsight: see *Bad Medicine*, 189–97 for his response.
56 Smith, *Hippocratic Tradition*, 125–6. Some ancient authors thought it was by a different 'Hippocrates', the grandfather of the famous one; Langholf, 'Structure and genesis of some Hippocratic texts', 248.
57 Smith, *Hippocratic Tradition*, 32.
58 Francis Adams, *The Genuine Works of Hippocrates* (London, Printed for the Sydenham Society, 1849), 2 vols, Vol. 1, v and 3.
59 Ibid., 6.
60 Wootton, *Bad Medicine*, 7–8; Adams, *The Genuine Works of Hippocrates*, vol. 1, 20–1.
61 Elizabeth M. Craik, 'The teaching of surgery' in Manfred Horstmanshoff (ed.), *Hippocrates and Medical Education: Selected papers presented at the XIIth International Hippocrates Colloquium, Universiteit Leiden, 24–26 August 2005* (Leiden: Brill, 2010), 232.
62 Ibid., 233.
63 Anon., 'Review of Houdart', 493.
64 Or, less likely, that the way to understand the whole is by understanding all the parts. Plato, *Protagoras* 311b–d; *Phaedrus* 270c. See Mansfeld, 'Plato and the method of Hippocrates', in the context of challenging Smith's attribution of the treatise *On Regimen* to Hippocrates. On the 'very generality of the alleged Hippocratic statement' in *Phaedrus*, see Rocca, 'Present at the creation', 289. I shall return to these passages in Chapter 7, where I discuss holism.
65 Volker Langholf, *Medical Theories in Hippocrates: Early texts and the 'Epidemics'* (Berlin and New York: de Gruyter, 1990), 197.
66 Jouanna, *Hippocrates*, 6 on Aristotle, *Politics* 1326a15–17. See further below, p. 37, on the use of this in an early biography of Hippocrates. The site https://notednames.com/Medical-Doctors/Physician/Hippocrates-Birthday-Real-Name-Age-Weight-Height/ misses an opportunity here, leaving Hippocrates' height blank. However, https://hippocrates.carrd.co/ accessed 20 February 2019 puts him at 5 foot 6 inches; its Hippocrates is 'not a healer. He's like a human version of biological warfare.'
67 On the meaning of 'Asclepiad', see the discussion in Smith, *Pseudepigraphic Writings*, 9–17, concluding that it could be a generic term for physician and that some – not all – physicians also claimed descent from Asclepius himself.
68 Iain M. Lonie, 'Literacy and the development of Hippocratic medicine', in François Lasserre and Philippe Mudry (eds), *Formes de pensée dans la collection*

hippocratique: Actes du Colloque hippocratique de Lausanne 1981 (Geneva: Droz, 1983), 145–61; Lloyd, *In the Grip of Disease*, 41.

69 Smith, *Pseudepigraphic Writings*, 7.

70 Lesley Dean-Jones, 'Identifying the Hippocratic' in DJR, 14; Pérez Cañizares, 'The treatise *Affections*', 93.

71 Jouanna, *Hippocrates*, xii. On the now-unfashionable attempt to divide up the Corpus into Coan/Cnidian texts, see Antoine Thivel, *Cnide et Cos? Essai sur les doctrines médicales dans la collection hippocratique* (Paris: Eds Belles Lettres, 1981) and Iain M. Lonie, 'Cos versus Cnidus and the historians: Part I', *History of Science*, 16 (1978).

72 Aristeas, *Letter to Philocrates*, 9; R.J.H. Shutt, 'Letter of Aristeas: a new translation and introduction' in J. Charlesworth (ed.), *The Old Testament Pseudepigrapha*, vol. 2: *Expansions of the 'Old Testament' and Legends, Wisdom and Philosophical Literature, Prayers, Psalms and Odes, Fragments of Lost Judeo-Hellenistic Works* (London: Darton, Longman & Todd, 1985), 12. Roger S. Bagnall, 'Alexandria: Library of dreams', *Proceedings of the American Philosophical Society*, 146.4 (2002), 356 points out that 200,000 volumes is the number held in the British Library in 1830. Bearing in mind that the papyrus rolls which would have been used in the second-century BCE took up far more space than a nineteenth-century book, the figures are simply impossible. I owe my knowledge of the reception history of this library to Joanna Paul's discussion of it for The Open University's Classical Studies MA.

73 Bagnall, 'Alexandria: Library of dreams', 348; 356 (noting not least the point that – even if something of this size really existed – it would be impossible to catalogue it with the pre-index card technology available); Susan Stephens, 'The new Alexandrian library' in Susan Stephens and Phiroze Vasunia (eds) *Classics and National Cultures* (Oxford: Oxford University Press, 2010), 272.

74 Smith, *Hippocratic Tradition*, 38, citing Max Wellmann, 'Hippokrates des Herakleides Sohn', *Hermes*, 64 (1929), 16–21.

75 Ibid., 34.

76 Ibid., 39. Ilberg's theory was accepted by W.H.S. Jones, when he began to translate the Corpus for the Loeb edition (Jones, 'General introduction', xxix–xxx), and was popularized by such works as Blaxland Stubbs and E.W. Bligh, *Sixty Centuries of Health and Physick* (London: Sampson Low, Marston & Co., 1931), 54.

77 Jones, 'General introduction', xxix; copied almost verbatim by Paterson, 'Hippocrates'.

78 Also in Pliny, *Natural History*, 29.2, citing Varro; Pinault, *Hippocratic Lives and Legends*, 7 (quotation from p. 12). See Marie-Helene Marganne, *L'ophtalmologie dans l'Égypte gréco-romaine d'après les papyrus littéraires grecs* (Leiden: Brill, 1994) on evidence for a medical library in Antinoopolis.

79 Jouanna, *Hippocrates*, 18; 26–7; Pinault, *Hippocratic Lives and Legends*, 11.
80 Smith, *Pseudepigraphic Writings*, 9.
81 Rocca, 'Present at the creation', 291.
82 Page DuBois, *Sappho is Burning* (Chicago, IL: University of Chicago Press, 1995), 31 and 63.
83 Philip van der Eijk, 'On "Hippocratic" and "non-Hippocratic" medical writings' in DJR, 43.
84 Ibid., 26 rejects as too revisionist the claim that the texts of the Corpus 'had little else in common except that they were concerned with medicine and written in the Ionic dialect'; Ann Ellis Hanson, 'The Hippocratic *Aphorisms* in Ptolemaic and Roman times' in DJR, 48 notes that 'Hippocratic papyri display Attic forms at least as frequently as Ionic ones', showing that the matter of dialect was less clear in antiquity; compare Paul Demont, 'Remarques sur le tableau de la médecine et d'Hippocrate chez Platon' in DJR.
85 Hanson, 'Hippocratic *Aphorisms*', 51. I shall address the modern authority of Hippocrates further in Chapter 6.
86 Ibid.
87 Van der Eijk, 'On "Hippocratic" and "non-Hippocratic" medical writings'; George Weisz, 'Hippocrates, holism and humanism in interwar France' in Cantor (ed.), *Reinventing Hippocrates*, 260. On Littré's edition of the Hippocratic Corpus, see Jacques Jouanna, 'Littré, éditeur et traducteur d'Hippocrate' in *Actes du Colloque Emile Littré, 1801–1881. Paris, 1–9 octobre 1981* (Paris: Eds Albin Michel, 1983), 285–301.
88 Craik, *'Hippocratic' Corpus*; Lloyd, *In the Grip of Disease*, 41; Kenneth Walker, *The Story of Medicine* (Tiptree: Arrow Books, 1959), 44.
89 Gerhard Fichtner, *Corpus Hippocraticum: Verzeichnis der hippokratischen und pseudohippoktratischen Schriften* (Tübingen: Institut für Geschichte der Medizin, 1995).
90 On the first three treatises and their connections, see Iain M. Lonie, *The Hippocratic Treatises 'On Generation', 'On the Nature of the Child', 'Diseases IV'* (Berlin and New York: De Gruyter, 1981). Elizabeth M. Craik, *The Hippocratic Treatise* On Glands, *edited and translated with introduction and commentary* (Leiden: Brill, 2009) extends the argument to a further treatise and possibly also to two of the gynaecological works, and proposed that these are all by a significant thinker of the early fourth century BCE.
91 On *Fractures/Joints*, see Smith, *Hippocratic Tradition*, 125–6. Craik, *The 'Hippocratic' Corpus* describes the combined treatise as 'magisterial' (287); she regards the case for them being by Hippocrates as 'strong' and lists a number of other treatises for which she regards Hippocrates' authorship as likely (289).

92 Littré (VIII, 532–4) regarded the main gynaecological texts, with *Diseases of Young Girls*, as one 'ouvrage entier' going from virginity to infertility, which had the merit of explaining those sweeping introductory remarks; Rebecca Flemming and Ann E. Hanson, 'Hippocrates' *Peri Parthenion* (*Diseases of Young Girls*): text and translation', *Early Science and Medicine*, 3 (1998). In the 2010 Loeb English translation, Paul Potter called it simply 'Girls', glossing as 'Literally the title means "On Girlish Matters"' (Loeb, *Hippocrates* IX, 359).
93 Elizabeth M. Craik, *Two Hippocratic Treatises* On Sight *and* On Anatomy (Leiden: Brill, 2006), 15 (also preferring 'compiler' to 'composer'); Langholf, 'Structure and genesis of some Hippocratic texts', 257.
94 Elizabeth M. Craik, *The Hippocratic Treatise* On Glands, 1.
95 Paul Potter, *Hippocrates* IX, 11: Galen referred to its contents fourteen times, but under different titles. *Excision* features twice in one of the early manuscripts of the Corpus (M, Marcianus graecus 269) under two titles.
96 In Chapter 3 I shall discuss a treatise that is often named today, but which never existed.
97 Pérez Cañizares, 'The treatise *Affections*', 89–90; Craik, On Sight *and* On Anatomy, 17–18.
98 Craik, *'Hippocratic' Corpus*, 291.
99 Ann Hanson, 'Diseases of women in the *Epidemics*' in Gerhaad Baader and Rolf Winau (eds), *Die hippokratischen Epidemien: Theorie-Praxis-Tradition*, *Sudhoffs Archiv*, 27 (Stuttgart: Franz Steiner, 1989), 38–51.
100 Craik, *'Hippocratic' Corpus*, 196 puts the three together as 'consecutive components in a loosely connected compilation'; Potter in Loeb, *Hippocrates* X, 331.
101 Hermann Grensemann, *Knidische Medizin Teil I: Die Testimonien zur ältesten knidischen Lehre und Analysen knidischer Schriften im Corpus Hippocraticum* (Berlin and New York: de Gruyter, 1975) and *Hippokratische Gynäkologie: die gynäkologischen Texte des Autors C nach den pseudohippokratischen Schriften De Muliebribus I, II und De Sterilibus* (Wiesbaden: Franz Steiner, 1982). The presentation of layer 'C' as a lost text has been challenged; e.g. the review by Vivian Nutton, *Classical Review*, 34 (1984), 55.
102 Craik, *The 'Hippocratic' Corpus*, 290–1.
103 Pérez Cañizares, 'The treatise *Affections*', 93; Craik, *'Hippocratic' Corpus*, 291: 'The writers and compilers [of the Hippocratic Corpus] are generally assertive, confident of their own place in an advancing scientific tradition. The convention that they claim authority, originality and superiority without stating their origins and identity may be due to medical collegiality, but still seems strangely restrictive.'

104 Van der Eijk, 'On "Hippocratic" and "non-Hippocratic" medical writings', 24.
105 *Diseases of Women* 1.63 (Loeb, *Hippocrates* XI, 133); 1.17 (61).
106 Langholf, 'Structure and genesis of some Hippocratic texts', 254–6.
107 Aline Rousselle, 'Images médicales du corps. Observation féminine et idéologie masculine: le corps de la femme d'après les médecins grecs', *Annales E.S.C.*, 35 (1980), 1094; *Porneia* (Paris: Presses Universitaires de France, 1983), 39 (tr. Felicia Pheasant, *Porneia: On desire and the body in antiquity* (Oxford: Blackwell, 1988)).
108 Paola Manuli, 'Fisiologia e patologia del femminile negli scritti ippocratici dell'antica ginecologia greca' in Mirko D. Grmek (ed.), *Hippocratica. Actes du Colloque hippocratique de Paris 1978* (Paris: Eds de CNRS, 1980), 402 and 'Donne mascoline, femmine sterili, vergini perpetue. La ginecologia greca tra Ippocrate e Sorano' in Silvia Campese, Paola Manuli and Giulia Sissa, *Madre Materia. Sociologia e biologia della donna greca* (Turin: Boringhieri, 1983).
109 Nancy Demand, *Birth, Death and Motherhood in Classical Greece* (Baltimore, MD and London: Johns Hopkins University Press, 1994), xvi; Lesley Dean-Jones, *Women's Bodies in Classical Greek Science* (Oxford: Clarendon Press, 1994), 27.
110 Gian A. Ferrari and Mario Vegetti, 'Science, technology and medicine in the classical tradition' in Pietro Corsi and Paul Weindling (eds), *Information Sources in the History of Science and Medicine* (London and Boston: Butterworth Scientific, 1983), 202.
111 *Diseases of Women*, 1.62 (Loeb, *Hippocrates* XI, 131); Helen King, 'From *parthenos* to *gynê*: the dynamics of category', PhD thesis, University of London, 1985; on the 'woman of experience', see Ann Hanson, 'The medical writers' woman' in David Halperin et al., *Before Sexuality: The construction of erotic experience in the ancient Greek world* (Princeton, NJ: Princeton University Press, 1990), 309.
112 *Diseases of Women*, 1.62 (Loeb, *Hippocrates* XI, 131).
113 Helen King, 'Medical texts as a source for women's history' in Anton Powell (ed.), *The Greek World* (London: Routledge, 1995).
114 Pinault, *Hippocratic Lives and Legends*, 1; Smith, *Hippocratic Tradition*, 30, 'an analytical scheme dressed up as a narrative of events'.
115 Heinrich von Staden, '"In a pure and holy way": personal and professional conduct in the Hippocratic Oath?', *JHM*, 51.4 (1966): translation p. 406. On the use of the family to account for differences between treatises, see Smith, *Pseudepigraphic Writings*, 8.
116 Adams, *Genuine Works*, 9.

117 Nelson, 'Tracking the Hippocratic Woozle', 131 and ibid., 'Hippocrates, Heraclids, and the "Kings of the Heracleidai": Adaptations of Asclepiad history by the author of the *Presbeutikos*', *Phoenix*, 61.3/4 (2007), 235. See also Nelson's argument that the *Probomios* is a fragment of a lost history of Cos: 'Coan promotions and the authorship of the *Presbeutikos*', in Philip van der Eijk (ed.), *Hippocrates in Context. Papers Read at the XIth International Hippocrates Colloquium, University of Newcastle-upon-Tyne 27–31 August 2002* (Leiden: Brill, 2005). On the dating of the pseudepigrapha, various proposals have been made ranging from the mid-fourth to the early third century BCE, and I am following here the argument made by Smith, *Pseudepigraphic Writings*, 6–7.
118 Smith, *Pseudepigraphic Writings*, 5.
119 Nelson, 'Tracking the Hippocratic Woozle'.
120 Adams, *Genuine Works*, 9; Edelstein, 'Genuine works', 138–9; Pinault, *Hippocratic Lives and Legends*; Smith, *Hippocratic Tradition*, 30, 'an etiological myth'.
121 Jouanna, *Hippocrates*, 8–9.
122 In 1849, Adams challenged the traditional birth year, on the grounds that Aulus Gellius (*Attic Nights* 17.21) – who wrote that Hippocrates was an older contemporary of Socrates – was more reliable than Soranus, on whose authority the date of 460 depends; *Genuine Works*, 9–10.
123 https://www.panaynews.net/money-or-life/ accessed 20 February 2019.
124 Johannes Ilberg (ed.), *Vita Hippocratis secundum Soranum* (CMG IV; Berlin: Teubner, 1927). Smith, *Pseudepigraphic Writings*, 49; 51 n.2; 53 n.3 on how this was not by the Soranus who wrote *Gynaecology* and *Lives of the Physicians*.
125 Ada Adler (ed.), *Suidae Lexicon*, 5 vols (Leipzig: Teubner, 1928–38).
126 Tzetzes, *Historiae* 7.155.936–50; Petrus Aloisius Leone (ed.), *Ioannis Tzetzes Historiae* (Naples: Libreria Scientifica, 1968).
127 Temkin, *Hippocrates in a World of Pagans and Christians*, 242; Pinault, *Hippocratic Lives and Legends*, 19.
128 Tzetzes 7.155.970; Pinault, *Hippocratic Lives and Legends*, 22.
129 Brussels ms. 1342–1350; Pinault, *Hippocratic Lives and Legends*, 25 and 131 on the Brussels 'Life'.
130 Thomas Rütten, 'Hippocrates', in Anthony Grafton, Glenn W. Most and Salvatore Settis (eds), *The Classical Tradition* (Cambridge MA: Harvard University Press, 2010), 438–9, building on Pinault, *Hippocratic Lives and Legends*. The projection image recalls James Davidson's comments on ancient Greek sexuality, when he challenged the modern view that it was all about who was penetrated and who did the penetration: 'The Greeks did not award points for penetration ... they

certainly did not structure the whole of society let alone the entire world according to a coital schema. The whole theory is simply a projection of our own gender nightmares on to the screen of a very different culture' (*Courtesans and Fishcakes: The consuming passions of classical Athens* (London: HarperCollins, 1997), 176).

131 https://asthma.net/living/how-did-hippocrates-diagnose-asthma/ accessed 20 February 2019.

132 F.N.L. Poynter and K.D. Keele, *Short History of Medicine* (London: The Scientific Book Club, 1961), 21; Guthrie, *History of Medicine*, 76 and 74.

133 *Assassin's Creed: Odyssey*, episode 'First Do No Harm'. This is an imaginary treatise and it will be interesting to see if its creation is taken up by others. I explore imaginary treatises in Chapter 3.

134 Warner, 'Making history in American medical culture', 203, quoting Victor J. Fourgeaud, 'An introductory lecture on the history of medicine, delivered on the 23rd December, 1845, before the Medico-Chirugical [sic] Society of St Louis, Mo.', *Saint Louis Medical and Surgical Journal*, 4 (1847), 482.

135 Roger J. Bulger and Anthony L. Barbato, 'On the Hippocratic sources of Western medical practice', *The Hastings Center Report*, 30.4 (July–Aug 2000), 4.

136 Poynter and Keele, *Short History of Medicine*, 17.

137 Stubbs and Bligh, *Sixty Centuries of Health and Physick*, 60–1.

138 Ibid., 67.

139 Vivien Longhi, 'Hippocrate a-t-il inventé la médecine d'observation?', *Cahiers Mondes Anciens*, 11 (2018), 9: 'L'image d'un Hippocrate inventeur et maître de l'observation clinique, forgée par une certaine histoire moderne de la médecine voulant trouver son origine chez les Grecs, est trompeuse.'

140 William Osler, *The Evolution of Modern Medicine: A series of lectures delivered at Yale University on the Silliman Foundation in April, 1913* (New Haven CT: Yale University Press, 1921), 62–3. Petersen, *Hippocratic Wisdom*, xvii uses 'sharp-minded'.

141 Fielding Garrison, *An Introduction to the History of Medicine* (second edition, Philadelphia, PA: W.B. Saunders, 1917), 83: originally 1913, 66. Fourth edition, 1929, 94.

142 Loeb, *Hippocrates* VII, 256; Winfried Schleiner, *Medical Ethics in the Renaissance* (Washington DC: Georgetown University Press, 1995), 9 in a discussion of the comments made by Rodrigo a Castro (1546–1627) on this passage. I reached a similar conclusion in *Hippocrates' Woman: Reading the female body in ancient Greece* (London: Routledge, 1988), 46–7.

143 Amneris Roselli, '"According to both Hippocrates and the truth": Hippocrates as witness to the truth, from Apollonius of Citium to Galen', in DJR.

144 Galen, *Commentary on Hippocrates' Epidemics* 6.5.13, 17B.266–269 K; Jacques Jouanna, 'Galen's reading of Hippocratic ethics' in Philip van der Eijk (ed.), *Greek Medicine from Hippocrates to Galen. Selected papers* (Leiden and Boston: Brill, 2012), 272.

145 Daniela Manetti and Amneris Roselli, *Ippocrate, Epidemie, libro sesto. Introduzione, testo critico, commento e traduzione*, Biblioteca di studi superiori, 66 (Florence: La nuova Italia editrice, 1982), 111–13.

146 Pinault, *Hippocratic Lives and Legends*, 79–94 explores the interaction between these texts.

147 Ibid., 88.

148 Thomas Crow, *Emulation: David, Drouais, and Girodet in the Art of Revolutionary France* (New Haven: Yale University Press, 1995), 140–4.

149 Lloyd, *Methods and Problems*, 194.

150 Cantor, 'Introduction', 3.

151 Helen King, 'The power of paternity: The Father of Medicine meets the Prince of Physicians' in Cantor (ed.), *Reinventing Hippocrates*, 23.

152 Rosalind Coward, *The Whole Truth: The myth of alternative health* (London: Faber & Faber, 1989), 2.

153 Benjamin Rush, 'Lecture 12', 292.

154 Thomas Rütten, 'Hippocrates and the construction of "progress" in sixteenth- and seventeenth-century medicine' in Cantor (ed.), *Reinventing Hippocrates*, 46–7.

Chapter 3

1 An earlier version of this chapter appears as 'Hippocratic Whispers: Telling the story of the life of Hippocrates on the internet' in Laurence Totelin and Rebecca Flemming (eds), *Medicines and Markets: Essays on Ancient Medicine in Honour of Vivian Nutton* (London and New York: Classical Press of Wales/Bloomsbury, 2019).

2 Warner, 'Making history', 201–2.

3 http://www.rethinkingcancer.org/resources/articles/who-was-hippocrates.php accessed 20 February 2019.

4 Sandra Cabot, *The Juice Fasting Bible: Discover the power of an all-juice diet to restore good health, lose weight and increase vitality* (Berkeley CA: Ulysses Press, 2007), 107.

5 John S. Haller, *American Medicine in Transition 1840–1910* (Urbana, Chicago and London: University of Illinois Press, 1981), 272; Weisz, 'Hippocrates, holism and humanism', 261.

6 Cabot, *Juice Fasting Bible*.
7 Alan Levinovitz, *The Gluten Lie: And other myths about what you eat* (New York: Regan Arts, 2015) includes a chapter on 'The Sin of Salt'; https://www.npr.org/sections/thesalt/2016/05/08/477057872/what-is-natural-food-a-riddle-wrapped-in-notions-of-good-and-evil, 8 May 2016, accessed 20 February 2019; https://mag.uchicago.edu/law-policy-society/eating-habits, July–August 2015, accessed 20 February 2019.
8 Here I have in mind Max Weber's concept of 'charismatic authority' outlined in 'The three types of legitimate rule' (1922, translated into English by Hans Gerth in 1958, Berkeley Publications in Society and Institutions, 4.1, 1–11). The other two were traditional authority and rational-legal authority. Some users of the name of Hippocrates are clearly leaders in the charismatic mode: most importantly, Brian Clement, founder of the Hippocrates Institute, who will be discussed further in Chapter 7.
9 'The Greek Physician Hippocrates, said in his scriptures …': http://www.digitaljournal.com/pr/3864905#ixzz5N0Ch04jI accessed 20 February 2019.
10 Armour, *It All Started with Hippocrates*, 28.
11 http://www.wpsdlocal6.com/2018/06/18/equine-assisted-therapy-may-help-autism-ptsd-and-pain/ 18 June 2018 referencing https://americanhippotherapy association.org/about-aha-inc/ where it is a 'chapter' rather than 'a thesis', accessed 20 February 2019. Whatever its origin, *Natural Exercise* is widely mentioned online, but more commonly as a 'chapter'. Sometimes it is instead that 'Hippocrates called riding "Natural Exercise"'; http://www.mentalhealthnewsradionetwork.com/right-from-the-horses-mouth-equine-assisted-therapy-with-mental-health-patients-works1/.
12 *AWP* 21 (Loeb, *Hippocrates* I, 125): 'the constant jolting on their horses unfits them for intercourse'. The confusion possibly derives from two other writers called Hippocrates, who in the fifth or sixth century CE – not BCE – wrote on veterinary medicine for horses and who are referenced in Arabic medicine: Anne McCabe, *A Byzantine Encyclopaedia of Horse Medicine: The sources, compilation and transmission of the* Hippiatrica (Oxford: Oxford University Press, 2007), 245–58. The name 'Hippocrates' combines the ancient Greek for 'horse' and 'rule'.
13 *Fistulas* 1 (Loeb, *Hippocrates* VIII, 391).
14 For a short guide to how Wikipedia works, and a discussion of whether or not it provides 'real history', see Petros Apostolopoulos, 'Producing historical knowledge on Wikipedia', *Madison Historical Review*, 16 (2019): https://commons.lib.jmu.edu/mhr/vol16/iss1/4 accessed 30 April 2019.
15 https://en.wikipedia.org/wiki/Talk%3AHippocrates.
16 https://en.wikipedia.org/wiki/Wikipedia:Featured_articles, accessed 20 February 2019.

17 Contributor using IP address 69.87.199.175, writing in 2008, on https://en.wikipedia.org/wiki/Talk:Hippocrates/Archive_2#Fever_benefits accessed 20 February 2019.
18 E.g. 'In general, the Hippocratic medicine was very kind to the patient.'
19 For the statistics on the page, see https://xtools.wmflabs.org/articleinfo/en.wikipedia.org/Hippocrates and https://tools.wmflabs.org/pageviews/?project=en.wikipedia.org&platform=all-access&agent=user&range=latest-20&pages=Hippocrates accessed 20 February 2019.
20 http://www.scielo.org.za/pdf/saoj/v10n4/v10n4a03.pdf accessed 20 February 2019.
21 https://en.wikipedia.org/w/index.php?title=Hippocrates&diff=next&oldid=602126560.
22 Jon Solomon, 'The Apician sauce: *ius apicianum*' in Wilkins et al. (eds), *Food in Antiquity*, 122. http://www.historicfood.com/Hippocras%20Recipes.htm accessed 20 February 2019; 'Peppermongers' Hippocras recipe', *The Telegraph*, 17 October 2013: https://www.telegraph.co.uk/foodanddrink/recipes/10383032/Peppermongers-Hippocras-recipe.html.
23 Sir Arthur Conan Doyle, *A Study in Scarlet, and, The Sign of the Four* (New York and London: Harper & Brothers, 1904), 197. On this feature in Raymond Chandler's novels, see Glenn W. Most, 'The Hippocratic Smile: John le Carré and the traditions of the detective novel' in Glenn W. Most and William W. Stowe (eds), *The Poetics of Murder* (San Diego, CA: Harcourt Brace Jovanovich, 1983), 347.
24 *Prognostics* 2 (Loeb, *Hippocrates* II, 9–11). Both the *facies Hippocratica* and the *risus sardonicus* are often described alongside each other in medical texts, e.g. John Elliotson, *The Principles and Practice of Medicine* (Philadelphia, PA: Carey and Hart, 1844), 57: on the *facies Hippocratica*, 'Hippocrates gave a most accurate description of it'. For a modern take on the *facies* in relation to the masks of Greek tragedy, see Chiara Thumiger, 'The tragic *prosopon* and the Hippocratic *facies*: face and individuality in classical Greece', *Maia*, 68 (2016), 637–64.
25 *Prognostics* 2 (Loeb, *Hippocrates* II, 11).
26 https://en.wikipedia.org/w/index.php?title=Hippocrates&diff=prev&oldid=406595060 accessed 20 February 2019.
27 https://en.wikipedia.org/wiki/Hippocrates.
28 Ben Witherington, *A Week in the Life of Corinth* (Downer's Grove IL: InterVarsity Press, 2012), 81. Aimed at a Christian readership, this book was welcomed as 'historically accurate ... a beach read for the lay person', http://www.jeremybouma.com/saturday-book-review-a-week-in-the-life-of-corinth-by-ben-witherington/. The Wikipedia section reads 'Hippocratic medicine was humble and passive. The

therapeutic approach was based on "the healing power of nature" ("*vis medicatrix naturae*" in Latin)', https://en.wikipedia.org/wiki/Hippocrates.
29 Garrison, *Introduction to the History of Medicine*, 98.
30 Elizabeth MacLeod and Frieda Wishinsky, *A History of Just About Everything: 180 events, people and inventions that changed the world* (Toronto, ON: Kids Can Press, 2013), 22; Steve Parker, *Kill or Cure. An Illustrated History of Medicine* (London: Dorling Kindersley, 2013), 36.
31 For the original wording proposed by this editor, see https://en.wikipedia.org/w/index.php?title=Hippocrates&diff=prev&oldid=599952657.
32 Added from IP address 76.217.165.168.
33 E.g. the 25 May 2018 revision by Randykitty, reverted as possible vandalism on 5 July 2018: https://en.wikipedia.org/w/index.php?title=Hippocrates&type=revision&diff=848954117&oldid=842864513 accessed 20 February 2019.
34 https://en.wikipedia.org/w/index.php?title=Vinegar&type=revision&diff=599951433&oldid=599904327.
35 E.g. Carol S. Johnston and Cindy A. Gaas, 'Vinegar: medicinal uses and antiglycemic effect', *Medscape General Medicine*, 8.2 (2006), 61 mention Hippocrates using vinegar in general 'to manage wounds' and 'to fight infections'.
36 http://pothos.org/forum/viewtopic.php?t=3825 accessed 20 February 2019.
37 Responses included two on the lines of 'Does it matter?', from supporters of the benefits of fermented foods who did not see why the type of vinegar was important. I would respond that, for the manufacturers of ACV, it most certainly does matter.
38 https://bragg.com/products/bragg-organic-apple-cider-vinegar-drink-honey.html and https://bragg.com/zencart/index.php?main_page=product_info&cPath=8&products_id=22&zenid=acaa1tt6s75495dcdceb52l014 accessed 20 February 2019.
39 'Vinegar: An ancient medicine and popular home remedy', *Connections Quarterly* https://www.pitt.edu/~cjm6/s98vinegar.html accessed 20 February 2019. The editor added at the end of the short article, 'We will print it on colored paper and place copies of it on our literature rack in the Self-Care Center for our students to enjoy. I invite you all to do the same.'
40 Thacker's work features, for example, on the site of the industry's Vinegar Institute: https://versatilevinegar.org/reference-library/ accessed 20 February 2019.
41 http://naturalmentor.com/why-apple-cider-vinegar-should-be-in-your-medicine-cabinet/, 21 October 2015, accessed 20 February 2019.
42 http://www.preventionandhealing.com/articles/Apple_Cider_Vinegar.pdf by 'Simon Yu MD', no date, accessed 20 February 2019.

43 Edwin LeFevre, 'Making vinegar in the home and on the farm', *Farmers' Bulletin*, 1424, U.S. Department of Agriculture, 1924.
44 J.J. Schommer, *Manufacture of Pure Cider Vinegar in the United States* (B.Sc. thesis in Chemical Engineering, Armour Institute of Technology, 1912), 1.
45 At the time of writing, this has been amended to 'Historians agree that Hippocrates was born around the year 460 BC on the Greek island of Kos; other biographical information, however, is likely to be untrue [6]'. The note still takes the reader to Sherwin B. Nuland, *Doctors: The biography of medicine* (New York: Vintage Books, 1988); the first chapter, 'The Totem of Medicine: Hippocrates', includes a largely balanced account of the myths about Hippocrates, apart from too much weight being put on the alleged Cos/Cnidos division (17–18).
46 Das, 'New material', 305.
47 Fichtner, *Corpus Hippocraticum*, 70 (treatise 79 of 170).
48 https://en.wikipedia.org/wiki/Wikipedia:FAQ/Schools#What_prevents_someone_from_contributing_false_or_misleading_information.3F describes how the 'content control mechanisms' work. It mentions that, in rare cases, errors may survive for 'months after the fact'; four years is exceptional.
49 For example, the change of 'figures' to 'willy models' by user 2.127.65.47 on 26 June 2015, https://en.wikipedia.org/w/index.php?title=Hippocrates&type=revision&diff=668812115&oldid=668810961 or, on the same day, altering the same word to 'cat rapists' by IP address 151.231.50.60. On 25 October 2014 user 173.69.46.128 was unable to resist the urge to insert '"""HEY GUYS CALIA MARSO WAS HERE. I WAS ON THIS PAGE BECAUSE IM WRITING A REPORT ON THIS STUFF SO YEAH, THATS ALL"""'. This was immediately picked up by a bot and reverted. 'was infact [sic] gay' was added on 25 March 2011 by Jamielee111, who was immediately blocked from Wikipedia 'with an expiry time of indefinite'; https://en.wikipedia.org/w/index.php?title=Hippocrates&diff=next&oldid=420070590 and https://en.wikipedia.org/wiki/User:Jamielee111; the reversion was made by a bot. 'I love you joslyn' briefly featured at the start of the article in November 2011; https://en.wikipedia.org/w/index.php?title=Hippocrates&diff=prev&oldid=461194932. On ClueBots see for example http://www.bbc.co.uk/news/magazine-18892510.
50 The suspect was using IP address 91.124.144.90; https://en.wikipedia.org/wiki/Talk:Hippocrates.
51 David Crystal, *Language and the Internet*, second edition (Cambridge: Cambridge University Press, 2006), 16.
52 P.D. Magnus, 'Early response to false claims in *Wikipedia*', *First Monday* 13.9 (2008); https://firstmonday.org/article/view/2115/2027 accessed 20 February 2019.

53 See for example the Internet Archive's Wayback Machine, which has to date saved over 341 billion web pages.
54 http://alex.halavais.net/the-isuzu-experiment, 29 August 2004, accessed 20 February 2019.
55 http://alex.halavais.net/please-dont-do-this, 5 September 2004, accessed 20 February 2019.
56 José van Dijck, *The Culture of Connectivity: A critical history of social media* (Oxford: Oxford University Press, 2013), 201–2, n.21.
57 P.D. Magnus, 'Early response to false claims' and 'Fibs in the Wikipedia (Supplemental Data)', *Philosophy Faculty Scholarship* (University of Albany, SUNY) 9 (2008) http://scholarsarchive.library.albany.edu/cas_philosophy_scholar/9.
58 For a valuable account of a student editing a page, see https://dynamicecology.wordpress.com/2014/05/05/using-wikipedia-in-the-classroom-a-cautionary-tale/. On 6 October 2015, Karl Steel, a medievalist at Brooklyn College of CUNY, tweeted 'Nobody touch the wikipedia plot summary for Oroonoko because we are going to tear that shit apart in class tomorrow' (https://twitter.com/KarlSteel/status/651554604916834304). On 7 October, he tweeted 'Much praise to my English 4113 students; Oroonoko wikipedia page is so much better. keep at it', https://twitter.com/KarlSteel/status/651787201563508736. See also the article on student contributions to Wikipedia on https://wikiedu.org/blog/2018/10/16/student-says-more-universities-need-to-participate-in-editing-wikipedia/, 16 October 2018, accessed 20 February 2019, which stresses 'the robust digital literacy skills' students need to develop.
59 https://blog.wikimedia.org.uk/2018/05/wikipedia-in-the-history-classroom/
60 Quotation from Barry Robson and O.K. Baek's *The Engines of Hippocrates: From the dawn of medicine to medical and pharmaceutical informatics* (Hoboken NJ: Wiley, 2009), 57. NB this is not the most reliable of pages; for example, it has 'Celus' for Celsus. See the discussions of Quentin J. Schultze and Randall L. Bytwerk, 'Plausible quotations and reverse credibility in online vernacular communities', *ETC: A Review of General Semantics*, 69.2 (2012), 224; René König, 'Wikipedia. Between lay participation and elite knowledge representation', *Information, Communication & Society*, 16.2 (2013), 162.
61 https://en.wikipedia.org/wiki/User:Yunshui/About accessed 20 February 2019.
62 Personal communication, Yun Shui, 7 October 2014.
63 https://en.wikipedia.org/wiki/Talk:Hippocrates.
64 http://oer2go.org/mods/en-wikipedia_for_schools-static/wp/h/Hippocrates.htm accessed 20 February 2019; this site is run by SOS Children's Villages 'to make Wikipedia content more accessible'. Their versions contain no references.

65 https://en.wikipedia.org/wiki/Hippocrates 12 April 2017 was running with 'Modern Medicine'; currently 'Father of Medicine' with a weak citation (a page of the Encarta online encyclopaedia); 'Father of Clinical Medicine' made a brief appearance on 14 September 2011, but was reverted three hours later; https://en.wikipedia.org/w/index.php?title=Hippocrates&diff=next&oldid=450528365. 'Western' has come and gone several times.

66 E.g. Patricia Davis, *Aromatherapy. An A–Z* (Saffron Walden: C.W. Daniel, 1988), 158; Vicki Pitman, *The Nature of the Whole: Holism in ancient Greek and Indian medicine* (Delhi: Motilal Banarsidass Publishers, 2005), 1. See Chapter 7 below.

67 Warner, 'Making history', 201.

68 https://en.wikipedia.org/wiki/List_of_people_considered_father_or_mother_of_a_scientific_field#Medicine_and_physiology accessed 20 February 2019. On local 'fatherhood', e.g. Dumitru Bagdasar, 'father of Romanian neurosurgery, see King, 'The power of paternity', 26. I shall return to Imhotep in Chapter 4.

69 https://www.urbandictionary.com/define.php?term=Who%27s%20the%20daddy%3F and https://www.whozthedaddy.com/ accessed 20 February 2019.

70 King, 'The power of paternity', 25.

71 Jan Sapp, 'The nine lives of Gregor Mendel' in Homer E. Le Grand, *Experimental Inquiries* (Dordrecht: Reidel, 1990), 137-66; http://www.mendelweb.org/MWsapp.html.

72 Jan Sapp, *Where the Truth Lies: Franz Moewus and the origins of molecular biology* (Cambridge: Cambridge University Press, 1999), 28–9. On science as the rape of Nature, see Ludmilla Jordanova, *Sexual Visions: Images of gender in science and medicine between the eighteenth and twentieth centuries* (London: Harvester Wheatsheaf, 1989).

73 Helen King, 'Women and doctors in ancient Greece' in Rebecca Flemming, Nick Hopwood and Lauren Kassell (eds), *From Generation to Reproduction* (Cambridge: Cambridge University Press, 2018), 39–52.

74 *On Generation/Nature of the Child* 10 (Loeb, *Hippocrates* X, 58). In earlier editions of these texts, such as that of Littré, this chapter is no. 21.

75 Jonathan Sawday, *The Body Emblazoned: Dissection and the human body in Renaissance culture* (London and New York: Routledge, 1995), 41: 'a doubly fathered masculine western knowledge of Greek medicine married to the passive, eastern tradition of transmission'.

76 On the uterine mole, see Helen King and Cathy McClive, 'When is a foetus not a foetus? Diagnosing false conceptions in early modern France' in V. Dasen (ed.), *L'Embryon humain à travers l'histoire: Images, savoirs et rites*, Actes du colloque international de Fribourg, 27–29 octobre 2004 (Gollion: Infolio, 2008).

77 Macfie, *Romance of Medicine*, 15; Withington, *Medical History*, 48; Stubbs and Bligh, *Sixty Centuries of Health and Physick*, 52.
78 Douglas Guthrie, *A History of Medicine* (London: Thomas Nelson, 1945), 39. The claims of Imhotep to the title are discussed but dismissed on 21–2 and 29, at least 'as far as mortals are concerned'.
79 Poynter and Keele, *Short History of Medicine*, 17–18.
80 Marco Fabio Calvi, *Hippocratis Coi medicorum omnium longe principis, Octoginta volumina . . .* (Rome: Franciscus Minitius, 1525); Janus Cornarius, *Hippocratis Coi medicorum omnium longe principis, opera quae ad nos extant omnia* (Basel: Froben, 1546); King, 'The power of paternity', 28–9.
81 https://en.wikipedia.org/w/index.php?title=Hippocrates&diff=401937923&oldid=399915431. Inserted from IP address 217.43.247.50 at 11:27 with the spelling 'embassador' (https://en.wikipedia.org/w/index.php?title=Hippocrates&diff=prev&oldid=401937923). The spelling was altered on 15 December 2010 from IP address 90.216.252.197. For 'The Complicated boy', see https://en.wikipedia.org/w/index.php?title=Hippocrates&diff=next&oldid=455206770. Among other changes made over a few hours, someone using the same IP address, 97.67.180.74, also changed the title to 'The Odessy' [sic]. The insertion of 'bullying' went with changing Hippocrates' date of birth to 1993 and Cos with Kuss; https://en.wikipedia.org/w/index.php?title=Hippocrates&diff=next&oldid=479316104. The attempt to insert 'don't' was made by IP address 50.128.191.40 on 9 February 2012 but rejected as 'possible vandalism', https://en.wikipedia.org/w/index.php?title=Hippocrates&diff=next&oldid=475864207. A further act of vandalism occurred on 13 May 2012 when the opening of this paragraph became instead 'Historians agree sex is fun', https://en.wikipedia.org/w/index.php?title=Hippocrates&diff=prev&oldid=492382799. 'Hippocrates liked to race turtles' was inserted briefly after the reference to *The Complicated Body* in September 2013, as was 'he is the first person to advocate people for harm reduction', https://en.wikipedia.org/w/index.php?title=Hippocrates&diff=next&oldid=574203450.
82 Change made on 8 October 2012. Paige Durkin is named online from 2013–17 as a player in girls' softball teams; http://www.senatorblake.com/blake-farina-applaud-aaa-girls-state-softball-champs-valley-view-hs/ and http://www.lackawannafalcons.com/sports/sball/2016-17/bios/durkin_paige_20ga accessed 20 February 2019. That does not of course mean that she was involved in the attempted change to the page.
83 https://en.wikipedia.org/w/index.php?title=Hippocrates&diff=next&oldid=523085847.
84 Attempt made by 98.155.17.93, who appears to have been using the Sandbox feature to experiment with editing, on 16 December 2013: reverted by a bot within

seconds. A few minutes later, this editor also changed Hippocrates' designation as 'physician' to 'fast food restaurant owner'.
85 Roshen Dalal, *The Puffin History of the World*, vol. 1 (London: Penguin Books, 2013); MacLeod and Wishinsky, *A History of Just About Everything*, 22; the reference to 'soothing balms' also exposes its origin in Wikipedia. It remains possible that the person who inserted the prison story into the page found it in a print source which has not yet been digitized, and I remain open to finding this.
86 Taylor, *Hippocrates Cried*, xiii.
87 http://totallyhistory.com/hippocrates/ published in 2014, accessed 20 February 2019. See also 'However, the years of incarceration were not wasted because it was during that time that he wrote his best know [sic] work "The complicated body"', http://www.actforlibraries.org/hippocrates-lived-in-460bc-and-is-still-considered-today-the-greek-father-of-the-of-western-medicine/ accessed 20 February 2019.
88 Ian Mueller, 'Greek arithmetic, geometry and harmonics: Thales to Plato' in C.C.W. Taylor (ed.), *Routledge History of Philosophy, Vol. I: From the Beginning to Plato* (London and New York: Routledge, 1997), 280; Plutarch, *On Exile* 17 (*Moralia* 607f).
89 Taylor, *Hippocrates Cried*, xiii.
90 Plutarch, *Life of Alcibiades*, 30.1.
91 Killis Campbell, *The Seven Sages of Rome* (Boston: Ginn & Co., 1907), lines 1101–1270: 'Master Hypocras' slew his nephew, in one manuscript (H) named as Galen: Karla Mallette, 'The *Seven Sages of Rome*: narration and silence' in Marion Vuagnoux-Uhlig and Yasmina Foehr-Janssens (eds), *D'Orient en Occident: Les Recueils de fables enchâssées avant les 'Milles et une nuits' de Galland* (Turnhout: Brepols, 2014).
92 As of 20 February 2019.
93 https://en.wikipedia.org/w/index.php?title=Hippocrates&diff=prev&oldid=407709694 accessed 20 February 2019. On the site infoplease.com, http://www.infoplease.com/biography/var/hippocrates.html gives 377 while http://www.infoplease.com/encyclopedia/people/hippocrates.html gives *c*. 370.
94 From IP address 72.199.67.48; https://en.wikipedia.org/w/index.php?title=Hippocrates&diff=next&oldid=449186664.
95 Schultze and Bytwerk, 'Plausible quotations and reverse credibility', 228.
96 http://www.answers.com/Q/FAQ/8893 and http://www.answers.com/Q/Did_Hippocrates_get_put_in_prison accessed 20 February 2019.
97 http://www.geni.com/people/Hippocrates/6000000011410012323, page updated 21 November, 2016; accessed 20 February 2019.

98 http://www.answers.com/Q/How_important_was_the_influence_of_Hippocrates_on_Roman_and_medieval_medicine accessed 20 February 2019.
99 There is an attempt to link Hippocrates to the Bible on http://www.bethelcog.org/church/church-of-god-articles/understanding-divine-healing, where Hippocrates is credited with spreading the belief in a 'life force' formerly revealed by God to Moses, but this wording is not used. The 'Right to Life' movement often emphasizes alleged similarities between the Bible and Hippocratic medicine, for example linking the serpent of Asclepius and the snake on Moses' staff in *Numbers* 21, as on http://americanrtl.org/Hippocratic-Oath-Serpent-Staff.
100 Vivian Nutton, 'What's in an oath?', *Journal of the Royal College of Physicians of London*, 29.6 (1995), 521.
101 http://classicalwisdom.com/hippocrates-the-father-of-medicine/ Classical Wisdom Weekly, accessed 20 February 2019.
102 http://totallyhistory.com/hippocrates/ accessed 20 February 2019; my request in the Comment feature for the source of the story remains unanswered.
103 http://eeever.com/en/hippocrates accessed 20 February 2019: according to this site, 'he performed the first known endoscopy', another claim deriving from the Wikipedia Hippocrates page and presumably based on the description of examining the rectum with a speculum, as referenced in the Wikipedia Hippocrates citations: J. Shah, 'Endoscopy through the ages', *BJU International*, 89.7 (2002), '464–10': these page numbers are incorrect, and should be 645–52, with the Hippocratic reference on p.645. On the instrument (the *katopter*), described in the treatises *Haemorrhoids* 5 and *Fistulas* 3, and which may have been simply two large spoons, see Lawrence J. Bliquez, *The Tools of Asclepius. Surgical instruments in Greek and Roman times* (Leiden: Brill, 2015), 48–9.
104 King, 'The power of paternity', 24; Philip van der Eijk, '"Airs, Waters, Places" and "On the Sacred Disease": two different religiosities?', *Hermes*, 119 (1991), 168.
105 Isabelle C. Torrance, 'The Hippocratic Oath' in Alan H. Sommerstein and Isabelle C. Torrance, *Oaths and Swearing in Ancient Greece* (Berlin and Boston, MA: De Gruyter, 2014), 373.
106 Nuland, *Doctors*, 10. 'Theurgy' also currently features in the Wikipedia 'Hippocrates' article: 'This intellectual school revolutionized medicine in ancient Greece, establishing it as a discipline distinct from other fields with which it had traditionally been associated (theurgy and philosophy), thus establishing medicine as a profession', https://en.wikipedia.org/wiki/Hippocrates.
107 E.g. Pliny, *Natural History*, 29.2; Strabo, *Geography*, 14.2.19. The earlier tradition, that Hippocrates was 'really a priest physician' who wrote *Prognostics* by using the notes compiled by the priests, survives: Precope, *Hippocrates on Diet and Hygiene*, 13 and 16; Eleni Tsiompanou and Spyros G. Marketos, 'Hippocrates:

timeless still', *Journal of the Royal Society of Medicine*, 106 (2013), 288. On burning libraries, see above, p. 30.
108 Temkin, *Hippocrates in a World of Pagans and Christians*, 54.
109 http://weeksmd.com/2012/10/hippocrates-did-20-years-in-prison/ written on October 23, 2012, accessed 20 February 2019.
110 On some receptions of this story, see Cantor, 'Western medicine since the Renaissance', 380–1.
111 https://books.google.co.uk/books?id=pC11fC7Pi60C&printsec=frontcover&source=gbs_ge_summary_r&cad=0#v=onepage&q=hippocrates&f=false.
112 Online version; no page numbers.
113 http://www.sciography.com/hippocrates.htm accessed 20 February 2019.
114 http://www.rethinkingcancer.org/resources/articles/who-was-hippocrates.php accessed 20 February 2019.
115 https://historiarex.com/e/en/121-hippocrates-ca-460-370-b-c accessed 20 February 2019.
116 http://en.infoglobe.cz/traveller-guide/greece-kos-following-the-steps-of-hippocrates-i/ accessed 20 February 2019; perhaps this information was given by a tour guide who had read the Wikipedia page?
117 http://weeksmd.com/2012/10/hippocrates-did-20-years-in-prison/ published 23 October 2012, accessed 20 February 2019.
118 http://bookstore.dorrancepublishing.com/dr-william-hobbys-the-promiscuous-kings-promiscuous-doctor/ accessed 20 February 2019.
119 *Dr William Hobbys*, 197. 'Drumstick fingers' (clubbed fingers), linked to empyema, are indeed known as 'Hippocratic fingers'. *Prognostic* 17 (Loeb, *Hippocrates* II, 35) says that in empyema 'the finger-nails are bent and the fingers grow hot, especially at the tips'.
120 http://thehealthmoderator.com/the-great-hippocrates-father-of-modern-medicine/ posted 14 January 2014, accessed 20 February 2019. This is an American site with a focus on the pharmaceutical industry's 'destructive influence on the U.S. medical system', http://thehealthmoderator.com/about-us/ accessed 20 February 2019. Unlike most sites copying the story, The Health Moderator names its sources, here 'Wikipedia, Encyclopedia Britannica, International Hippocratic Foundation, infoplease.com, Encyclopedia of World Biographies, discoveriesinmedicine.com, bbc.co.uk/dna, complete-herbal.com/history, Britannica Great Books, Vol. 10, Hippocrates/Galen'.
121 http://totallyhistory.com/hippocrates/ written 2014, accessed 20 February 2019.
122 http://chloe-chambers.blogspot.co.uk/2012/07/the-egyptians-greeks-and-hippocrates.html 'Global health education' blog, written 26 July 2012, accessed 20 February 2019.

123 Nuland, *Doctors*, 15. I shall return to the role of nature in Chapter 7.
124 http://www.mixbook.com/photo-books/interests/hippocrates-pursuit-to-the-truth-7035001.
125 http://www.notablebiographies.com/He-Ho/Hippocrates.html. The date of composition of the article is not given, but it includes a reference to a book published in 2002.
126 Paraphrasing Wikipedia's 'Medicine at the time of Hippocrates knew almost nothing of human anatomy and physiology because of the Greek taboo forbidding the dissection of humans.'
127 http://www.882m.com/questions/asthma/201512110531360-0-Did-Hippocrates-discover-asthma.html; http://ezinearticles.com/?Who-Discovered-Asthma-Hippocrates-Or-Galen?&id=1381520; http://hardluckasthma.blogspot.co.uk/2011/07/360-460-bc-what-did-hippocrates-think.html; https://asthma.net/living/how-did-hippocrates-diagnose-asthma/ accessed 20 February 2019.
128 https://monq.com/eo/herbs-spices/what-difference-between-herb-spice/ accessed 20 February 2019.
129 Nikolaos Angelou, *Cures of the Body and Cures of the Soul: From Hippocrates to the Early Eastern Christian Fathers* (Trinity St David, University of Wales, 2012), 10, http://repository.uwtsd.ac.uk/438/1/NIKOLAOS%20ANGELOU.pdf.
130 http://www.sciography.com/hippocrates.htm published 13 August 2014, 20 February 2019. It is a feature of Lepton's site that the final section of each biography is the *'rumor has it'* part and there is a particularly bad joke at the end about Hippocrates' younger brother Ted, the 'Hippocratic Oaf'; the majority of the biography simply plods through familiar material. Cantor draws our attention to an episode of a children's cartoon series, *Baby Huey*, also called 'The Hippocratic Oaf'; Cantor, 'Western medicine since the Renaissance', 303.
131 Pers. comm.
132 https://www.ultralingua.com/onlinedictionary/dictionary#src_lang=Latin&dest_lang=English&query=corpus accessed 20 February 2019.
133 Armour, *It All Started with Hippocrates*, 31.
134 Episode 'First Do No Harm'. See also the wiki, http://assassinscreed.wikia.com/wiki/Hippokrates accessed 20 February 2019; which currently suggests that Hippocrates had to treat some patients in secret due to local resistance to his methods.
135 http://thehealthmoderator.com/about-us/.
136 http://thehealthmoderator.com/the-great-hippocrates-father-of-modern-medicine/.

137 Warner, 'Making history', 200.
138 Dale C. Smith, 'The Hippocratic Oath and modern medicine', *JHM*, 51 (1996), 493.
139 Wesley J. Smith, 'Defending the Hippocratic Oath; the importance of conscience in health care', *Human Life Review*, 35.1/2 (2009), 64.
140 Smith, 'Defending the Hippocratic Oath', 65.
141 https://web.archive.org/web/20130925081055/http://www.reversingvaccineinduceddiseases.com/services accessed 20 February 2019.
142 http://gomerblog.com/2014/04/hippocratic-oath/.
143 https://www.panaynews.net/money-or-life/ 28 October 2018, accessed 20 February 2019. On the Act, see http://apps.who.int/medicinedocs/en/d/Jh2943e/9.13.html#Jh2943e.9.13 accessed 20 February 2019.
144 http://www.rethinkingcancer.org/resources/articles/who-was-hippocrates.php accessed 20 February 2019.
145 http://weeksmd.com/2012/10/hippocrates-did-20-years-in-prison/ accessed 20 February 2019.

Chapter 4

1 Whoever untied the knot would rule Asia: Alexander either cut it with his sword or took out the pin which kept the knot together so that he could remove the yoke from the pole; sources discussed in N.G.L. Hammond, *Sources for Alexander the Great: An analysis of Plutarch's* Life *and Arrian's* Anabasis Alexandrou (Cambridge: Cambridge University Press, 1993), 217–8, on Arrian 2.3.7.
2 J.C. McKeown and Joshua M. Smith, *The Hippocrates Code: Unravelling the ancient mysteries of modern medical terminology* (Indianapolis and Cambridge: Hackett Publishing Company, 2016), ix. At other points, the book is more willing to accept the myths of Hippocrates as truth (e.g. 22: the myth that Hippocrates picked up his cures from the temple of Asclepius).
3 The Loeb Classical Library, which continues to expand its coverage of Hippocratic treatises, is behind a paywall, but open access online texts include: the Perseus Project, http://www.perseus.tufts.edu/hopper/collection?collection=Perseus:collection:Greco-Roman; Corpus Medicorum Graecorum, although few of the translations are into English, http://galen.bbaw.de/epubl/online/editionen.html; extracts from texts concerning women and medicine on Diotima, http://www.stoa.org/diotima/anthology/wlgr/wlgr-medicine.shtml; Internet Classics Archive, Francis Adams' translations of selected Hippocratic treatises, http://classics.mit.edu/Browse/index.html, all accessed 20 February 2019.

4   Medline is one component of PubMed, which currently contains 'more than 28 million citations for biomedical literature', many of these full-text; it includes the Brill monograph series 'Studies in Ancient Medicine'. Scopus, founded in 2004, claims to have a wider range in terms of subjects. Since 2013, it has been expanding its coverage of monographs and of edited volumes other than those published in a series. Simply checking on my own publications, Scopus will take the user only to a letter and a short piece I wrote for *The Lancet* and a review essay for *Culture, Medicine and Psychiatry*. PubMed includes, in addition to these, several very short pieces I published in *The Practising Midwife* and a letter to which I contributed in *Isis* in 2004. With Monica Green, I have discussed this phenomenon in 'On the misuses of medical history'.

5   Schultze and Bytwerk, 'Plausible quotations', 226.

6   https://www.ref.ac.uk/2014/panels/assessmentcriteriaandleveldefinitions/ accessed 20 February 2019. Impact is defined as 'an effect on, change or benefit to the economy, society, culture, public policy or services, health, the environment or quality of life, beyond academia'; http://www.hefce.ac.uk/rsrch/REFimpact/ accessed 20 February 2019.

7   For Gaea Products' claim, see https://www.pinterest.co.uk/pin/172122016978930465/?lp=true accessed 20 February 2019.

8   'Help the world discover dear leader's accomplishments!', 15 May 2012, http://thepeoplescube.com/peoples-blog/barack-obama-history-s-party-crasher-t9000.html accessed 20 February 2019: http://thepeoplescube.com/ presents itself as 'America through the eyes of a former Soviet agitprop artist'.

9   Jodi Owen (@JodiOwen16) on twitter, 2 October 2018. Operation Hypocritical Oath, explained as 'a play on the Hippocratic oath taken by doctors', was reported in https://www.latimes.com/local/lanow/la-me-ln-doctors-opioid-arrests-20190221-story.html accessed 25 February 2019.

10 Carlo Giansanti, @carlocopper, believes that 'Breathing copper clears lungs from any bacteria that enters the body', https://twitter.com/carlocopper, and he regularly repeats variations on this tweet. On rectal examination, Dave Steele, @hullodave. Since April 2018 someone has tweeted as 'Hippocrates', @FirstlyDoNoHarm.

11 Asked by @stuartwilks. All tweets from 31 May 2012.

12 Stubbs and Bligh, *Sixty Centuries of Health and Physick*, 53; Withington, *Medical History from the Earliest Times*, 46.

13 Steven H. Miles, *The Hippocratic Oath and the Ethics of Medicine* (Oxford: Oxford University Press, 2004), 2. The *Oath* is now invoked far more frequently than, for example, in 2004, when Nutton was still able to write that 'Its provisions, however, are usually invoked only in debates about abortion and euthanasia' (*Ancient Medicine*, 333 n.2).

14 Smith, *Pseudepigraphic Writings*, 10–11, n.28. The best recent article on the *Oath* by a historian of ancient medicine remains von Staden, '"In a pure and holy way"'.
15 I owe this reference to Cantor, 'Introduction,' 4; the script for 'Round Springfield' and discussion of the episode is now at https://www.simpsonsarchive.com/episodes/2F32.html accessed 20 February 2019.
16 https://forensicoutreach.com/library/the-deadly-doctor-the-poisonous-pattern-that-gave-harold-shipman-away/ 13 June 2016, accessed 20 February 2019; David Ward and Helen Carter, 'The doctor Jekyll of Hyde', *The Guardian*, 1 February 2000, https://www.theguardian.com/uk/2000/feb/01/shipman.health16 accessed on 20 February 2019. The *Panorama* programme, 'The Man Who Played God', first broadcast on 31 January 2000, is currently available on YouTube, https://www.youtube.com/watch?v=5jHbWGmXcQE accessed 20 February 2019.
17 E.g. http://www.pbs.org/wgbh/nova/body/hippocratic-oath-today.html#modern accessed 20 February 2019.
18 Miles, *Hippocratic Oath*, 2.
19 Nutton, 'What's in an oath?', 518; see also ibid., 'Hippocratic morality and modern medicine' in Helmut Flashar and Jacques Jouanna (eds.), *Médicine et morale dans l'Antiquité: dix exposés suivis de discussions, Genève, Vandoeuvres 1996* (Geneva: Fondation Hardt, Entretiens, 43, 1997).
20 'Hippocratic oath' (2015). *The Hutchinson Unabridged Encyclopedia with Atlas and Weather Guide* (Abington, United Kingdom: Helicon, 2015), online version accessed 20 February 2019.
21 http://www.aegeanislands.gr/islands/kos/KostheHippocraticOath.html; https://prezi.com/ykuf5o7atuz8/hippocrates/; http://www.actforlibraries.org/hippocrates-lived-in-460bc-and-is-still-considered-today-the-greek-father-of-the-of-western-medicine/ all accessed 20 February 2019.
22 Nutton, 'What's in an oath?', 518–19 showed in 1995 that a formal ceremony involving the *Oath* 'is a feature largely of this century'; http://www.amednews.com/article/20060220/profession/302209962/6/ accessed 20 February 2019. The encyclopaedia published under the auspices of the Royal Society of Medicine has it right: 'Although by no means universally used in graduation ceremonies, it is still taken by the graduates of many medical schools' (Robert Youngson, *The Royal Society of Medicine Health Encyclopedia* (London: Bloomsbury, 2000), s.v. 'Hippocratic oath').
23 Wootton, *Bad Medicine*, 2–3.
24 Ibid., 5–6.
25 Ibid., 7–8, 11, 34.
26 Nigel Cameron, 'A future for medicine?' (first published in 1991), in Guinan, *Hippocrates is Not Dead*, 65.

27 Ann Blair, *Too Much to Know: Managing scholarly information before the modern age* (New Haven and London: Yale University Press, 2010), 241.
28 Ibid., 251–6.
29 On 'first do no harm' and *primum non nocere*, see Cedric Smith, 'Origin and uses of *primum non nocere* – above all, do no harm!', *Journal of Clinical Pharmacology*, 45.4 (2005) and Daniel K. Sokol, '"First do no harm" revisited', *BMJ*, 347 (6426) (2013). Diana Cardenas, 'Let not thy food be confused with thy medicine: The Hippocratic misquotation', *e-SPEN Journal* 8 (2013), cites Gerald de Lacey, Carol Record and Jenny Wade, 'How accurate are quotations and references in medical journals?', *BMJ (Clinical Research Ed.)*, 291 (6499) (1985), whose work on a sample of these journals found that 'the original author was misquoted in 15% of all references, and most of the errors would have misled readers' (de Lacey et al., 'How accurate are quotations?', 884).
30 De Lacey et al. 'How accurate are quotations?', 885.
31 Nutton, 'What's in an oath?', 522.
32 Howard Markel, '"I swear by Apollo" – On taking the Hippocratic Oath', *New England Journal of Medicine*, 350.20 (2004), 2026. He further writes (2028), 'as I rise to take the oath with my peers, my heart grows full with reverence for the profession I have chosen'.
33 J. Aaron Johnson, 'The vanishing oath', *Journal of the Medical Society of New Jersey*, 61 (1964); also cited by Dale C. Smith, 'The Hippocratic Oath and modern medicine', *JHM*, 51 (1996), 497.
34 Justin Morgenstern, 'The medical oath: honorable tradition or ancient ritual?', *University of Western Ontario Medical Journal*, 78.1 (2008), 27; rather than abandon all oaths, he suggested that a new one be drawn up to focus on 'the physician's altruistic dedication to his patients' (29).
35 D.C. Smith, 'The Hippocratic Oath and modern medicine', 484–5.
36 Johnson, 'The vanishing oath', 514. On the different versions of the Hippocratic *Oath* currently in use, see http://www.amednews.com/article/20060220/profession/302209962/6/ accessed 20 February 2019; in addition to the 1964 Lasagna version this has one produced in 2005 by the Weill Cornell Medical College. A number of these oaths are collected on http://www.aapsonline.org/ethics/oaths.htm accessed 20 February 2019. Further variants feature in Erich H. Loewy, 'Oaths for physicians: necessary protection or elaborate hoax?', *Medscape General Medicine*, 9.1 (2000), 7. Many studies of regional variation in taking the *Oath* exist; for example, Robert D. Orr, Norman Pang, Edmund D. Pellegrino, D. and Mark Siegler, 'Use of the Hippocratic Oath: A review of twentieth century practice and a content analysis of oaths administered in medical schools in the U.S. and Canada in 1993,' *Journal of Clinical Ethics*, 8 (1997).

37 At the time of writing, Imhotep does not feature in the article, but on 12 October 2011 the article included the line 'There are also claims that point to Imhotep of ancient Egypt as history's first physician'.
38 The Astrochologist presents his form of astrology as 'classic astrology ... a glorious form of astrology that steps away from many of the lousy principles of modern astrology and uses the proven wisdom of the ancients', https://astro-chologist.com/store-2/road-space-find-21st-century-ebook/ accessed 20 February 2019.
39 E.g. Marco Rossi, 'Homer and Herodotus to Egyptian medicine', *Vesalius* Congress Supplement (2010); http://www.vesalius.org.uk/images/issues/specialdic2010.PDF accessed 20 February 2019. Rossi was then in a department of anaesthesia, intensive care and pain medicine.
40 Jacques Jouanna, 'Egyptian medicine and Greek medicine' in Philip van der Eijk (ed.), *Greek Medicine from Hippocrates to Galen. Selected papers* (Leiden and Boston: Brill, 2012), 11 and 18–19; he traces this misguided notion to G. Lefebvre and J.F. Porge, 'La médecine égyptienne' in René Taton (ed.), *La science antique et médiévale. Des origines à 1450* (Paris: Presses Universitaires de France, 1966).
41 18 January 2019, using the hashtags #colonhealthisimportant and #getclean.
42 https://www.ancient.eu/timeline/imhotep/ accessed 20 February 2019.
43 James H. Breasted, *The Edwin Smith Surgical papyrus (facsimile and hieroglyphic transliteration with translation and commentary, in two volumes)* (Chicago: The University of Chicago Press, 1930) repeated for example (without attribution) on https://www.pastmedicalhistory.co.uk/imhotep-the-first-physician/ accessed 20 February 2019.
44 https://www.journeytothesource.info/black_athena.html accessed 20 February 2019. This site's purpose is to show that 'Black Africans were the creators of the entire world's major ancient civilisations', https://www.journeytothesource.info/about.html accessed 4 October 2018.
45 https://en.wikipedia.org/wiki/Imhotep accessed 20 February 2019.
46 James P. Allen, *The Art of Medicine in Ancient Egypt* (New York: Metropolitan Museum of Art and New Haven CT, and London: Yale University Press, 2005), 69; László Kákosy, 'Some problems of the magical healing statues', in Alessandro Roccati and Alberto Siliotti (eds.), *La Magia in Egitto ai tempi dei Faraoni* (Milan: Rassegna Internazionale di Cinematografia Archeologica Arte e Natura Libri, 1987); Campbell Price, 'On the function of "healing" statues' in Campbell Price, Roger Forshaw, Andrew Chamberlain, and Paul Nicholson (eds), *Mummies, Magic and Medicine in Ancient Egypt: Multidisciplinary Essays for Rosalie David* (Manchester: Manchester University Press, 2016).

47 Friedhelm Hoffman, 'Ancient Egypt' in David J. Collins (ed.), *The Cambridge History of Magic and Witchcraft in the West: From antiquity to the present* (Cambridge: Cambridge University Press, 2015), 64.
48 Stubbs and Bligh, *Sixty Centuries of Health and Physick*, 67. Stubbs and Bligh had access to the English translations of the Corpus from the then-unpublished early volumes of the Loeb Classical Library (see Preface, x).
49 Edward T. Withington, *Medical history from the Earliest Times: A popular history of the healing art* (London: The Scientific Press, 1894), 22–3.
50 Garrison, *Introduction to the History of Medicine*, 41.
51 From the title of George G.M. James, *Stolen Legacy: The Egyptian origins of western philosophy* (New York: Philosophical Library, 1954), described by Mary Lefkowitz, *Not Out of Africa: How Afrocentrism Became an Excuse to Teach Myth as History* (New York: Basic Books, 1996), 125 as a nationalistic myth offering 'an explanation for past suffering' and 'a source of ethnic pride'.
52 http://www.blackathena.com/outline.php accessed 20 February 2019. The response of the academy can be summarized in Lefkowitz, *Not Out of Africa*; Mary R. Lefkowitz and Guy Maclean Rogers (eds), *Black Athena Revisited* (Chapel Hill, NC and London: University of North Carolina Press, 1996); and Jacques Berlinerblau, *Heresy in the University: The Black Athena controversy and the responsibilities of American intellectuals* (New Brunswick, NJ: Rutgers University Press, 1999).
53 'Imhotep: the true Father of Medicine', posted 12 July 2015: http://www.afrikanheritage.com/imhotep-the-true-father-of-medicine/ accessed 20 February 2019. The story has been much copied. The source given is 'oakwood.edu' and the Wayback Machine provides evidence of its use up to the end of 2016: http://www.oakwood.edu/historyportal/Research/otherside/imhotep.htm accessed 20 February 2019. A respondent on Quora on 11 October, 2015, referencing the Oakwood piece, states 'Even Hippocrates considered Imhotep to be his mentor' https://www.quora.com/What-are-some-things-invented-by-Africans accessed 20 February 2019. This idea that Hippocrates knew the work of Imhotep is widely shared, for example Jide Uwechia's 'Even Hippocrates so called Greek Father of modern medicine was a devotee of Imhotep the Prince of Peace', https://www.africaresource.com/rasta/sesostris-the-great-the-egyptian-hercules/medical-science-africas-gift-to-the-world/ written 8 June 2007, accessed 20 February 2019.
54 Osler, *Evolution of Modern Medicine*, 10.
55 James H. Brien, 'Imhotep: The real father of medicine? An iconoclastic view', https://www.healio.com/pediatrics/news/blogs/%7B475f0fed-3f4c-4767-9cd7-0725a4e1034d%7D/james-h-brien-do/imhotep-the-real-father-of-medicine-an-iconoclastic-view published 6 October 2014; accessed 20 February 2019. Osler

calls Hippocrates 'Father of Medicine' in *Evolution of Modern Medicine*, 60 and 66. I have found no evidence of him applying the title to Imhotep. Possibly this comes via a casual reading of Ruthie Johnson, *An Abridged History: Africa and her history* (Bloomington IN: Xlibris Corporation, 2014), 96: '[Imhotep] was the real Father of Medicine. He is, says Sir William Osler, "The first figure of a Physician to stand out clearly from the mists of antiquity"'. 'Imhotep the first physician', https://www.pastmedicalhistory.co.uk/imhotep-the-first-physician/ 28 May 2016, accessed 20 February 2019, clearly depends on the same source.

56 http://www.acwbinc.org/icm.html accessed 20 February 2019; a link takes the reader direct to a translation of the Hippocratic *Oath*.

57 Anthony C. Pickett, 'The oath of Imhotep: in recognition of African contributions to Western medicine', *Journal of the National Medical Association*, 84.7 (1992); https://www.ncbi.nlm.nih.gov/pmc/articles/PMC2571702/?page=2 accessed 20 February 2019.

58 The 2005 announcement of £180k in funding and Rosalie David's January 2009 report, 'Pharmacy in ancient Egypt' in 'Awards in focus', are currently not on the Leverhulme Trust site, but the intention is to put up pdf versions in due course. My thanks to Bahia Dawatly for supplying me with the relevant documents.

59 This is an award-winning sustainability project working with the Bedouin community, focused on the 102 medicinal plants grown in the area: a full description following a 2012 award from a United Nations fund can be found on file://userdata/documents5/hk2455/Downloads/ST.%20CATHERINE%20MEDICINAL%20PLANTS%20ASSOCIATION.pdf accessed 20 February 2019. It does not mention the Manchester link.

60 https://www.manchester.ac.uk/discover/news/egyptians-not-greeks-were-true-fathers-of-medicine/ accessed 20 February 2019. There was also a Radio 4 programme on the 'discovery', http://www.bbc.co.uk/radio4/science/thematerialworld_20070503.shtml accessed 20 February 2019.

61 https://web.archive.org/web/20180611171455/http://www.knhcentre.manchester.ac.uk/research/previousandcompletedresearch/pharmacyproject/ accessed 20 February 2019.

62 For my response to similar claims for medieval European medicine, see 'Why I wasn't excited about the medieval remedy that works against MRSA', https://theconversation.com/why-i-wasnt-excited-about-the-medieval-remedy-that-works-against-mrsa-39719, 9 April 2015, accessed 20 February 2019.

63 Roger Highfield, 'How Imhotep gave us medicine', https://www.telegraph.co.uk/news/science/science-news/3293164/How-Imhotep-gave-us-medicine.html, 10 May 2007, accessed 20 February 2019.

64 Ibid. The first phrase here is new; the second two are from the Manchester press release, https://www.manchester.ac.uk/discover/news/egyptians-not-greeks-were-true-fathers-of-medicine/ accessed 20 February 2019: 'Classical scholars have always considered the ancient Greeks, particularly Hippocrates, as being the fathers of medicine but our findings suggest that the ancient Egyptians were practising a credible form of pharmacy and medicine much earlier.'
65 Above, n.58.
66 Highfield, 'How Imhotep gave us medicine'.
67 Ibid.
68 http://www.colourfulradio.com/about accessed 20 February 2019.
69 https://www.africaresource.com/rasta/sesostris-the-great-the-egyptian-hercules/medical-science-africas-gift-to-the-world/, 8 June 2007, accessed 20 February 2019.
70 http://deborahgabriel.com/wp-content/uploads/2013/09/ancient-egyptians-were-fathers-of-medicine15may2007.pdf accessed 20 February 2019. This was written for the Black Britain site, launched in 1998 but no longer operational: https://www.independent.co.uk/arts-entertainment/web-sites-light-and-darkness-underground-and-out-of-the-window-1172339.html.
71 http://deborahgabriel.com/wp-content/uploads/2013/09/ancient-egyptians-were-fathers-of-medicine15may2007.pdf accessed 20 February 2019.
72 Evilena Anastasiou, Anastasia Papathanasiou, Lynne A. Scheparz and Piers D. Mitchell, 'Infectious disease in the ancient Aegean: Intestinal parasitic worms in the Neolithic to Roman Period inhabitants of Kea, Greece', *Journal of Archaeological Science: Reports*, 17 (2018); online version published 14 December 2017.
73 Anastasiou et al., 'Infectious disease in the ancient Aegean', 864.
74 Ibid., 861.
75 Ibid., 860, 861.
76 This reference is Totelin, 'Old recipes, new practices?', which mentions neither humoral medicine, nor the humours. On the humours, see my 'Female fluids in the Hippocratic corpus: how solid was the humoral body?' in Peregrine Horden and Elisabeth Hsu (eds), *The Body in Balance* (New York: Berghahn, 2013).
77 Anastasiou et al., 'Infectious disease in the ancient Aegean', 860. The researchers (862) note that pig roundworm and human roundworm are difficult to distinguish; so it has to be possible that pig dung was present at the sites. The oddly late dating for 'Hippocrates' is on p. 864.
78 Constantinos Trompoukis, Vasilios German and Matthew E. Falagas, 'From the roots of parasitology: Hippocrates' first scientific observations in helminthology', *Journal of Parasitology*, 93.4 (2007).

79 Ibid., 971.
80 https://www.cam.ac.uk/research/news/ancient-faeces-reveal-parasites-described-in-earliest-greek-medical-texts accessed 20 February 2019.
81 https://www.forbes.com/sites/kristinakillgrove/2017/12/15/archaeologists-find-intestinal-worms-in-burials-from-the-time-of-hippocrates/#ea6ebda6c4e6, 15 December 2017, accessed 20 February 2019; tweet from @greekhistorypod, 16 December 2017.
82 @MicrobesInfect and @clasicasIEDA, both tweeted 16 December 2017.
83 Crystal, *Language and the Internet*, 144.
84 https://www.livescience.com/61198-hippocrates-poop-parasites-proof.html, 14 December 2017, accessed 20 February 2019.
85 https://www.newsweek.com/parasitic-worms-described-hippocrates-2500-years-ago-identified-ancient-poop-748949, 15 December 2017, accessed 20 February 2019.
86 https://www.sciencealert.com/hippocrates-worms-confirmed-ancient-greek-faeces, 18 December 2017, accessed 20 February 2019.
87 http://www.dailymail.co.uk/sciencetech/article-5179559/Scientists-discover-parasites-described-Hippocrates.html, 15 December 2017, accessed 20 February 2019.
88 https://www.forbes.com/sites/kristinakillgrove/2017/12/15/archaeologists-find-intestinal-worms-in-burials-from-the-time-of-hippocrates/#39b9e9996c4e, 15 December 2017, accessed 20 February 2019.
89 https://www.newhistorian.com/faeces-reveals-hippocrates-parasites-history-news-week/8427/, 19 December 2018, accessed 20 February 2019.
90 http://mentalfloss.com/article/521052/ancient-poop-contains-first-evidence-parasites-described-hippocrates, 14 December 2017, accessed 20 February 2019.
91 https://www.livescience.com/61198-hippocrates-poop-parasites-proof.html 14 December 2017, accessed 20 February 2019.
92 Loeb, *Hippocrates* X, 165.
93 Loeb, *Hippocrates* VIII, 277; Loeb, *Hippocrates* II, 23.
94 Rush, *Sixteen introductory lectures*, 292; above, p. 40.
95 Cecilia Tasca, Mariangela Rapetti, Mauro Giovanni Carta and Bianca Fadda, 'Women and hysteria in the history of mental health', *Clinical Practice and Epidemiology in Mental Health*, 8 (2012), 111: https://www.ncbi.nlm.nih.gov/pmc/articles/PMC3480686/; blog post by Nadine Ducca, http://www.nadineducca.cat/2016/04/why-women-are-hysterical-etymology.html, 11 April 2016, accessed 20 February 2019 and using as a source Marquette University student Vanessa Traniello's undated report https://academic.mu.edu/meissnerd/hysteria.html accessed 20 February 2019; Robert A. Woodruff, 'Hysteria: an

evaluation of objective diagnostic criteria by the study of women with chronic medical illnesses', *British Journal of Psychiatry*, 114 (1974), 118. I have written elsewhere, on https://mistakinghistories.wordpress.com/2018/08/25/quote-unquote-basic-errors-in-using-the-internet-for-doing-history/, 25 August 2018, accessed 20 February 2019, about the way in which the internet gives authority to simple errors in a student essay.

96 As acknowledged for example by Jean-Philippe Catonné, 'Femmes et hystérie au XIXe siècle', *Annales médico-psychologiques*, 150.10 (1992).

97 King, *Hippocrates' Woman*, 34.

98 The title of a piece for Listverse by Mark Oliver, 3 January 2017, https://listverse.com/2017/01/03/10-disgusting-facts-about-ancient-greek-life/ accessed 20 February 2019, which makes explicit the contrast between the 'fathers of democracy, men of a more civilized time who lived lives of meaning in the pursuit of truth' and the 'difficult, dirty, and often truly disgusting' realities of those lives.

99 Sabine Arnaud, *On Hysteria: The invention of a medical category between 1670 and 1820* (Chicago IL: University of Chicago Press, 2015), 13.

100 Jean-Pierre Luauté, Olivier Saladini, Olivier Walusinski, 'L'arc de cercle des hystériques. Histoire, interprétations', *Annales Médico-Psychologiques*, 173 (2015), 391. The authors discussed their work with an expert on ancient medicine, Danielle Gourevitch. The arc shape, present in a second-century CE description, did not move to the foreground until the medieval period, when it was linked with demonic possession. For a review of the historiography of hysteria, see Mark Micale, *Approaching Hysteria: Disease and its interpretations* (Princeton NJ: Princeton University Press, 1995).

101 Jeffrey M.N. Boss, 'The seventeenth-century transformation of the hysteric affection, and Sydenham's Baconian medicine', *Psychological Medicine*, 9 (1979), 232.

102 Arnaud, *On Hysteria*, 1 and 29.

103 Ibid., 30.

104 Edward Shorter, 'Paralysis – the rise and fall of a "hysterical" symptom', *Journal of Social History*, 19 (1986), 549.

105 Natalie L. Dinsdale and Bernard J. Crespi, 'Revisiting the wandering womb: oxytocin in endometriosis and bipolar disorder', *Hormones and Behavior*, 96.11 (2017), 69.

106 Micale, *Approaching Hysteria*, 220.

107 See my 'Once upon a text: the Hippocratic origins of hysteria' in Sander Gilman, Helen King, Roy Porter, George S. Rousseau and Elaine Showalter, *Hysteria Beyond Freud* (Berkeley CA: University of California Press, 1993), 14–25. On later references to female desire in the history of hysteria, see Arnaud, *On Hysteria*, 73–6.

108 Rachel Maines, *The Technology of Orgasm: "Hysteria", the vibrator and women's sexual satisfaction* (Baltimore, MD: Johns Hopkins University Press, 1999); Felicity Jones quoted in 'Felicity Jones and the buzz about hysteria'. *The Guardian*, 10 September 2012, https://www.theguardian.com/film/2012/sep/10/felicity-jones-hysteria-interview accessed 20 February 2019.

109 Laurinda Dixon, *Perilous Chastity: Women and illness in pre-Enlightenment art and medicine* (Ithaca and London: Cornell University Press, 1995), 240; see my review in *Medical History*, 40 (1996).

110 Discussed in more detail in Helen King, 'Galen and the widow. Towards a history of therapeutic masturbation in ancient gynaecology', *EuGeStA: Journal on Gender Studies in Antiquity*, 1 (2011), 206 citing http://www.austinchronicle.com/books/1999-09-10/73756/, 10 September 1999, accessed 20 February 2019.

111 Lesley Hall, (n.d.). 'Doctors masturbating women as a cure for hysteria/"Victorian vibrators", http://www.lesleyahall.net/factoids.htm#hysteria accessed 20 February 2019.

112 Hallie Lieberman and Eric Schatzberg, 'A failure of academic quality control: *The Technology of Orgasm*', *Journal of Positive Sexuality*, 4.2 (2018), http://journalofpositivesexuality.org/wp-content/uploads/2018/08/Failure-of-Academic-Quality-Control-Technology-of-Orgasm-Lieberman-Schatzberg.pdf accessed 20 February 2019.

113 Discussed in detail in King, 'Galen and the widow'.

114 Charles Daremberg, *Oeuvres anatomiques, physiologiques et médicales de Galien* vol. 2 (Paris: Baillière, 1856); Henri Cesbron, *Histoire critique de l'hystérie* (Paris: Asselin et Houzeau, 1909); Ilza Veith, *Hysteria: The history of a disease* (Chicago: University of Chicago Press, 1965), 38; Andrew Scull, *Hysteria: The disturbing history* (Oxford: Oxford University Press, 2009), 211 on Veith as merely 'a charming relic of an earlier age' on account of the narrowly Freudian approach and 'anachronistic lens'.

115 Vern L. Bullough, 'Masturbation: a historical overview' in Walter O. Bockting and Eli Coleman (eds), *Masturbation as a Means of Achieving Sexual Health* (New York: Haworth Press, 2003), 22.

116 King, 'Galen and the widow', 232.

117 Ibid., 222.

118 https://www.thesun.co.uk/news/6800693/papyrus-mystery-solved-ancient-roman-medical-scroll/, 17 July 2018 accessed 20 February 2019.

119 http://www.dailymail.co.uk/sciencetech/article-5969799/A-mysterious-2-000-year-old-papyrus-finally-decoded-sex-starved-women.html, 19 July 2018 accessed 20 February 2019.

120 https://metro.co.uk/2018/07/19/ancient-scroll-reveals-bonkers-roman-theory-happens-women-starved-sex-7735071/, 19 July 2018 accessed 20 February 2019.
121 https://arstechnica.com/science/2018/07/after-500-years-a-uv-lamp-solves-the-mystery-of-the-basel-papyrus/, 19 July 2018 accessed 20 February 2019.
122 https://www.smithsonianmag.com/smart-news/researchers-unlock-secrets-basel-papyrus-now-identified-late-antiquity-medical-document-180969625/, 13 July 2018 accessed 20 February 2019.
123 Tasca et al., 'Women and hysteria'.
124 Ruth Beier, 'Science and medicine in the social construction of woman: from Aristotle to the corpus callosum', *Transactions and Studies of the College of Physicians of Philadelphia*, 9.4 (1987), 272. As a lecture, this has very few references and none to the Hippocratic treatises.
125 Plinio Prioreschi, *A History of Medicine*, Vol. III, *Roman Medicine* (Omaha: Horatius Press, 1998), 475–8.
126 Mark Bridge, 'Ancient proof of Roman hysteria over too little sex', *The Times*, 24 July 2018.
127 https://arstechnica.com/science/2018/07/after-500-years-a-uv-lamp-solves-the-mystery-of-the-basel-papyrus/, 19 July 2018 accessed 20 February 2019.
128 Original press release, 12 July 2018, https://www.unibas.ch/en/News-Events/News/Uni-Research/Mystery-of-the-Basel-papyrus-solved.html.
129 Blair, *Too Much to Know*, 93.
130 Leah Graham and P. Takis Metaxas, 'Of course it's true; I saw it on the Internet: critical thinking in the Internet era', *Communications of the ACM,* 46.5 (2003), 72.
131 Ibid., 72–3.
132 Susan Gerhart, 'Do Web search engines suppress controversy?', *First Monday*, 9.1 (2004), https://firstmonday.org/article/view/1111/1031 accessed 20 February 2019 citing Steve Lawrence and C. Lee Giles, 'Accessibility and Distribution of Information on the Web,' *Nature*, 400 (6740) (1999). See also Graham and Metaxas, 'Of course it's true', 73.
133 https://eu.tennessean.com/story/money/tech/2014/05/02/jj-rosen-popular-search-engines-skim-surface/8636081/ accessed 20 February 2019.
134 Loeb, *Hippocrates* XI, 301–3; http://www.stoa.org/diotima/anthology/wlgr/wlgr-medicine345.shtml.
135 King, 'Hysteria from Hippocrates', 15.
136 Nancy Scheper-Hughes and Margaret M. Lock, 'The mindful body: a prolegomenon to future work in medical anthropology', *Medical Anthropology Quarterly*, 1 (1987).

137 Edward H. Reynolds, 'Review Article. Hysteria in ancient civilisations: A neurological review. Possible significance for the modern disorder', *Journal of the Neurological Sciences*, 388 (15 May 2018).
138 Ibid., 208.
139 Ibid., 208.
140 Eliot Slater, 'Diagnosis of hysteria,' *BMJ* I (1965), 1399 and 1396.
141 Ibid., 1452 on Francis Walshe, 'Diagnosis of hysteria,' *BMJ*, II (1965).
142 Jon Stone, Charles Warlow, Alan Carson and Michael Sharpe, 'Eliot Slater's myth of the non-existence of hysteria,' *Journal of the Royal Society of Medicine*, 98.12 (2005), 547–8.
143 'Translation and analysis of a cuneiform text forming part of a Babylonian treatise on epilepsy', *Medical History*, 34 (1990). They met in 1987 at a symposium celebrating Kinnier Wilson's father; Reynolds and J.V. Kinnier Wilson, 'Neurology and psychiatry in Babylon', *Brain*, 137 (2014), 2612.
144 Reynolds and Kinnier Wilson, 'Translation and analysis', 193.
145 Ibid., 194–5.
146 Ibid., 195.
147 Ibid., 195.
148 JoAnn Scurlock, 'Marginalia to Mesopotamian malevolent magic', *Journal of the American Oriental Society*, 133.3 (2013), 537.
149 Marten Stol, *Epilepsy in Babylonia* (Groningen: Styx, 1993), preface.
150 Reynolds and Kinnier Wilson, 'Neurology and psychiatry'.
151 Ibid., 2613. JoAnn Scurlock, 'Physician, exorcist, conjurer, magician: a tale of two healing professionals' in Karel van der Toorn and Tzvi Abusch (eds), *Mesopotamian Magic* (Groningen: Styx, 1999), 75–6; Scurlock, 'Marginalia to Mesopotamian malevolent magic', 537, 'I stick to my guns on this issue'.
152 Scurlock, 'Physician, exorcist, conjurer, magician', 77–8. She explicitly rejects the label 'exorcist'.
153 Reynolds and Kinnier Wilson, 'Neurology and psychiatry', 2614.
154 King, 'Once upon a text', 4.
155 Reynolds, 'Hysteria in ancient civilisations', 209.
156 http://emel-library.org/projects-2/ accessed 20 February 2019.
157 https://news.nationalgeographic.com/2017/07/hippocrates-manuscript-sinai-palimpsests-st-catherines-monastery-spd/ and http://www.ancient-origins.net/news-history-archaeology/hippocratic-medical-recipe-lost-famous-egyptian-monastery-finally-comes-021500; https://www.ancient-origins.net/news-history-archaeology/hippocratic-medical-recipe-lost-famous-egyptian-monastery-finally-comes-021500 has 'lost'; http://orthochristian.com/104984.html, 7 July 2017 used 'unknown'. All accessed 20 February 2019.

158 https://www.ancient-origins.net/news-history-archaeology/hippocratic-medical-recipe-lost-famous-egyptian-monastery-finally-comes-021500 accessed 20 February 2019.

159 https://news.nationalgeographic.com/2017/07/hippocrates-manuscript-sinai-palimpsests-st-catherines-monastery-spd/, 11 July 2017, accessed 20 February 2019; in another version, this is 'a few centuries after his death' and he 'penned' the *Oath*, https://allthatsinteresting.com/hippocrates-ancient-text, 12 July 2017, updated 4 May 2018, accessed 20 February 2019.

160 https://eng-archive.aawsat.com/waleed-abdul-rahman/lifestyle-culture/egypt-rare-manuscript-discovered-saint-catherine-monastery accessed 20 February 2019; https://www.realmofhistory.com/2017/07/08/hippocrates-medical-recipe-st-catherines-monastery/ accessed 20 February 2019. http://orthochristian.com/104984.html uses 'palmezit'.

161 https://allthatsinteresting.com/hippocrates-ancient-text, 12 July 2017 updated 4 May 2018, accessed 20 February 2019.

162 https://eng-archive.aawsat.com/waleed-abdul-rahman/lifestyle-culture/egypt-rare-manuscript-discovered-saint-catherine-monastery accessed 20 February 2019.

163 https://www.thetimes.co.uk/article/latest-detox-diet-from-hippocrates-3gmg3g2x6, 14 July 2017, accessed 20 February 2019.

164 http://sinaipalimpsests.org/palimpsests-and-scholarship and http://emel-library.org/meet-us/ both accessed 20 February 2019.

165 https://www.biblicalarchaeology.org/scholars-study/did-morton-smith-forge-secret-mark/, 14 October 2009, accessed 20 February 2019.

166 https://www.livestrong.com/article/316511-homemade-detox-for-weight-loss/ accessed 20 February 2019.

167 Healing Arts Press, 2002. On the author see http://www.carrielesperance.com/ accessed 20 February 2019.

168 https://hippocratesinst.org/ accessed 8 October 2018.

169 For a discussion of the origin of the term 'meme', see Schultze and Bytwerk, 'Plausible quotations and reverse credibility', 226–7.

Chapter 5

1 https://every48.com/2014/09/05/fitness-meme-of-the-week-hippocrates-was-right/ accessed 20 February 2019.

2 Vivian Nutton, 'Review of A. Anastassiou and D. Irmer, *Testimonien zum Corpus Hippocraticum*, Teil I,' *Gnomon*, 80 (2008), cited in van der Eijk, 'On "Hippocratic" and "non-Hippocratic" medical writings', 19.

3   https://www.drjohnlapuma.com/chefmd-video-wall/ and https://www.drjohnlapuma.com/about/ accessed 20 February 2019. Dr La Puma has confirmed to me that he is not responsible for the addition of the quotes (pers. comm.).
4   Daniel E. Moerman, 'Minding the body: the placebo effect unmasked' in Maxine Sheets-Johnstone (ed.), *Giving the Body Its Due* (Albany NY: SUNY Press, 1992), 74. The sensory aspects of medication are picked up in a Science Daily feature on how the colour and shape of pills 'affects how patients feel about their medication', 19 January 2011, accessed 20 February 2019; https://www.sciencedaily.com/releases/2010/11/101115110959.htm.
5   E.g. http://thejourneytogoodhealth.blogspot.com/2013/02/let-your-food-be-your-medicine.html accessed 20 February 2019.
6   https://www.snopes.com/fact-check/the-doctor-of-the-future/, 25 January 2015, accessed 20 February 2019.
7   https://drhyman.com/, accessed 20 February 2019. The banner version is 'Your fork, the most powerful tool to transform your health and change the world.'
8   Martha Stewart's *Whole Living* magazine closed in 2012; https://www.wsj.com/articles/SB10001424127887324640104578163763713103532 accessed 20 February 2019.
9   In the interests of the reader's sanity, from this point I shall drop the scare quotes around 'quote'; they are still in my mind, and I hope in yours too.
10 Blair, *Too Much to Know*, 256.
11 Earle Havens, *Commonplace Books: A history of manuscripts and printed books from antiquity to the twentieth century* (New Haven CT: Yale University Press, 2001), the catalogue of an exhibition described at http://beinecke.library.yale.edu/exhibitions/commonplace-books-manuscripts-and-printed-books-antiquity-twentieth-century accessed 20 February 2019.
12 Erasmus, *De Copia*, 636 and 638, cited by Heidi Brayman Hackel, *Reading Material in Early Modern England: Print, gender, and literacy* (Cambridge: Cambridge University Press, 2005), 147.
13 Ann Moss, *Printed Commonplace-Books and the Structuring of Renaissance Thought* (Oxford: Oxford University Press, 1996), 114.
14 Victoria E. Burke, 'Recent studies in commonplace books', *English Literary Renaissance*, 43.1 (2013), 158 on Rebecca W. Bushnell's discussion of the metaphor of the garden, which appears in her 'Harvesting books' in Bushnell, *A Culture of Teaching: Early modern humanism in theory and practice* (Cornell University Press, 1996), 135–6.
15 Burke, 'Recent studies in commonplace books', 156.
16 John Bartlett, *A Collection of Familiar Quotations: With complete indices of authors and subjects* (Cambridge: the author, 1856), 288.

17 Blair, *Too Much to Know*, 14–15; Seneca considered that one should stick with a small number of books and re-read them, whereas Francis Bacon used the same tag to suggest the benefits of the accumulation of knowledge.
18 M. Prefontaine, *The Big Book of Quotes: Funny, inspirational and motivational quotes on life, love and much else* (Isle of Man: MP Publishing, 2015).
19 https://www.amazon.com/Big-Book-Quotes-Inspirational-Motivational-ebook/dp/B015UM59T4 accessed 20 February 2019.
20 Schultze and Bytwerk, 'Plausible quotations', 219.
21 Gary Saul Morson, *The Words of Others: From quotations to culture* (New Haven and London: Yale University Press, 2011), 24 and 49.
22 Kate Eichhorn, 'Archival genres: gathering texts and reading spaces', *Invisible Culture: An electronic journal for visual culture*, 12 (2008). Burke, 'Recent studies in commonplace books', provides a very useful overview. Commonplace books as blogs also feature on http://webcentre.co.nz/kk/commonplace.htm accessed 20 February 2019.
23 Blair, *Too Much to Know*.
24 Ralph Keyes, 'The quote verifier', *The Antioch Review*, 64.2 (2006), 263.
25 Crystal, *Language and the Internet*, 216.
26 Milton Mayer, *They Thought They Were Free: The Germans, 1933–45* (Chicago: University of Chicago Press, 1966) famously coined the word 'contextomy' – using the image of surgical excision – to describe how Julius Streicher, editor of the 1930s and 1940s anti-Semitic newspaper *Der Stürmer*, would take decontextualized lines from the Jewish Talmud, and print them in his paper to claim that the Jewish people intended to embark upon mass murder. Matthew S. McGlone, 'Quoted out of context: contextomy and its consequences', *Journal of Communication*, 55.2 (2005), 332 demonstrated how, 'although rarely employed to this malicious extreme, contextomy is a common method of misrepresentation in contemporary mass media.'
27 Marjorie Garber, *Quotation Marks* (London and New York: Routledge, 2003), 42. She also notes that Austen's title, *Pride and Prejudice*, now means 'more or less the opposite of what it did' when 'pride' meant privilege (207–8).
28 https://todayinsci.com/H/Hippocrates/Hippocrates-Quotations.htm accessed 20 February 2019; this has forty-one Hippocratic quotes on science, fourteen on medicine, and so on, although there is duplication within and between the lists.
29 https://en.wikiquote.org/wiki/Hippocrates accessed 11 October 2018.
30 Examples of these sites include www.brainyquote.com, https://www.goodreads.com/quotes/search?utf8=%E2%9C%93&q=hippocrates&commit=Search (where 'Let food be thy medicine and medicine be thy food' is currently running at 936 likes), www.quotegarden.com, https://en.wikiquote.org/wiki/Main_Page all

accessed 20 February 2019. On print media, see Ruth Finnegan, *Why Do We Quote? The culture and history of quotation* (Cambridge: Open Book Publishers, 2011), 116–20 on the creation and development of the *Oxford Dictionary of Quotations*.
31 Keyes, 'The quote verifier', 257.
32 Marc Galanter, *Cults: Faith, healing, and coercion*, second edition (Oxford and New York: Oxford University Press, 1999), 214.
33 Herbert H. Clark and Richard J. Gerrig, 'Quotations as demonstrations', *Language*, 66.4 (1990), 769 and 792.
34 Garber, *Quotation Marks*, 2 and 11.
35 Finnegan, *Why Do We Quote?*, 241; also widely quoted online.
36 Prefontaine, *The Big Book of Quotes*, 365.
37 https://www.brainyquote.com/quotes/hippocrates_125445 accessed 20 February 2019, attributes the Chaucer wording to Hippocrates.
38 Keyes, 'The quote verifier', 256.
39 Jim Holt, 'Science resurrects God', *Wall Street Journal* (24 December 1997), https://www.wsj.com/articles/SB882911317496560000 accessed 20 February 2019; because Holt is 'an American philosopher and a best-selling author, others think he must be reliable, e.g. Amna, 'Did Einstein really believe in God?', https://gadgtecs.com/2017/01/02/einstein-believed-god/ asserting that 'not every quote that is hard to believe is a false attribution', or http://2012daily.com/?q=node/16 citing 'Holt 1997' as its source, both accessed 20 February 2019.
40 Schultze and Bytwerk, 'Plausible quotations', 220.
41 https://en.wikipedia.org/wiki/Standing_on_the_shoulders_of_giants and http://wiki.c2.com/?ShouldersOfGiants, accessed 20 February 2019; see also, e.g., https://www.brainyquote.com/quotes/isaac_newton_135885 and Finnegan, *Why Do We Quote?* 241.
42 Morson, *Words of Others*, 130–1.
43 Ibid., 94.
44 Ibid., 18.
45 Ibid., 79 and 91.
46 Ibid., 57 and 65.
47 http://www.washingtontimes.com/news/2014/may/16/ammon-obamacare-versus-the-hippocratic-oath/, 16 May 2014, accessed 20 February 2019.
48 Quotation from Tony Briffa, 'Intersex variations: Western medicine and the Hippocratic Oath', 28 September 2018, http://archermagazine.com.au/2018/09/intersex-variations-western-medicine-and-the-hippocratic-oath/ accessed 20 February 2019. The problem is acknowledged by Miles, *Hippocratic Oath*, 143.
49 http://www.answers.com/Q/what_did_the_hippocrates_do accessed 20 February 2019.

50 This is from Michael North's 2002 translation on https://www.nlm.nih.gov/hmd/greek/greek_oath.html accessed 20 February 2019.

51 Almost correctly attributed at https://en.wikiquote.org/wiki/Hippocrates accessed 20 February 2019 although it gives Chapter 2 not Chapter 11 which links to the Adams translation on Wikisource, here given as 'have two special objects in view with regard to disease, namely, to do good or to do no harm', https://en.wikisource.org/wiki/Of_the_Epidemics#Section_Two accessed 20 February 2019.

52 Parsons, *Doing Harm*, 39.

53 Ibid., 40.

54 Elizabeth Vandiver, *Stand in the Trench, Achilles: Classical receptions in British poetry of the Great War* (Oxford: Oxford University Press, 2010), 45.

55 https://www.imdb.com/title/tt8490842/ accessed 20 February 2019: the 'trivia' for the episode on IMdb read 'The episode title, "Primum Non Nocere", is Latin for "First, do no harm", an important ethical rule in the medical profession, meaning "even if you can't make the patient any better, at least make sure you don't make him any worse"'. *Assassin's Creed: Odyssey*, episode 'First Do No Harm': extract on http://www.ign.com/videos/2018/08/08/assassins-creed-odyssey-12-minutes-of-exclusive-mission-gameplay, accessed 20 February 2019.

56 John Fabre, 'Medicine as a profession: Hip, Hip, Hippocrates: extracts from *The Hippocratic Doctor*,' *BMJ*, 315 (7123) (1997), 1669–70.

57 Cedric M. Smith, 'Origin and uses of *primum non nocere* – above all, do no harm!' *Journal of Clinical Pharmacology*, 45.4 (2005). While only the abstract is currently outside the paywall, this alone dates the first print use to 1860, with the phrase attributed to Thomas Sydenham. An online account of the non-Hippocratic nature of the phrase is available at https://www.thoughtco.com/first-do-no-harm-hippocratic-oath-118780 accessed 20 February 2019.

58 Smith, 'Origin and uses of *primum non nocere*', 371. In Parsons' *Doing Harm*, 40, Galen is claimed as the one who 'coined the Latin variation'.

59 Smith, 'Origin and uses of *primum non nocere*', 375.

60 Ibid., 376.

61 Richards is a retired editor who worked with a medical journal. Reprinted on https://piedtype.com/2011/08/15/first-do-no-harm-is-not-in-the-hippocratic-oath/, 15 August 2011, accessed 20 February 2019.

62 https://www.thoughtco.com/first-do-no-harm-hippocratic-oath-118780, 20 September 2018, accessed 20 February 2019.

63 Sokol, '"First do no harm" revisited', 347. Smith is not listed in the references but they are the ones used by him. See pp. 103 and 120 for the hazards of doing this sort of survey work, as applied to Google Books.

64 Reviewed on https://www.theguardian.com/books/2014/mar/19/do-no-harm-brain-surgery-henry-marsh-review accessed 20 February 2019.
65 Miles, *Hippocratic Oath*, 144; https://www.health.harvard.edu/blog/first-do-no-harm-201510138421, 13 October 2015, accessed 20 February 2019. Similar points are made in Parsons, *Doing Harm*, 40–1.
66 Miles, *Hippocratic Oath*, 144.
67 https://www.imdb.com/title/tt0118526/ accessed 20 February 2019.
68 On how the diet works see for example Jong M. Rho, 'How does the ketogenic diet induce anti-seizure effects?', *Neuroscience Letters*, 637.1 (2017).
69 Reviewer ryanlupin, 10 December 2004, https://www.imdb.com/title/tt0118526/reviews?ref_=tt_ov_rt accessed 20 February 2019. Another reviewer also talks about how the story encourages 'people who need to take back responsibility for their families' health'.
70 Von Staden, '"In a pure and holy way"'; compare Nutton, 'What's in an oath?', 519 on early variants on the *Oath* which omitted the references so that 'The doctor no longer has any obligations, financial or otherwise, to his [sic] colleagues.'
71 Full movie currently available on https://www.youtube.com/watch?v=HyeC9IiFKpw accessed 20 February 2019. For a collection of versions of the *Oath* which could lie behind this creation, see http://www.aapsonline.org/ethics/oaths.htm accessed 20 February 2019.
72 Discussed by Lederer, 'Hippocrates American style', 252–3; the film was based on the best-selling novel of 1935, by Lloyd C. Douglas.
73 Julia Hubbel, 'How doctors manage to make us even sicker: the problem with being female and needing healthcare,' https://medium.com/@jhubbel/how-doctors-manage-to-make-us-even-sicker-a3c83d1d3d96, 31 July 2018 accessed 20 February 2019.
74 'How to be good in restaurants,' *Sunday Times Magazine*, 27 October 2018, 72.
75 https://academic.oup.com/occmed/article/62/5/320/1490801 accessed 20 February 2019.
76 https://food.unl.edu/documents/family-fun/2014%20August%20Newsletter%20Cardiac%20Walking.pdf; http://sites.macewan.ca/sportandwellness/2014/05/01/walking-is-mans-best-medicine-hippocrates/ published 1 May 2014; http://www.geneva-fit.com/Walking-is-mans-best-medicine---Hippocrates published 2 June 2017; all accessed 20 February 2019.
77 https://www.naturalnews.com/Quote-Walking-Best-Medicine-Hippocrates.html# accessed 20 February 2019.
78 https://www.psychologytoday.com/gb/blog/the-athletes-way/201506/hippocrates-was-right-walking-is-the-best-medicine, posted 12 June 2015, accessed 20 February 2019.

79 https://en.wikipedia.org/wiki/Talk:Hippocrates, 8 October 2017, accessed 20 February 2019.
80 https://every48.files.wordpress.com/2014/09/9_05_14_hippocrates-meme.gif accessed 20 February 2019. The ellipsis is not in the original; there are no words omitted here. On the relationship between food and exercise in the Hippocratic Corpus, see Hynek Bartoš, *Philosophy and Dietetics in the Hippocratic* On Regimen: *A delicate balance of health* (Leiden and Boston: Brill, 2015).
81 Galen, *Alim. Fac.* 1.1 (Helmreich 213.6–8), trans. Grant.
82 Tipton, 'The history of "Exercise Is Medicine" in ancient civilizations', *Advances in Physiology Education*, 38.2 (2014); https://www.ncbi.nlm.nih.gov/pmc/articles/PMC4056176/ accessed 20 February 2019. On the EIM initiative, see https://www.exerciseismedicine.org/support_page.php/about-eim5/ and the 2017 conference site of the European version of the scheme, http://exerciseismedicine.eu/ accessed 20 February 2019.
83 Jack W. Berryman, 'Exercise is Medicine: A historical perspective', *Current Sports Medicine Reports*, 9.4, July-August 2010; https://depts.washington.edu/bhdept/facres/CurrSports%20Med%20Reports.pdf accessed 20 February 2019.
84 Tipton, 'Exercise Is Medicine', 109.
85 https://www.ncbi.nlm.nih.gov/pmc/articles/PMC4056176/ accessed 20 February 2019.
86 Adams, *Genuine Works* Vol. 1, 285 (*Regimen in Acute Diseases*, part 3); http://classics.mit.edu/Hippocrates/acutedis.3.3.html accessed 20 February 2019.
87 *Regimen in Acute Diseases*, 9 (the division of sections is entirely different to that used by Littré and then by Adams); Loeb, *Hippocrates* II, 71.
88 *Diseases* 2, 48 and 49 (Loeb, *Hippocrates* V, 281).
89 *Internal Affections*, 10 (Loeb, *Hippocrates* VI, 105).
90 *Internal Affections*, 12 (Loeb, *Hippocrates* VI, 111). One stade is 185 metres.
91 Nikitas Nomikos, C. Trompoukis, Chris Lamprou, and G. Nomikos, 'The role of exercise in Hippocratic medicine', *American Journal of Sports Science and Medicine*, 4 (2016); http://pubs.sciepub.com/ajssm/4/4/6/ accessed 20 February 2019. The standard of English in this article is poor, and cries out for the intervention of an editor.
92 There is also '*Regimen* VII' which does not exist; this confusion arises because here the VII is a chapter number rather than a treatise identifier. The authors appear to think that all the Hippocratic texts with 'Regimen' in the title are part of one treatise.
93 Nomikos et al., 'The role of exercise', 115 and 117.
94 *Regimen* 2, 63 (Loeb, *Hippocrates* IV, 353–5). See also the advice on 'plenty of natural exercises and long runs with the cloak worn' in *Regimen* 4, 69 (Loeb, *Hippocrates* IV, 431).

95 Lesley Dean-Jones, 'Too much of a good thing: the health of Olympic athletes in ancient Greece', in Susan E. Brownell (ed.), *From Athens to Beijing: West Meets East in the Olympic Games*, Vol. I: *Sport, the Body and Humanism in Ancient Greece and China* (New York: Greekworks, 2013).
96 *Places in Man*, 35 (Loeb, *Hippocrates* VIII, 77).
97 Nomikos et al., 'The role of exercise', 116; *Regimen* 2, 62 (Loeb, *Hippocrates* IV, 351).
98 *Regimen* 2, 61 (Loeb, *Hippocrates* IV, 349).
99 Bernard Jensen, *Foods That Heal: A guide to understanding and using the healing powers of natural foods* (New York: Penguin Books, 1988), xii and 3.
100 Ibid., 4.

Chapter 6

1 The dietician and wellness nutritionist Kristin Kirkpatrick, '9 amazing benefits of coffee', https://www.huffingtonpost.com/kristin-kirkpatrick-ms-rd-ld/coffee-health-benefits_b_2962490.html?guccounter=1, 4 April 2013, accessed 20 February 2019: widely copied online.
2 Merchandise offered on https://www.zazzle.co.uk/let+food+be+thy+medicine+gifts accessed 20 February 2019.
3 http://www.digitaljournal.com/pr/3864905#ixzz5N0Ch04jI accessed 20 February 2019.
4 http://wiki.answers.com/Q/Did_Hippocrates_say_let_food_by_thy_medicine_and_medicine_by_thy_food accessed 20 February 2019.
5 Adidas Wilson, *The Alkaline Diet CookBook: The alkaline meal plan to balance your pH, reduce body acid, lose weight and have amazing health* (self-published, 2013), 1.
6 https://hermeticahealth.me/2012/09/06/the-doctor-aka-my-dad/ 6 September 2012 accessed 20 February 2019. The spelling error also appears on, *inter alia*, https://www.sacredsparklez.com/nutrition-and-food/ and https://holmanhealthconnections.com/let-food-be-thy medicine/ accessed 20 February 2019 but this page is not dated, so it is unclear who is copying whom or whether this is just a common mistake.
7 https://agnostic.com/post/173278/i-am-into-the-hippocrates-maxim-make-food-your-medicine-and-make-medicine-your-food-if-you-can accessed 25 October 2018.
8 Juliana Adelman and Lisa Haushoffer, 'Introduction: Food as medicine, medicine as food', *JHM*, 73.2 (2018).
9 Ibid., 130.
10 Richard Caton, 'Hippocrates and the newly-discovered health temple of Cos', *BMJ*, 10 March (1906), 572.

11 Jacques Jouanna, 'Regimen in the Hippocratic corpus: *diaita* and its problems', in DJR, 214.
12 Bartoš, *Philosophy and Dietetics*, 34; Manetti, *Anonymus Londinensis*. For *On Ancient Medicine*, see most recently Ralph Rosen, 'Towards a Hippocratic anthropology: *On Ancient Medicine* and the origins of humans', in DJR. On the range of meanings of the Greek *diaita*, see Jouanna, 'Regimen in the Hippocratic corpus', 211–16.
13 Celsus, *On Medicine*, preface 9; discussed by Totelin, 'When foods become remedies in ancient Greece: The curious case of garlic and other substances', *Journal of Ethnopharmacology*, 167 (2015), 34 as 'not quite present in the Hippocratic treatises themselves'.
14 Saumell, 'New lights on the *Anonymus Londiniensis*', 133–4, n.68; Jouanna, 'Regimen in the Hippocratic corpus', 224.
15 Anon. Lond. 7.15–24. See Manetti, *Anonymus Londiniensis* and, for an English translation, W.H.S. Jones, *The Medical Writings of Anonymus Londinensis* (Cambridge: Cambridge University Press, 1947).
16 Bartoš, *Philosophy and Dietetics in the Hippocratic* On Regimen, 16.
17 Totelin, 'When foods become remedies', 32 citing the ps-Aristotelian *Problems* 842b.
18 Use of 'our'; e.g. an academic site for an Institute of Nutrition Science, https://www.nyas.org/media/14916/sackler-institute-brochure.pdf but also on fitness quotes sites such as http://www.theiflife.com/top-health-fitness-quotes/; 'Eat your food like your medicines or else you will eat your medicines like food', https://www.practo.com/healthfeed/eat-your-food-like-medicine-27500/post; https://nhchaltonoakville.wordpress.com/, 1 October 2017: also on https://www.amazingdietsolutions.com/just-one-tablespoon-of-extra-virgin-olive-oil-every-morning-is-super-healthy-for-you-here-is-why/, 20 February 2018, all accessed 20 February 2019.
19 Lindsay M. Jaacks and Alexandra L. Bellows, 'Let food be thy medicine: linking local food and health systems to address the full spectrum of malnutrition in low-income and middle-income countries', *BMJ Global Health*, 2.4 (2017); http://gh.bmj.com/content/2/4/e000564 accessed 20 February 2019.
20 http://healthyhomecafe.com/let-food-be-thy-medicine/ accessed 20 February 2019. The 'let food by thy medicine' version is also that used by Brian Clement, *Supplements Exposed: The truth they don't want you to know about vitamins, minerals, and their effects on your health* (Franklin Lakes NJ: The Career Press, 2010), 88; is the typo a clue to who copied whom?
21 Curry soup: https://bestwinterhavencoffeehouse.wordpress.com/2017/01/17/curry-soup-and-glaucoma-let-food-by-thy-medicine-and-medicine-thy-food-hippocrates/ accessed 20 February 2019. Celery: '"Let food be thy medicine and

medicine be thy food." So goes the well-known quote attributed to Hippocrates, the ancient Greek physician who is sometimes referred to as the father of Western medicine. Whenever we include celery in our meals, we are doing just what Hippocrates advised', http://www.theepochtimes.com/n3/75933-celery-the-balancer/ accessed 20 February 2019.

22 https://sciencebasedmedicine.org/let-food-be-thy-medicine-and-medicine-be-thy-food-the-fetishism-of-medicinal-foods/ accessed 20 February 2019. The article is introduced by: 'Let food be thy medicine and medicine be thy food – attributed to Hippocrates. Who said anything about medicine? Let's eat! – attributed to one of Hippocrates forgotten (and skeptical) students'.

23 *Vegetarian Times*, January 1988, 19.

24 Martin Luther Holbrook, *Eating for Strength, or, Food and Diet in Their Relation to Health and Work* (New York: M.L. Holbrook and Co, 1888), Preface and 34.

25 https://christyharrison.com/foodpsych/4/how-to-leave-the-religion-of-dieting-with-alan-levinovitz accessed 20 February 2019.

26 Louis Rosenfeld, 'Vitamine—vitamin. The early years of discovery', *Clinical Chemistry*, 43.4 (1997).

27 https://draxe.com/food-is-medicine/ accessed 20 February 2019.

28 See for example https://www.practo.com/healthfeed/eat-your-food-like-medicine-27500/post accessed 20 February 2019. In a recent online article, 'Hippocrates would have wanted you to eat cake', 15 February 2019, Sarah Scullin examined 'appeals to antiquity in fad dieting': https://eidolon.pub/hippocrates-would-have-wanted-you-to-eat-cake-d5127ca40e09 accessed 20 February 2019.

29 Jouanna, 'Regimen in the Hippocratic corpus,' 225–6.

30 http://www.answers.com/Q/FAQ/8893 accessed 20 February 2019.

31 'A note from Steven Gundry' on https://goop.com/wellness/health/uncensored-a-word-from-our-doctors/?utm_source=impactradius&utm_medium=affiliate&utm_campaign=10079_OnlineTrackingLink&irgwc=1 accessed 20 February 2019.

32 Rob Kutch, 'A weight loss idea on the edge . . . Part One', 6 February 2013, https://renovatingyourmind.com/2013/02/06/a-weight-loss-ideas-on-the-edge-part-one/ accessed 20 February 2019.

33 Rob Kutch, 'Imagine doctors writing out a prescription for healthy foods to prevent disease', 11 April 2004, https://renovatingyourmind.com/2014/04/11/imagine-doctors-writing-out-a-prescriptions-for-healthy-foods-to-prevent-disease/ accessed 20 February 2019.

34 'Dr Hip Pocrates' was the nickname of Eugene Schoenfeld, a 1960s advice columnist, and there is a song entitled 'Dr Hip' by Country Joe McDonald; Cantor, 'Western medicine since the Renaissance', 383. Kutch also chats with Shakespeare

and Einstein: https://renovatingyourmind.com/2017/02/21/love-on-a-quantum-entanglement-scale-featuring-alcoholic-hallucinations-with-shakespeare-and-einstein/ accessed 20 February 2019.
35 Kutch, 'Imagine doctors writing out a prescription'.
36 'Let food be thy medicine: Nutrition for inflammation', http://www.fitnessnetwork.com.au/resources-library/let-food-be-thy-medicine-nutrition-for-inflammation accessed 20 February 2019.
37 ἐν τροφῇ φαρμακείη ἄριστον, ἐν τροφῇ φαρμακείη φλαῦρον, φλαῦρον καὶ ἄριστον πρός τι.
38 W.H.S. Jones, 'Introduction' to *On Nutriment* in Loeb, *Hippocrates I*, 338–9.
39 Heinrich von Staden, *Herophilus: the Art of Medicine in Early Alexandria: Edition, Translation and Essays* (Cambridge: Cambridge University Press, 1989), 77.
40 Totelin, 'When foods become remedies', 31.
41 Jones, 'Introduction', 337 and 340.
42 Adams, *The Genuine Works of Hippocrates*, 117.
43 John Chadwick and William Mann, *The Medical Works of Hippocrates* (Oxford: Blackwell, 1950), 2; currently online in the Penguin version in full at https://storage.googleapis.com/global-help-publications/books/help_hippocraticwritings.pdf accessed 20 February 2019.
44 Menahem Luz, 'The philosophical background of Hippocrates' *On Nutriment*' in Konstantine J. Boudouris (ed.), *Philosophy and Medicine Vol. I* (Alimos: Ionia Publications, 1998), 117–18.
45 Above, Chapter 2; Smith, *Hippocratic Tradition*, 13.
46 Smith, *Hippocratic Tradition*, 73.
47 Mark Grant, *Galen on Food and Diet* (London and New York: Routledge, 2000), 6.
48 Galen, *On the Powers of Foods* (K VI 467.14–468.4); Grant, *Galen on Food and Diet*, 73.
49 Ibid., 74.
50 Ibid., 73.
51 Diana Cardenas, 'Let Not Thy Food Be Confused with Thy Medicine: The Hippocratic misquotation,' *E-SPEN, The European e-Journal of Clinical Nutrition and Metabolism*, 8 (6) (December 1, 2013), 260; currently available as a free download from Researchgate.
52 Ibid., 261.
53 https://honey-guide.com/2017/10/31/hippocratic-misquotations-let-thy-quotations-not-be-by-hippocrates/ accessed 20 February 2019. The methodological problems of using Ngram in this way are addressed by Eitan Adam Pechenick, Christopher M. Danforth and Peter Sheridan Dodd, 'Characterizing the Google Books Corpus: Strong limits to inferences of socio-cultural and linguistic

54 *Public Opinion*, 130 (1921), 562.
55 Pers. comm.
56 Anon., 'To Correspondents,' *The People's Medical Journal, and Family Physician*, 8.1 (1850), 64.
57 Other references given by Popik include a story in the 22 July 1913 Kansas City, MO *Star*, without the name of Hippocrates: https://www.barrypopik.com/index.php/new_york_city/entry/let_food_be_your_medicine_and_medicine_be_your_food, 26 March 2013, accessed 20 February 2019.
58 Keating n.d. Chiropractors often use a Hippocratic 'quote' to lend authority to their theories: 'Oddly enough it was Hippocrates, widely regarded as the Father of (Western) Medicine who said, "First and foremost, look to the spine for the cause of disease". It seems that Hippocrates used to manipulate the joints of the spine while tractioning the spine to correct low back and leg pain. Does that make the Father of Medicine the Father of Chiropractic?' (https://drwells.net/history-development-of-chiropractic/ accessed 20 February 2019). This comes from *On Joints*, 45 (Loeb, *Hippocrates* III, 289; Jones's translation: 'One should first get a knowledge of the structure of the spine; for this is also requisite for many diseases').
59 Gustave Haas, *Health Through Sunshine and Diet* (Los Angeles: Gem Publishing Company, 1926), 1. Brian Clement of the Hippocrates Health Institute, discussed in Chapter 7 below, also has strong views about food ripened in the sun's rays.
60 Ibid., 5. This is one year earlier than Dalby's finding of the quote being 'first attributed to Hippocrates'.
61 Ibid., 6.
62 Ibid., 161. The ten Normalettes are described in full in *Health Secrets of the Desert* (Long Beach CA: Health Laboratories, 1925), 24, which advertises Haas's book: https://babel.hathitrust.org/cgi/pt?id=uc1.31822035082866;view=1up;seq=2 accessed 20 February 2019.
63 Haas, *Health Through Sunshine*, 162.
64 Gayelord Hauser, *Gayelord Hauser's Dictionary of Foods* (1932), New York: Benedict Lust Publications 1970), vii.
65 Ibid., 125.
66 Max Gerson, *A Cancer Therapy: Results of fifty cases* (New York: Dura Books, 1958), 79. On Gerson see American Cancer Society, 'Unproven Methods of Cancer Management: Gerson Method,' *CA: A Cancer Journal for Clinicians*, 40.4 (1990).
67 http://www.treating-cancer-alternatively.com/Hippocrates-Soup.html and https://juicing-for-health.com/hippocrates-soup accessed 20 February 2019.

68 https://topnaturalremedies.net/home-remedies/hippocrates-miraculous-soup-detoxification-cancer-chronic-diseases-weight-loss/ accessed 20 February 2019. The site dates Hippocrates to 550 BCE. Max Gerson, 'The cure of advanced cancer by diet therapy: a summary of 30 years of clinical experimentation,' *Physiological Chemistry and Physics*, 10.5 (1978); recipe (often specifying unpeeled vegetables and/or distilled water, e.g. on http://gerson-research.org/hippocrates-soup/ accessed 20 February 2019); see also https://topnaturalremedies.net/home-remedies/hippocrates-miraculous-soup-detoxification-cancer-chronic-diseases-weight-loss/ accessed 20 February 2019.

69 *Vegetarian Times*, 49 (September 1981), 82.

70 https://www.motherearthliving.com/food-and-recipes/vegetarian-recipes/hippocrates-famous-green-juice-recipe-zerz1506zdeb accessed 20 February 2019.

71 Further examples are discussed by Sarah Scullin, https://eidolon.pub/hippocrates-would-have-wanted-you-to-eat-cake-d5127ca40e09 accessed 20 February 2019.

72 http://www.answers.com/Q/Why_may_Hippocrates_be_called_the_father_of_western_medicine accessed 20 February 2019.

73 Loeb, *Hippocrates* IV, 332–6.

74 Galen, *On the properties of foodstuffs*, 21; Grant, *Galen on Food and Diet*, 126; Owen Powell, *Galen* On the Properties of Foodstuffs (Cambridge: Cambridge University Press, 2003), 87.

75 Von Staden, *Herophilus*, 425.

76 U. Satyanarayana and U. Chakrapani, *Biochemistry*, 4th edition (New Delhi: Elsevier, 2014), 118; also found in many online sites.

77 H.A. Hajar Al Binali, 'Night blindness and ancient remedy', *Heart Views*, 15.4 (2014). This picks up a similar observation that, in Java, the liver is often fed to the patient even though the description of the therapy omits any mention of this, made in a letter to the editor of *The American Journal of Clinical Nutrition*, 31.9 (1978), 1489. For more references to ancient sources, see D. Brouzas, A. Charokidas, M. Vasilakis, *et al.*, 'Nyctalopia in antiquity: a review of the ancient Greek, Latin, and Byzantine literature', *Ophthalmology*, 108 (2001) and Gerald A. Fishman, 'A historical perspective on the early treatment of night blindness and the use of dubious and unproven treatment strategies for patients with retinitis pigmentosa,' *Journal of Ophthalmology*, 58 (2013), 653, but citing Brouzas et al. as its only Hippocratic evidence.

78 This treatise appears to be an excerpt from a surgical manual; Elizabeth Craik, 'The Hippocratic treatise *Peri opsios* (*De videndi acie, On the origin of sight*)' in Philip J. van der Eijk (ed.), *Hippocrates in Context: Papers Read at the XIth International Hippocrates Colloquium (University of Newcastle upon Tyne, 27–31 August 2002)* (Leiden: Brill, 2005), 197 notes that squirting cucumber is more closely associated

with the gynaecological treatises, and there are several other linguistic links to those texts. On the remedy, see also Danielle Gourevitch, 'Le dossier philologique de nyctalope' in Mirko D. Grmek (ed.). *Hippocratica: Actes du colloque hippocratique de Paris (4–9 septembre 1978)* (Paris: Editions du CNRS, 1980).
79 Craik, '*Peri opsios*', 200.
80 Ibid.
81 Von Staden, *Herophilus*, 425–6.
82 Anon. *Garlic* (Pomeroy WA: Health Research Books, 1983), 7.
83 Ibid., 14.
84 C. Gary Hullquist, *Garlic: Nature's Perfect Prescription* (Brushton NY: TEACH Services, Inc., 1996), 7; first published in 1983.
85 Series 4, broadcast 18 August 2014.
86 'Watercress – *Nasturtium officinale*', April 2009; https://gardenofeaden.blogspot.com/2009/04/watercress-nasturtium-officinale.html accessed 20 February 2019.
87 https://www.bwqualitygrowers.com/watercress/history-and-facts/ accessed 20 February 2019.
88 https://www.healwithfood.org/articles/watercress-oldest-healing-food.php accessed 20 February 2019. See also https://lizearlewellbeing.com/top-5-health-benefits-of-watercress/ accessed 20 February 2019, which repeats 'cure of cures' but adds a little doubt with regard to the hospital: 'even went so far as to reputedly build his first hospital in Kos near a river so he could grow it specifically for his patients'. The 'cure of cures' is repeated in Jennifer Thompson, *Green Smoothies for Dummies* (Hoboken NJ: John Wiley & Sons, 2014), 49.
89 'Clean your body with watercress', 4 April 2014; http://www.headpositivemom.com/clean-your-body-with-watercress/ accessed 20 February 2019. Hoerner is an integrative nutritionist, aromatherapist and life coach; https://www.headpositivemom.com/work-with-me/recover-your-positiveness/ accessed 20 February 2019. 'Blood disorders' are mentioned in other discussions of Hippocrates and watercress, for example a growers' site, https://www.bwqualitygrowers.com/watercress/history-and-facts/ accessed 20 February 2019.
90 http://allaboutthekale.blogspot.com/ accessed 20 February 2019.
91 E.g. https://www.bwqualitygrowers.com/watercress/history-and-facts/ accessed 20 February 2019.
92 http://kitchenherbwife.blogspot.com/2009/06/summer-weeds-watercress-and-sorrel.html, 30 June 2009 accessed 20 February 2019. Either or both of these sentences are repeated on other sites e.g. https://www.britishleafysalads.co.uk/know/leaf-guide.shtml accessed 20 February 2009.
93 *Diseases of Women* 1, 44 (Loeb, *Hippocrates* XI, 106); 1, 88 (Loeb, *Hippocrates* XI, 226).

94 *Diseases of Women* 2, 24 (Loeb, *Hippocrates* XI, 330).
95 *Superfetation* 31 (Loeb, *Hippocrates* X, 344).
96 https://altnature.com/gallery/watercress.htm accessed 20 February 2019.
97 https://www.bwqualitygrowers.com/watercress/history-and-facts/; https://herbsarespecial.com.au/plant-information/herb-information/watercress/ both accessed 20 February 2019.
98 James C. Whorton, *Inner Hygiene: Constipation and the pursuit of health in modern society* (Oxford and New York: Oxford University Press, 2000), 253: see Barry's syndicated column which appeared, *inter alia*, in the *Chicago Tribune*, 21 March 1993, 59 (http://articles.chicagotribune.com/1993-03-21/features/9303200357_1_middle-class-middle-class-tax-relief; this site is currently not available in Europe).
99 Whorton, *Inner Hygiene*, 22–7.
100 Ibid., 246–57.
101 K.W. Heaton, 'Regular review: Dietary fibre', *BMJ*, 300 (6738) (1990), 1479–80. He noted that feeding people small bits of plastic increased intestinal transit speed in the same way as wheat bran, suggesting that stimulating the lining of the colon was the reason for relieving constipation. On the role of Denis Burkitt – 'Fibre Man' – in the creation of the fibre hypothesis, see John H. Cummings and Amanda Engineer, 'Denis Burkitt and the origins of the dietary fibre hypothesis', *Nutrition Research Reviews*, 31.1 (2018).
102 Louisa Lyon, '"All disease begins in the gut": was Hippocrates right?' *Brain*, 141.3 (2018), 4; https://neoskosmos.com/en/43228/hippocrates-was-right-let-food-be-thy-medicine-mind-gut-connection/ accessed 20 February 2019.
103 Ibid.
104 http://positivemed.com/2016/03/15/colon-cleanse/ accessed 20 February 2019.
105 https://www.youtube.com/watch?v=tJieeGxQO38 accessed 20 February 2019; http://www.drfrances.co.nz/probiotics.html accessed 20 February 2019; on Mechnikov, see https://www.nobelprize.org/nobel_prizes/medicine/laureates/1908/mechnikov-bio.html accessed 20 February 2019.
106 Gary R. Lichtenstein, 'Letter from the editor', *Gastroenterology & Hepatology*, 9.9 (2013), 552: https://www.ncbi.nlm.nih.gov/pmc/articles/PMC3983972/.
107 Rolf Stuhmer, *The Big Book of Health* (Zurich: PSM Publishing, 2000), 143.
108 https://www.barrypopik.com/index.php/new_york_city/entry/death_begins_in_the_colon, 12 September 2011, accessed 23 November 2017.
109 Whorton, *Inner Hygiene*, 182.
110 John Harvey Kellogg, 'The rise of bran', *Good Health* 63.5 (1928), 36–7, summarized in William Shurtleff and Akiko Aoyagi, *History of Seventh-Day Adventist Work with Soyfoods, Vegetarianism, Meat Alternatives, Wheat Gluten,*

Dietary Fiber and Peanut Butter (1863–2013) (Lafayette, CA: Soyinfo Center, 2014), 179.

111 Sylvester Graham, *A Treatise on Bread, and Breadmaking* (Boston, MA: Light and Stearns, 1837), 59. On Graham, see James C. Whorton, 'Patient, heal thyself: popular health reform movements as unorthodox medicine' in Norman Gevitz (ed.), *Other Healers: Unorthodox medicine in America* (Baltimore, MD: Johns Hopkins University Press, 1988), 60–7 and Levinovitz, *The Gluten Lie*, 79. Both Graham and Kellogg believed that sweet foods and spices led to masturbation; Levinovitz, *The Gluten Lie*, 110. Recipes for the Graham cracker are still available online, made with Graham flour (wholewheat, unbleached, unrefined: https://www.hodgsonmill.com/products/homemade-graham-crackers accessed 20 February 2019).

112 The phrase turns up in the 1970s in the work of Peter G. Lindner, with a feature in various local newspapers in 1978 citing an editorial by him in the journal *Obesity/Bariatric Medicine*; e.g. https://newspaperarchive.com/ottumwa-courier-aug-12-1978-p-5/ accessed 20 February 2019.

113 Hugh Trowell, 'The development of the concept of dietary fiber in human nutrition', *American Journal of Clinical Nutrition*, 31.10 (1974).

114 Denis P. Burkitt and Gene A. Spiller, 'Dietary fiber: from early hunter-gatherers to the 1980s' in Gene A. Spiller (ed.), *CRC Handbook of Dietary Fiber in Human Nutrition* (Boca Raton, FL: CRC Press, 3rd edition, 2001: first edition 1986), 3; see in the same volume Hans Englyst and Geoffrey Hudson, 'Dietary fiber analysis as non-starch polysaccharides (NSPS)', 69.

115 Joanne L. Slavin and Beate Lloyd, 'Health benefits of fruit and vegetables', *Advances in Nutrition* 3.4 (2012) (https://www.ncbi.nlm.nih.gov/pmc/articles/PMC3649719/); https://wholegrainscouncil.org/sites/default/files/atoms/files/SlavinArticle0504.pdf both accessed 20 February 2019.

116 Maurice H. Lessof, *Food Intolerance* (London: Chapman and Hall, 1992), 11 citing Royal College of Physicians, 'Medical aspects of dietary fibre' (London: Pitman Medical, 1980).

117 Loeb, *Hippocrates* IV, 307–9. This is not *On Regimen in Acute Diseases* II, XL, 1 (which does not exist) as is claimed by Hara Procopiou, 'Barley meal processing in the ancient world: a look at diversity' in Annelou van Gijn, John Whittaker, Patricia C. Anderson (eds), *Exploring and Explaining Diversity in Agricultural Technology* (Oxford: Oxbow Books, 2014), 245, although Procopiou correctly has barley rather than wheat as the context of the *Regimen* passage.

118 K.D. White, 'Cereals, bread and milling in the Roman world' in John Wilkins, David Harvey and Mike Dobson (eds), *Food in Antiquity* (Exeter: University of Exeter Press, 1995), 43 n.7.

119 Petronius, *Satyricon* 66.1; *et cum mea re [causa] facio, non ploro*; in the 1913 Loeb translation by Michael Heseltine, 'it puts strength into you, and is good for the bowels'.
120 Athenaeus 3, 110e: Alexis mentions the bread in his play *The Man from Cyprus*.
121 Celsus, *On Medicine* 2.18.4.
122 Galen, *Method of Medicine to Glaucon* 2.
123 Loeb, *Hippocrates* VI, 139.
124 Loeb *Hippocrates* VI, 145. The term translated here as 'cavity' is *koiliê*, intestines.
125 Loeb, *Hippocrates* VI, 177.
126 https://www.prnewswire.com/news-releases/herbal-tea-experience-store-opens-in-nyc-offering-ancient-remedies-for-modern-living-300723375.html, 3 October 2018, accessed 20 February 2019. Also found on quotes sites, e.g. https://quotefancy.com/quote/829265/Hippocrates-Foolish-the-doctor-who-despises-the-knowledge-acquired-by-the-ancients; https://www.azquotes.com/quote/949377 accessed 20 February 2019; Greek Medicine (a site I will discuss more in Chapter 7), http://www.greekmedicine.net/therapies/Herbal_Medicine.html accessed 20 February 2019; and a letter to the *BMJ* by Kevin Ong, listing ten medical quotes, on 5 February 2018: https://www.bmj.com/rapid-response/2011/10/29/10-quotes-being-good-doctor accessed 20 February 2019.
127 Peter McDonald, *Oxford Dictionary of Medical Quotations* (Oxford: Oxford University Press, 2005), 47 gives as his source Michel Odent's *Entering the World: The way to gentle, loving birth* (Harmondsworth: Penguin, 1985), 6 (first published 1976), and this attribution is repeated on https://www.azquotes.com/quote/949377. It is used as one of Odent's four opening quotations, but without further attribution.
128 http://historum.com/general-history/32642-sourcing-hippocratic-quote.html accessed 20 February 2019. It is not only found on such websites; it also features, for example, in Kathie Madonna Swift and Gerard E. Mullin, *The Inside Tract: Your good gut guide to great digestive health* (New York: Rodale, 2011), 16.
129 http://www.southbaytotalhealth.com/Nutrition.htm accessed 20 February 2019.
130 http://theshineonhealth.com/index.php?p=1_16 accessed 21 November 2017; account now suspended.
131 E. Shyong Tai and Peter J. Gillies (eds), *Nutrigenomics: Opportunities in Asia* (2007), 67; this book opens with a chapter mentioning LFBTM (p. 1).
132 Gunther B. Paulien, *The Divine Prescription and Science of Health and Healing* (Fort Oglethorpe, GA: TEACH Services Inc, 1995). Paulien comes from a prominent SDA family and worked at their Canadian Union College, now Burman University.

133 Edward Hopper, *The Dutch Pilgrim Fathers, and other poems, humorous and not humorous* (New York, Hurd and Houghton; Boston, E.P. Dutton and company, 1865), 42; https://archive.org/details/dutchpilgrimfath00hopp accessed 20 February 2019. A possible correlation is with the Louis Lasagna version of the *Oath*, in which the doctor is asked to 'remember that … warmth, sympathy and understanding may outweigh the surgeon's knife or the chemist's drug', https://www.pbs.org/wgbh/nova/article/hippocratic-oath-today/ accessed 20 February 2019.

Chapter 7

1 Quotation from Vanessa Heggie, 'Specialization without the hospital: the case of British Sports Medicine', *Medical History*, 54.4 (2010), 458.
2 Above, p. 37.
3 Whorton, *Nature Cures*, 3 and 6.
4 See for an overview Max Neuburger, 'An historical survey of the concept of Nature from a medical viewpoint', *Isis*, 35.1 (1944); see also John Harley Warner, *The Therapeutic Perspective: Medical practice, knowledge, and identity in America, 1820–1885* (Cambridge MA: Harvard University Press, 1986), 21 on the reluctance of some physicians to give Nature a 'personality', and John Harley Warner, '"The nature-trusting heresy": American physicians and the concept of the healing power of nature in the 1850's and 1860's', *Perspectives in American History*, 11 (1977–8). For the *mediatrix* variant, within alternative medicine journals see for example Robert B. Jackson, 'Vis mediatrix naturae, vital force to innate intelligence and concepts for 2000', *Journal of Chiropractic Humanities*, 10 (2001), 41 or Mike Money, 'Shamanism as a healing paradigm for complementary therapy', *Complementary Therapies in Nursing & Midwifery*, 7 (2001), 126. Naturopathic sites often just repeat the (correct) phrase as if we all knew what it meant; e.g. 'Hippocrates, 460BC–370 BC, who is considered to be the father of medicine, introduced Vis Medicatrix Naturae — the concept of the healing power of nature', https://eatbreathegarden.com/horticulture-and-health-according-to-three-wise-men/, 6 January 2016, accessed 20 February 2019.
5 G. Munro Smith, 'Vis Medicatrix Naturae: Inaugural Address at the Annual Meeting of the Bath and Bristol Branch of the British Medical Association', *Bristol Medico-Chirurgical Journal*, 27 (106) (1909), 321 attributes ('as far as I can discover') the Latin phrase to William Cullen.
6 Pamela Snider and Roger Newman Turner, 'Nature cure in Europe: the transatlantic journey from pragmatism to principles,' *Naturopathic Doctor News*

and Reviews, October 2010, 8–9, http://www.foundationsproject.com/documents/NDNR-reprint%20oct2010%20Turner-Snider.pdf accessed 20 February 2019. The mistaken claims about *nature* probably derive from the Wikipedia article which states that *vis medicatrix naturae* is 'also known as *natura medica*' accessed 20 February 2019.

7 https://en.wikipedia.org/wiki/Vis_medicatrix_naturae accessed 20 February 2019.
8 Hosimi Hiroshi, 'On Vis medicatrix naturae and Hippocratic idea of physis', *Memoirs of School of Health Sciences, Faculty of Medicine, Kanazawa University*, 22 (1998) is often cited as evidence that 'The power, called vis medicatrix naturae, has been traditionally asociated [sic] with Hippocrates in spite of the fact that he did never mention it anywhere clearly in his writings', https://web.archive.org/web/20080610160955/http://sciencelinks.jp/j-east/article/199907/000019990799A0162403.php accessed 20 February 2019. For once, I think there is more Hippocratic justification for the phrase than has been acknowledged.
9 *Epidemics* 6.5.1; Loeb, *Hippocrates* VII, 255 note a.
10 Whorton, *Nature Cures*, 6–7.
11 http://www.naturalwellbeing.com/blog/the-history-of-holistic-medicine-the-ancient-greeks-and-holistic-medicine/ accessed 20 February 2019.
12 Coward, *The Whole Truth*, 15.
13 Ibid., 35.
14 Gevitz, 'Osteopathic medicine', 125.
15 Whorton, *Nature Cures*, 4.
16 Coward, *Whole Truth*, 28.
17 Jessica Hughes, 'Fragmentation as metaphor in the classical healing sanctuary', *Social History of Medicine*, 21.2 (2008).
18 270c1–4, suggesting that both for the soul and for the body one cannot know their nature unless one learns 'the nature of the whole'. Damianos Tsekourakis, 'Plato's *Phaedrus* and the holistic viewpoint in Hippocrates' therapeutics', *Bulletin of the Institute of Classical Studies*, 38 (1991–3), 164 suggests that any attempt to tie this passage to a single Hippocratic treatise is doomed, as Plato was referring instead to Hippocratic medicine in general.
19 Robson and Baek, *The Engines of Hippocrates*, 57.
20 Tsekourakis, 'Plato's *Phaedrus*'.
21 Wellmann, 'Hippokrates des Herakleides Sohn', 16–21, cited in W.D. Smith, *Hippocratic Tradition*, 38 n.40.
22 W.D. Smith, *Hippocratic Tradition*, 46; see also 48, 'Plato left "the whole" ambiguous because both "man as a whole" and "cosmos" are comprehended in the Hippocratic science.'
23 *On Ancient Medicine* 7; Jouanna, 'Regimen in the Hippocratic corpus', 228–9.

24 Rosen, 'Towards a Hippocratic anthropology', 253.
25 Weisz, 'Hippocrates, holism and humanism', 264.
26 http://www.hippocrate.net/en/ accessed 20 February 2019.
27 https://greekcitytimes.com/2018/07/22/greeces-leading-natural-cosmetics-brand-taking-the-world-by-storm/ accessed 20 February 2019.
28 W.C. Sellars and R.J. Yeatman, *1066 And All That: A Memorable History of England, comprising all the parts you can remember, including 103 Good Things, 5 Bad Kings and 2 Genuine Dates* (London: Methuen, 1930) used the capitalized phrase 'A Good Thing' to describe historical events universally accepted in schoolbook history as positive. So, for example, the Magna Carta was A Good Thing.
29 Whorton, *Nature Cures*, 247.
30 Mike Saks, *Orthodox and Alternative Medicine. Politics, professionalization and health care* (London: Sage Publications, 2003), 107–8; Whorton, *Nature Cures*, 246; Saks, *Orthodox and Alternative Medicine*, 114–5.
31 Coward, *Whole Truth*, 181–2.
32 Whorton, *Nature Cures*, 271–2.
33 http://www.greekmedicine.net/whos_who/Hippocrates.html accessed 20 February 2019; https://www.ukessays.com/essays/history/a-brief-history-into-greek-medicine-history-essay.php, 5 December 2016, accessed 20 February 2019; presented as an essay by a student rather than 'our professional academic writers', this does quote its source here.
34 http://www.greekmedicine.net/blog/events/celebrating-ten-great-years.html accessed 20 February 2019.
35 http://www.discovergreece.com/en/greek-islands/dodecanese/kos/hippocrates-asclepeion-a-holistic-healing-centre accessed 20 February 2019.
36 Fritz Graf, 'Heiligtum und Ritual: Das Beispiel der griechisch-römischen Asklepieia', in A. Schachter (ed.), *Le sanctuaire grec* (Geneva: Fondation Hardt, 1992), 199; Ido Israelowich, *Patients and Healers in the High Roman Empire* (Baltimore, MD: Johns Hopkins University Press, 2015), 111.
37 http://www.greekmedicine.net/whos_who/Hippocrates.html accessed 20 February 2019.
38 http://www.greekmedicine.net/blog/events/celebrating-ten-great-years.html accessed 20 February 2019.
39 Whorton, *Nature Cures*, 305. This 'strives to embody the healing wisdom and techniques of all civilizations from antiquity onward and to overcome the spiritual poverty of the biomedical model of disease'; Nomikos et al., 'Exercise in Hippocratic medicine', 115.
40 http://www.greekmedicine.net/blog/events/celebrating-ten-great-years.html accessed 20 February 2019.

41 Sylvie Chermet-Carroy, *L'Astrologie Médicale* (Paris: Editions Guy Trédaniel, 1998).
42 Ghulam M. Chishti, *The Traditional Healer's Handbook: A classic guide to the medicine of Avicenna* (Rochester, VT: Healing Arts Press, 1988), 11.
43 http://doctorscrubs.blogspot.co.uk/2009/04/hatred-of-tmb-and-tma-against.html accessed 20 February 2019.
44 https://coltonspointtimes.blogspot.co.uk/2017/01/ accessed 20 February 2019.
45 https://www.testednutrients.com/en/about/; in the author's response to a comment on http://jamesmalloy.blogspot.co.uk/2013/07/nietzscheaphorism-120-gay-science.html. Both accessed 20 February 2019.
46 Much of the page of greekmedicine.net is copied without attribution in Francesco Perono Cacciafoco, 'Food as therapy: elements of the history of nutrition in ancient Greece and Rome' (Pollenzo: Università degli Studi di Scienze Gastronomiche – University of Gastronomic Sciences, 2012), 20–2 where, bizarrely, the words 'band' and 'renegade physicians' are marked by quotation marks when the rest of the plagiarized text is not.
47 http://www.unani.com/hipporcates.htm accessed 20 February 2019; the lyrics are on http://users.ox.ac.uk/~archery/old/hood.html accessed 20 February 2019.
48 http://www.redhouseaustralia.org/hippocrates accessed 20 February 2019, the updated website of 2017, which also claims that the philosophy owes something to 'Louis Pasture'.
49 https://en.wikipedia.org/wiki/Hippocrates as of 20 July 2017.
50 Acknowledged as the source for the 'humble and passive' on http://www.isabellehutton.com/Hippocrates.FatherOfMedicine.html (domain now expired).
51 Chishti, *The Traditional Healer's Handbook*, 12.
52 https://edzardernst.com/2013/10/alternative-practitioners-treat-the-whole-person-not-the-disease/. See also the earlier post, 'Integrated medicine makes no sense', https://edzardernst.com/2012/12/integrated-medicine-makes-no-sense/ and the later post, https://edzardernst.com/2014/10/the-disgraceful-abduction-of-holism/ which dates 'clinical holistic medicine' 'as far back as Hippocrates'; all accessed 20 February 2019.
53 Online quotes pages: e.g. https://quotereel.com/tag/hippocrates/ accessed 20 February 2019. See http://www.osler.org.uk/osleriana-2/oslers-aphorisms/; claimed as the key principle of Chinese medicine on https://www.chinesemedicineliving.com/acupuncture/cancer-chinese-medicine-part-3 or used on the website of a natural healer in several traditions on https://www.drlaurenpolm.com/; all accessed 20 February 2019.
54 I owe this reference to Dr Mary Hague-Yearl, Head Librarian of the Osler Library at McGill University, pers. comm. 24 September 2018; the source is William Osler,

'Address to the students of the Albany Medical College', *Albany Medical Annals*, 20 (1899), 307–9. Dr Hague-Yearl checked with one of the compilers of Mark E. Silverman, T. Jock Murray and Charles S. Bryan, *The Quotable Osler* (American College of Physicians, 2003), Charley Bryan, who 'wrote that he was 99% sure that it was merely attributed to Osler, and agreed that an investigation of these attributions would be very interesting indeed'. Those attributing the words to Osler sometimes date them to 1895, but the best I have been able to find here is Edward Shorter, 'Primary care' in Roy Porter (ed.), *Cambridge Illustrated History of Medicine* (Cambridge: Cambridge University Press, 1996), 144, with 381 n.45 citing the aphorism as being quoted by Clarence B. Farrar in a 1959 article. Shorter later repeated this footnote, in his 'The history of the biopsychosocial approach in medicine: before and after Engel' in Peter White (ed.), *Biopsychosocial Medicine: An integrated approach to understanding illness* (Oxford: Oxford University Press, 2005), 9–10.

55 http://www.pbs.org/wgbh/nova/body/hippocratic-oath-today.html#modern accessed 20 February 2019.
56 On how 'dis-ease can become disease if left unresolved': https://www.amazon.com/Healing-Groovy-Realistic-Holistic-Self-Care/dp/1505613256 accessed 20 February 2019.
57 http://windermeresun.com/2016/03/08/natural-healing-with-sandra-sigur/ accessed 20 February 2019. Sigur supports other myths about Hippocrates, such as 'Hippocrates said "let food be thy medicine and medicine be thy food". So, since food is your medicine, I would say there are many deficiencies leading to illness in America.'
58 This is discussed, with other modern versions, by Hurwitz and Richardson, 'Swearing to care'.
59 http://www.naturalwellbeing.com/blog/the-history-of-holistic-medicine-the-ancient-greeks-and-holistic-medicine/ accessed 20 February 2019.
60 https://wildrosecollege.com/; https://wildrosecollege.com/product/wholistic-therapist-diploma/ both accessed 20 February 2019.
61 https://wildrosecollege.com/product/thesis-wholistic-therapist/ accessed 20 February 2019.
62 https://wildrosecollege.com/home/wild-rose-college-about-page/ accessed 20 February 2019.
63 http://www.naturalwellbeing.com/blog/the-history-of-holistic-medicine-the-ancient-greeks-and-holistic-medicine/ accessed 20 February 2019.
64 https://medicine.llu.edu/about/our-mission accessed 20 February 2019.
65 https://www.redlandsdailyfacts.com/2008/01/09/wholistic-for-kids/ 9 January 2008, accessed 20 February 2019.

66 http://wholistickids.com/services/wholistic-integrative-services/ accessed 20 February 2019.
67 https://www.adventist.org/en/vitality/health/ accessed 20 February 2019.
68 Ellen White, *The Desire of Ages* (Mountain View CA: Pacific Press Publishing Association, 1940: first published 1898), 824 and *The Ministry of Healing* (Mountain View CA: Pacific Press Publishing Association, 1942: first published 1905).
69 White, *The Desire of Ages*, 824.
70 White, *The Ministry of Healing*, 127; this was based on a vision she had in June 1863, and included the use of 'simple herbs and roots'. See Ronald L. Numbers, *Prophetess of Health: A Study of Ellen G. White* (3rd edition) (Grand Rapids MI: Wm. B. Eerdmans, 2008), 263.
71 The debate is summarized on http://dedication.www3.50megs.com/David/index.html and https://www.adventistsaffirm.org/previous-issues/volume-15-number-1/ellen-g-white-prophet-or-plagiarist, both accessed 20 February 2019. On the six non-naturals, discussed most extensively in Galen's commentary on the Hippocratic *Epidemics*, Book 6, see Luis García-Ballester, 'On the origins of the six non-natural things in Galen,' in Jutta Kollesch and Diethard Nickel (eds), *Galen und das hellenistische* Erbe, special issue of *Sudhoffs Archiv*, 32 (1993).
72 https://www.redlandsdailyfacts.com/2008/01/09/wholistic-for-kids/ accessed 20 February 2019.
73 https://www.wholisticmedical.co.uk/mission-statement accessed 20 February 2019.
74 https://www.wholisticmedical.co.uk/food-therapy accessed 20 Februrary 2019.
75 https://www.wholisticmedical.co.uk/food-therapy and https://www.wholisticmedical.co.uk/pemf-ondamed-pmt-120 accessed 20 February 2019.
76 https://www.wholisticmedical.co.uk/food-therapy accessed 20 February 2019.
77 https://www.wholisticmedical.co.uk/breast-and-body-screening accessed 20 February 2019. This quote is used by those promoting thermography, who cite doctors in 400 BCE using mud on the body and seeing which area dried first in order to see where the hottest regions were; https://thermographymedicalclinic.com/the-history-of-thermography/ accessed 20 February 2019, a site which includes a well-known modern image of Hippocrates with a patient.
78 Weisz, 'Hippocrates, holism and humanism', 272.
79 F.G. Crookshank, 'The new psychology and the health of the people', *Purpose* (July–September 1932), 123 cited in David Cantor, 'The name and the word: neo-Hippocratism and language in interwar Britain' in David Cantor (ed.), *Reinventing Hippocrates* (Aldershot: Ashgate, 2002), 280.

80 Britain: Cantor, 'The name and the word', 284; France: Weisz, 'Hippocrates, holism and humanism', 268.
81 As for example on the 'History' page of the British Homeopathic Organization, https://www.britishhomeopathic.org/homeopathy/the-history-of-homeopathy/ accessed 20 February 2019; Weisz, 'Hippocrates, holism and humanism', 260.
82 Warner, 'Making history in American medical culture', 222–3.
83 https://www.paramnaturals.com/meet-paulina/ accessed 20 February 2019. The initial consultation costs $475, including one month's supply of the 'personalized' herbal remedy, then $185 per follow-up.
84 https://www.paramnaturals.com/services/online-consultations/ accessed 20 February 2019.
85 Weisz, 'Hippocrates, holism and humanism', 270 and 278 n.82.
86 Warner, '"The nature-trusting heresy"', 301–6.
87 Ibid., 307.
88 Robson and Baek, *The Engines of Hippocrates*, 267.
89 Sneha Mantri, 'Holistic medicine and the Western medical tradition', *Virtual Mentor*, 10.3 (2008), http://journalofethics.ama-assn.org/2008/03/mhst1-0803.html accessed 20 February 2019.
90 Cantor, 'The name and the word', 284 and 286.
91 Ibid., 289.
92 Heggie, 'Specialization without the hospital', 457. Sports medicine, Heggie showed, was a particularly unpromising area to become a specialism due to the breadth of what it covered: it is 'a holistic practice, covering everything from gross musculo-skeletal injuries to dietary advice to genetic testing. It has virtually no unique diseases or injuries (one can get tennis elbow cleaning floors) nor any unique treatment modalities or technologies.' On medical specialization more broadly, see George Weisz, 'The emergence of medical specialization in the nineteenth century', *Bulletin of the History of Medicine*, 77 (2003) and *Divide and Conquer: A comparative history of medical specialization* (Oxford: Oxford University Press, 2006).
93 Roger Cooter, 'The meaning of fractures: orthopaedics and the reform of British hospitals in the inter-war period', *Medical History*, 31.3 (1987), 306.
94 Ibid., 307.
95 Roger Cooter, 'The evolution of orthopaedic surgery (review)', *Bulletin of the History of Medicine*, 77.2 (2003), 467–8.
96 Heggie, 'Specialization without the hospital', 458.
97 Robert Jones, 'Lady Jones' lecture on crippling due to fractures: its prevention and remedy', *BMJ*, I: (1925), quoted in Cooter, 'The meaning of fractures', 314.

98 Robson and Baek, *Engines of Hippocrates*, 267. In 2009 they reported nearly 3 million hits for 'holistic + medicine', half a million for "holistic medicine". In August 2018 I had around 104 million for the first search, 4 million for the second. They had 154,000 hits for holistic + "managed care" (a key term in US medicine): I had 878,000. Even taking into account the vagaries of search engines, I suspect that this means the word is moving further into the mainstream.
99 Ibid., 20.
100 Barrett, Bruce et al., 'Themes of holism', 940–1.
101 Saks, *Orthodox and Alternative Medicine*, 109.
102 http://www.spiritofchange.org/Spring-2014/Let-Food-Heal-Your-Body--An-interview-with-Dr-Brian-Clement/, 23 February 2014, accessed 20 February 2019.
103 https://hippocratesinst.org/history accessed 20 February 2019.
104 https://www.tripadvisor.co.uk/ShowUserReviews-g34731-d223100-r92355354-Hippocrates_Health_Institute-West_Palm_Beach_Florida.html, reviewed 9 January 2011, accessed 20 February 2019.
105 https://sciencebasedmedicine.org/brian-clement-claims-hippocrates-treatments-reverse-multiple-sclerosis/, 26 November 2015, accessed 20 February 2019; he claims a PhD ('a degree in biochemistry') and an LN (Licensed Nutritionist), https://hippocratesinst.org/our-team/brianclement accessed 20 February 2019. https://www.huffingtonpost.ca/2015/02/24/brian-clement-hippocrate_n_6741786.html, updated 24 May 2015, accessed 20 February 2019, notes that the PhD is supposed to be from the University of Science Arts and Technology (USAT), based in Montserrat; for evidence that this is a diploma mill, see the 2014 report https://www.faimer.org/research/faimer-short-report-caribbean.pdf accessed 20 February 2019. Alternatively the PhD may be from Lady Malina Memorial Medical College, according to a 2010 discussion site (http://freerepublic.com/focus/news/2558811/posts?page=72 accessed 20 February 2019) referencing a website which is now dead.
106 https://hippocratesinst.org/our-team/brianclement accessed 20 February 2019, still mentions a biochemistry PhD. See the discussion on http://www.rawfoodsupport.com/read.php?2,267730,267759 accessed 20 February 2019 and McGill University's Office for Science and Society's 'Cancer quackery costs lives', https://www.mcgill.ca/oss/article/cancer-health-quackery/serious-nonsense, 20 March 2017 accessed 20 February 2019.
107 https://responsibleeatingandliving.com/favorites/brian-clement-8292012-interview/, 29 August 2012 accessed 20 February 2019.
108 Clement, *Supplements Exposed*, 88.

109 Brian Clement, *Hippocrates LifeForce: Superior health and longevity* (Summertown TN: Healthy Living Publications, 2007), Chapter 2.
110 https://hippocratesinst.org/history accessed 20 February 2019.
111 http://www.spiritofchange.org/Spring-2014/Let-Food-Heal-Your-Body--An-interview-with-Dr-Brian-Clement/, 23 February 2014, accessed 20 February 2019.
112 https://responsibleeatingandliving.com/favorites/brian-clement-8292012-interview/, 29 August 2012, accessed 20 February 2019.
113 https://ideamensch.com/brian-clement/, 21 August 2018, accessed 20 February 2019.
114 https://www.thestar.com/news/gta/2015/02/21/founder-of-hippocrates-health-institute-sued-successfully-twice.html, 21 February 2015, accessed 20 February 2019.
115 https://www.cbc.ca/news/indigenous/brian-clement-hippocrates-health-institute-head-ordered-to-stop-practising-medicine-1.2968780, updated 25 February 2015, accessed 20 February 2019.
116 https://sciencebasedmedicine.org/florida-tells-brian-clement-to-stop-practicing-medicine/ accessed 20 February 2019.
117 https://www.tripadvisor.co.uk/ShowUserReviews-g34731-d223100-r566995381-Hippocrates_Health_Institute-West_Palm_Beach_Florida.html, reviewed 17 March 2018 by 'tomsuemegmaur'; review subsequently removed. The HHI response was to insist that the detoxifying process was responsible for these symptoms. In alternative medicine in general, particularly in naturopathy, the sometimes serious discomfort associated with a violent change in diet and lifestyle is normalized as a 'healing crisis' by proponents; see Coward, *Whole Truth*, 89.
118 https://www.tripadvisor.co.uk/ShowUserReviews-g34731-d223100-r565346701-Hippocrates_Health_Institute-West_Palm_Beach_Florida.html, 8 March 2018, accessed 20 February 2019.
119 http://weeksmd.com/2012/10/hippocrates-did-20-years-in-prison/, written on 23 October 2012, accessed 20 February 2019.
120 Coward, *Whole Truth*, 64.
121 Ibid., 42.
122 Clement, *Hippocrates LifeForce*, Chapter 2.
123 https://www.tripadvisor.co.uk/ShowUserReviews-g34731-d223100-r38523258-Hippocrates_Health_Institute-West_Palm_Beach_Florida.html, reviewed 23 August 2009, accessed 20 February 2019.
124 https://www.tripadvisor.co.uk/ShowUserReviews-g34731-d223100-r92355354-Hippocrates_Health_Institute-West_Palm_Beach_Florida.html, reviewed 9 January 2011 by 'islandler', accessed 20 February 2019.

125 http://www.anticancermom.com/the-hippocrates-health-institute/ accessed 20 February 2019.
126 https://www.tripadvisor.co.uk/ShowUserReviews-g34731-d223100-r267304382-Hippocrates_Health_Institute-West_Palm_Beach_Florida.html, reviewed 22 April 2015 by 'zeezeebranson', accessed 20 February 2019.
127 https://www.tripadvisor.co.uk/ShowUserReviews-g34731-d223100-r290796443-Hippocrates_Health_Institute-West_Palm_Beach_Florida.html, reviewed 20 July 2015 by 'JuicegirlSouthampton', accessed 20 February 2019. Guests are also taught 'how to read a blood test', according to 'garrinh', https://www.tripadvisor.co.uk/ShowUserReviews-g34731-d223100-r331419859-Hippocrates_Health_Institute-West_Palm_Beach_Florida.html, reviewed 8 December 2015, accessed 20 February 2019, who also mentions Vitamin C IV therapy and Vitamin D shots.
128 https://ideamensch.com/brian-clement/, 21 August 2018, accessed 20 February 2019.
129 http://www.agreenroadjournal.com/2012/05/dr-rebecca-carley-md-now-holistic.html; on her suspension and the revoking of her licence, https://www.quackwatch.com/11Ind/carley1.html both accessed 20 February 2019.
130 https://web.archive.org/web/20130925081055/http://www.reversingvaccineinduceddiseases.com/services; also quoted on http://casewatch.net/board/med/carley/order_2004.shtml both accessed 20 February 2019.

Conclusion

1 Nutton, 'What's in an oath?' 519.
2 Ann F. La Berge, 'The rhetoric of Hippocrates at the Paris School' in David Cantor (ed.), *Reinventing Hippocrates* (Aldershot: Ashgate, 2002), 178 and 194–5.
3 Full text of the book on https://gallica.bnf.fr/ark:/12148/btv1b52505831s?rk=21459;2 accessed 20 February 2019.
4 I am grateful to Jacqueline Fabre-Serris for discussing this image with me.
5 Robert Goldberg, *Tabloid Medicine: How the Internet is being used to hijack medical science for fear and profit* (New York: Kaplan Publishing, 2010), 106.
6 Christopher Wanjek, *Bad Medicine: Misconceptions and Misuses Revealed, from Distance Healing to Vitamin O* (Hoboken NJ: John Wiley and Sons, 2003), 157.
7 Goldberg, *Tabloid Medicine*, 119.
8 Pinault, *Hippocratic Lives and Legends*, 126.
9 Miles, *Hippocratic Oath*, 1.
10 Levinovitz, *Gluten Lie*, 41.
11 Loeb, *Hippocrates* II, 67.

Bibliography

Adams, Francis (1849), *The Genuine Works of Hippocrates*, London: Sydenham Society, 2 vols.

Adelman, Juliana and Haushoffer, Lisa (2018), 'Introduction: Food as medicine, medicine as food', *JHM*, 73.2: 127–34.

Allen, James P. (2005), *The Art of Medicine in Ancient Egypt*, New York: Metropolitan Museum of Art and New Haven CT, and London: Yale University Press.

American Cancer Society (1990), 'Unproven methods of cancer management: Gerson Method', *CA: A Cancer Journal for Clinicians*, 40.4: 252–6.

Anastasiou, Evilena; Papathanasiou, Anastasia; Scheparz, Lynne A. and Mitchell, Piers D. (2018), 'Infectious disease in the ancient Aegean: Intestinal parasitic worms in the Neolithic to Roman Period inhabitants of Kea, Greece', *Journal of Archaeological Science: Reports*, 17: 860–4.

Angelou, Nikolaos (2012), *Cures of the Body and Cures of the Soul: From Hippocrates to the Early Eastern Christian Fathers* (Master's thesis, Trinity St David, University of Wales).

Anon. (1839), Review of M.S. Houdart, *Études historiques et critiques sur la vie et la doctrine d'Hippocrate, et sur l'état de la médecine avant lui*, Edinburgh Medical and Surgical Journal, 51: 493–9.

Anon. (1850), 'To Correspondents,' *The People's Medical Journal, and Family Physician*, 8.1: 64.

Anon. (1925), *Health Secrets of the Desert*, Long Beach CA: Health Laboratories.

Anon. (1983), *Garlic*, Pomeroy WA: Health Research Books.

Apostolopoulos, Petros (2019), 'Producing historical knowledge on Wikipedia', *Madison Historical Review*, 16: https://commons.lib.jmu.edu/mhr/vol16/iss1/4, accessed 30 April 2019.

Armour, Richard (1966), *It All Started with Hippocrates: A mercifully brief history of medicine*, New York: McGraw Hill.

Arnaud, Sabine (2015), *On Hysteria: The invention of a medical category between 1670 and 1820*, Chicago IL: University of Chicago Press.

Bagnall, Roger S. (2002), 'Alexandria: Library of dreams', *Proceedings of the American Philosophical Society*, 146.4: 348–62.

Barrett, Bruce et al. (2003), 'Themes of holism, empowerment, access, and legitimacy define complementary, alternative, and integrative medicine in relation to conventional biomedicine', *Journal of Alternative and Complementary Medicine*, 9.6: 937–47.

Barrow, Mark V. (1972), 'Portraits of Hippocrates', *Medical History*, 16.1: 85–8.

Bartlett, John (1856), *A Collection of Familiar Quotations: With complete indices of authors and subjects*, Cambridge: the author.

Bartoš, Hynek (2015), *Philosophy and Dietetics in the Hippocratic* On Regimen: *A Delicate Balance of Health*, Leiden and Boston: Brill.

Beier, Ruth (1987), 'Science and medicine in the social construction of woman: from Aristotle to the corpus callosum', *Transactions and Studies of the College of Physicians of Philadelphia*, 9.4: 267–88.

Berlinerblau, Jacques (1999), *Heresy in the University: The Black Athena controversy and the responsibilities of American intellectuals*, New Brunswick, NJ: Rutgers University Press.

Berryman, Jack (2010), 'Exercise is medicine: a historical perspective', *Current Sports Medicine Reports*, 9.4, July–August: 195–201.

Al Binali, H.A. Hajar (2014), 'Night blindness and ancient remedy', *Heart Views*, 15.4: 136–9.

Blair, Ann (2010), *Too Much to Know: Managing scholarly information before the modern age*, New Haven and London: Yale University Press.

Bliquez, Lawrence J. (2015), *The Tools of Asclepius. Surgical instruments in Greek and Roman Times*, Leiden: Brill.

Boss, Jeffrey M.N. (1979), 'The seventeenth-century transformation of the hysteric affection, and Sydenham's Baconian medicine', *Psychological Medicine*, 9: 221–34.

Boudon-Millot, Véronique (2016), 'Ce qu'"hippocratique" (ἱπποκράτειος) veut dire: la réponse de Galien' in DJR, 378–98.

Breasted, James H. (1930), *The Edwin Smith Surgical papyrus (facsimile and hieroglyphic transliteration with translation and commentary, in two volumes)*, Chicago: The University of Chicago Press.

Brehany, John F. (2011), 'The indispensability of Hippocrates' (originally 2007) in Patrick Guinan, *Hippocrates is Not Dead: An anthology of Hippocratic readings*, Bloomington IN: AuthorHouse, 19–24.

Brouzas, D., Charokidas, A., Vasilakis, M. *et al.* (2001), 'Nyctalopia in antiquity: a review of the ancient Greek, Latin, and Byzantine literature', *Ophthalmology*, 108: 1917–21.

Bulger, Roger J. and Barbato, Anthony L. (2000), 'On the Hippocratic sources of Western medical practice', *The Hastings Center Report*, 30.4: 4–7.

Bullough, Vern L. (2003), 'Masturbation: a historical overview' in Walter O. Bockting and Eli Coleman (eds), *Masturbation as a Means of Achieving Sexual Health*, 17–34, New York: Haworth Press.

Burke, Victoria E. (2013), 'Recent studies in commonplace books', *English Literary Renaissance*, 43.1: 153–77.
Burkitt, Denis P. and Spiller, Gene A. (2001), 'Dietary fiber: from early hunter-gatherers to the 1980s' in Gene A. Spiller (ed.), *CRC Handbook of Dietary Fiber in Human Nutrition*, 3–8, Boca Raton, FL: CRC Press (3rd edition, first edition 1986).
Bushnell, Rebecca (1996), *A Culture of Teaching: Early modern humanism in theory and practice*, Ithaca and London: Cornell University Press.
Cabot, Sandra (2007), *The Juice Fasting Bible: Discover the power of an all-juice diet to restore good health, lose weight and increase vitality*, Berkeley CA: Ulysses Press.
Cacciafoco, Francesco Perono (2012), 'Food as therapy: elements of the history of nutrition in ancient Greece and Rome', Pollenzo: Università degli Studi di Scienze Gastronomiche – University of Gastronomic Sciences.
Calvi, Marco Fabio (1525), *Hippocratis Coi medicorum omnium longe principis, Octoginta volumina...*, Rome: Franciscus Minitius.
Cameron, Nigel (2011), 'A future for medicine?' (originally published in 1991), in Patrick Guinan, *Hippocrates is Not Dead: An anthology of Hippocratic readings*, 63–77, Bloomington IN: AuthorHouse.
Campbell, Killis (1907), *The Seven Sages of Rome*, Boston: Ginn & Co.
Cañizares, Pilar Pérez (2016), 'The treatise *Affections* in the context of the Hippocratic Corpus' in DJR, 83–98.
Cantor, David (2002), 'Introduction: the uses and meanings of Hippocrates' in David Cantor (ed.), *Reinventing Hippocrates*, 1–18, Aldershot: Ashgate.
Cantor, David (2002), 'The name and the word: neo-Hippocratism and language in interwar Britain' in David Cantor (ed.), *Reinventing Hippocrates*, 280–301, Aldershot: Ashgate.
Cantor, David (2018), 'Western medicine since the Renaissance' in Peter Pormann (ed.), *The Cambridge Companion to Hippocrates*, 362–83, Cambridge: Cambridge University Press.
Cardenas, Diana (2013), 'Let not thy food be confused with thy medicine: The Hippocratic misquotation', *e-SPEN Journal*, 8: 260–2.
Caton, Richard (1906), 'Hippocrates and the newly-discovered health temple of Cos', *BMJ*, 10 March: 571–4.
Catonné, Jean-Philippe (1992), 'Femmes et hystérie au XIXe siècle', *Annales médico-psychologiques*, 150.10: 705–19.
Cesbron, Henri (1909), *Histoire critique de l'hystérie*, Paris: Asselin et Houzeau.
Chadwick, John and Mann, William (1950), *The Medical Works of Hippocrates*, Oxford: Blackwell.
Chermet-Carroy, Sylvie (1998), *L'Astrologie Médicale*, Paris: Editions Guy Trédaniel.

Chishti, Ghulam M. (1988), *The Traditional Healer's Handbook: A classic guide to the medicine of Avicenna*, Rochester, VT: Healing Arts Press.

Clark, Herbert H. and Gerrig, Richard J. (1990), 'Quotations as demonstrations', *Language*, 66.4: 764–805.

Clement, Brian (2007), *Hippocrates LifeForce: Superior health and longevity*, Summertown TN: Healthy Living Publications.

Clement, Brian (2010), *Supplements Exposed: The truth they don't want you to know about vitamins, minerals, and their effects on your health*, Franklin Lakes NJ: The Career Press.

Clifton, Francis (1734), *Hippocrates upon Airs, Water and Situation*, London: J. Watts.

Cooter, Roger (1987), 'The meaning of fractures: orthopaedics and the reform of British hospitals in the inter-war period', *Medical History*, 31.3: 306–32.

Cooter, Roger (2003), 'The evolution of orthopaedic surgery (review)', *BHM*, 77.2: 467–8.

Cornarius, Janus (1546), *Hippocratis Coi medicorum omnium longe principis, opera quae ad nos extant omnia*, Basel: Froben.

Coward, Rosalind (1989), *The Whole Truth: The myth of alternative health*, London: Faber & Faber.

Craik, Elizabeth M. (2005), 'The Hippocratic treatise *Peri opsios* (*De videndi acie*, *On the origin of sight*) in Philip J. van der Eijk (ed.), *Hippocrates in Context: Papers Read at the XIth International Hippocrates Colloquium (University of Newcastle upon Tyne, 27–31 August 2002)*, 191–207, Leiden: Brill.

Craik, Elizabeth M. (2006), *Two Hippocratic Treatises* On Sight *and* On Anatomy, Leiden: Brill.

Craik, Elizabeth M. (2009), *The Hippocratic Treatise* On Glands, *edited and translated with introduction and commentary*, Leiden: Brill.

Craik, Elizabeth M. (2010), 'The teaching of surgery' in Manfred Horstmanshoff (ed.), *Hippocrates and Medical Education: Selected papers presented at the XIIth International Hippocrates Colloquium, Universiteit Leiden, 24–26 August 2005*, 223–33, Leiden: Brill.

Craik, Elizabeth M. (2015), *The 'Hippocratic' Corpus: Content and context*, London: Routledge.

Crookshank, F.G. (1932), 'The new psychology and the health of the people', *Purpose*, July–September: 122–7.

Crow, Thomas (1995), *Emulation: David, Drouais, and Girodet in the art of revolutionary France*, New Haven: Yale University Press.

Crystal, David (2006), *Language and the Internet*, second edition, Cambridge: Cambridge University Press.

Cummings, John H. and Engineer, Amanda (2018), 'Denis Burkitt and the origins of the dietary fibre hypothesis', *Nutrition Research Reviews*, 31.1: 1-15.

Cunningham, Andrew (2002), 'The transformation of Hippocrates in seventeenth-century Britain' in David Cantor (ed.), *Reinventing Hippocrates*, 91–115, Aldershot: Ashgate.

Dalal, Roshen (2013), *The Puffin History of the World*, vol. 1, London: Penguin Books.

Daremberg, Charles (1856), *Oeuvres anatomiques, physiologiques et médicales de Galien* vol. 2, Paris: Baillière.

Das, Aileen R. (2018), 'New material from Galen's *On the Authentic and Spurious Works of Hippocrates*', *Classical Philology*, 113.3: 305–29.

Davidson, James (1997), *Courtesans and Fishcakes: The consuming passions of classical Athens*. London: HarperCollins.

Davis, Patricia (1988), *Aromatherapy. An A–Z*, Saffron Walden: C.W. Daniel.

Dean-Jones, Lesley (1994), *Women's Bodies in Classical Greek Science*, Oxford: Clarendon Press.

Dean-Jones, Lesley (2013), 'Too much of a good thing: the health of Olympic athletes in ancient Greece', in Susan E. Brownell (ed.), *From Athens to Beijing: West meets East in the Olympic Games*, Vol. I: *Sport, the Body and Humanism in Ancient Greece and China*, 49–65, New York: Greekworks.

Dean-Jones, Lesley (2016), 'Identifying the Hippocratic' in DJR, 1–14.

Demand, Nancy (1994), *Birth, Death and Motherhood in Classical Greece*, Baltimore, MD and London: Johns Hopkins University Press.

Demont, Paul (2016), 'Remarques sur le tableau de la médecine et d'Hippocrate chez Platon' in DJR, 61–82.

Dinsdale, Natalie L. and Crespi, Bernard J. (2017), 'Revisiting the wandering womb: oxytocin in endometriosis and bipolar disorder,' *Hormones and Behavior*, 96.11: 69–83.

Dixon, Laurinda (1995), *Perilous Chastity: Women and illness in pre-Enlightenment art and medicine*, Ithaca and London: Cornell University Press.

Doyle, Sir Arthur Conan (1904), *A Study in Scarlet, and, The Sign of the Four*, New York and London: Harper & Brothers.

DuBois, Page (1995), *Sappho is Burning*, Chicago, IL: University of Chicago Press.

Dusenbery, Maya (2018), *Doing Harm: The truth about how bad medicine and lazy science leave women dismissed, misdiagnosed, and sick*, London and New York: HarperCollins.

Edelstein, Ludwig (1939), 'The genuine works of Hippocrates', *BHM*, 7: 236–48; reprinted in Owsei and C. Lilian Temkin (eds), *Ancient Medicine: Selected papers of Ludwig Edelstein*, 133–44, Baltimore, MD and London: Johns Hopkins University Press.

Eichhorn, Kate (2008), 'Archival genres: gathering texts and reading spaces', *Invisible Culture: An electronic journal for visual culture*, 12: 1–10.
Elliotson, John (1844), *The Principles and Practice of Medicine*, Philadelphia, PA: Carey and Hart.
Englyst, Hans and Hudson, Geoffrey (2001), 'Dietary fiber analysis as non-starch polysaccharides (NSPS)', in Gene A. Spiller (ed.), *CRC Handbook of Dietary Fiber in Human Nutrition*, 67–82, Boca Raton, FL: CRC Press, 3rd edition, first edition 1986.
Fabre, John (1997), 'Medicine as a profession: Hip, Hip, Hippocrates: extracts from *The Hippocratic Doctor*,' *BMJ*, 315 (7123): 1669–70.
Ferrari, Gian A. and Vegetti, Mario (1983), 'Science, technology and medicine in the classical tradition' in Pietro Corsi and Paul Weindling (eds), *Information Sources in the History of Science and Medicine*, 197–220, London and Boston: Butterworth Scientific.
Fichtner, Gerhard (1995), *Corpus Hippocraticum: Verzeichnis der hippokratischen und pseudohippoktratischen Schriften*, Tübingen: Institut für Geschichte der Medizin.
Finlayson, James (1892), *Hippocrates: A bibliographical demonstration in the library of the Faculty of Physicians and Surgeons of Glasgow, 23rd November 1891*, Glasgow: Alex Macdougall.
Finnegan, Ruth (2011), *Why Do We Quote? The culture and history of quotation*, Cambridge: Open Book Publishers.
Fishman, Gerald A. (2013), 'A historical perspective on the early treatment of night blindness and the use of dubious and unproven treatment strategies for patients with retinitis pigmentosa', *Journal of Ophthalmology*, 58: 652–63.
Flemming, Rebecca (2002), 'The pathology of pregnancy in Galen's commentaries on the *Epidemics*' in Vivian Nutton (ed.), *The Unknown Galen*, Bulletin of the Institute of Classical Studies, 45: 101–12.
Flemming, Rebecca and Hanson, Ann Ellis (1998), 'Hippocrates' *Peri Parthenion* (*Diseases of Young Girls*): text and translation', *Early Science and Medicine*, 3: 241–52.
Fourgeaud, Victor J. (1847), 'An introductory lecture on the history of medicine, delivered on the 23d December, 1845, before the Medico-Chirugical [sic] Society of St Louis, Mo', *Saint Louis Medical and Surgical Journal*, 4: 481–96.
Galanter, Marc (1999), *Cults: Faith, Healing, and Coercion*, second edition, Oxford and New York: Oxford University Press.
Garber, Marjorie (2003), *Quotation Marks*, London and New York: Routledge.
García-Ballester, Luis (1993), 'On the origins of the six non-natural things in Galen', in Jutta Kollesch and Diethard Nickel (eds), *Galen und das hellenistische Erbe*, Special Issue of *Sudhoffs Archiv*, 32: 105–15.

Garrison, Fielding (1917), *An Introduction to the History of Medicine*, second edition, Philadelphia, PA: W.B. Saunders.
Gerson, Max (1958), *A Cancer Therapy: Results of fifty cases*, New York: Dura Books.
Gerson, Max (1978), 'The cure of advanced cancer by diet therapy: a summary of 30 years of clinical experimentation', *Physiological Chemistry and Physics*, 10.5: 449–64.
Gevitz, Norman (1988), 'Osteopathic medicine: from deviance to difference' in Norman Gevitz (ed.), *Other Healers: Unorthodox medicine in America*, 124–56, Baltimore, MD: Johns Hopkins University Press.
Goldberg, Robert (2010), *Tabloid Medicine: How the Internet is being used to hijack medical science for fear and profit*, New York: Kaplan Publishing.
Gourevitch, Danielle (1980), 'Le dossier philologique de nyctalope' in Mirko D. Grmek (ed.), *Hippocratica: Actes du colloque hippocratique de Paris (4–9 septembre 1978)*, 167–87, Paris: Editions du CNRS.
Graf, Fritz (1992), 'Heiligtum und Ritual: Das Beispiel der griechisch-römischen Asklepieia', in A. Schachter (ed.), *Le sanctuaire grec*, 159–99, Geneva: Fondation Hardt.
Graham, Leah and Metaxas, P. Takis (2003), 'Of course it's true; I saw it on the Internet: critical thinking in the Internet era', *Communications of the ACM*, 46.5: 71–5.
Graham, Sylvester (1837), *A Treatise on Bread, and Breadmaking*, Boston, MA: Light & Stearns.
Grant, Mark (2000), *Galen on Food and Diet*, London and New York: Routledge.
Grensemann, Hermann (1975), *Knidische Medizin Teil I: Die Testimonien zur ältesten knidischen Lehre und Analysen knidischer Schriften im Corpus Hippocraticum*, Berlin and New York: de Gruyter.
Grensemann, Hermann (1982), *Hippokratische Gynäkologie: die gynäkologischen Texte des Autors C nach den pseudohippokratischen Schriften De Muliebribus I, II und De Sterilibus*, Wiesbaden: Franz Steiner.
Guinan, Patrick (2011), *Hippocrates is Not Dead: An anthology of Hippocratic readings*, Bloomington IN: AuthorHouse.
Guthrie, Douglas (1945), *A History of Medicine*, London: Thomas Nelson.
Haas, Gustave (1926), *Health Through Sunshine and Diet*, Los Angeles: Gem Publishing Company.
Hackel, Heidi Brayman (2005), *Reading Material in Early Modern England: Print, gender, and literacy*, Cambridge: Cambridge University Press.
Haller, John S. (1981), *American Medicine in Transition 1840–1910*, Urbana, Chicago and London: University of Illinois Press.

Hammond, N.G.L. (1993), *Sources for Alexander the Great: An analysis of Plutarch's Life and Arrian's Anabasis Alexandrou*, Cambridge: Cambridge University Press.

Hankinson, R.J. (2016), 'Galen on Hippocratic physics' in DJR, 421–44.

Hanson, Ann Ellis (1989), 'Diseases of women in the *Epidemics*' in Gerhaad Baader and Rolf Winau (eds), *Die hippokratischen Epidemien: Theorie–Praxis–Tradition*, *Sudhoffs Archiv*, 27, 38–51, Stuttgart: Franz Steiner.

Hanson, Ann Ellis (1990), 'The medical writers' woman' in David Halperin et al., *Before Sexuality: The construction of erotic experience in the ancient Greek world*, 309–39, Princeton, NJ: Princeton University Press.

Hanson, Ann Ellis (2016), 'The Hippocratic *Aphorisms* in Ptolemaic and Roman times' in DJR, 48–60.

Harris, Charles Reginald Schiller (1973), *The Heart and the Vascular System in Ancient Greek Medicine from Alcmaeon to Galen*, Oxford: Clarendon Press.

Hauser, Gayelord (1932), *Gayelord Hauser's Dictionary of Foods*, 1970 reprint, New York: Benedict Lust Publications.

Havens, Earle (2001), *Commonplace Books: A history of manuscripts and printed books from antiquity to the twentieth century*, New Haven CT: Yale University Press.

Heaton, K.W. (1990), 'Regular review: Dietary fibre', *BMJ*, 300 (6738), 9 June: 1479–80.

Heggie, Vanessa (2010), 'Specialization without the hospital: the case of British sports medicine', *Medical History*, 54.4: 457–74.

Hiroshi, Hosimi (1998), 'On Vis medicatrix naturae and Hippocratic idea of physis', *Memoirs of School of Health Sciences, Faculty of Medicine, Kanazawa University*, 22: 45–54.

Hoedeman, Paul (1991), *Hitler or Hippocrates? Medical experiments in euthanasia in the Third Reich*, trans. Ralph de Rijke, Sussex: Book Guild.

Hoffman, Friedhelm (2015), 'Ancient Egypt' in David J. Collins (ed.), *The Cambridge History of Magic and Witchcraft in the West: From antiquity to the present*, 52–82, Cambridge: Cambridge University Press.

Holbrook, Martin Luther (1888), *Eating for Strength, or, Food and Diet in Their Relation to Health and Work*, New York: M.L. Holbrook and Co.

Hopper, Edward (1865), *The Dutch Pilgrim Fathers, and other poems, humorous and not humorous*, New York: Hurd and Houghton; Boston: E.P. Dutton and Company.

Houdart, M.-S. (1836), *Études historiques et critiques sur la vie et la doctrine d'Hippocrate, et sur l'etat de la médecine avant lui*, Paris: Baillière.

Hughes, Jessica (2008), 'Fragmentation as metaphor in the classical healing sanctuary', *Social History of Medicine*, 21.2: 217–36.

Hullquist, C. 1996 [1983] *Garlic: Nature's perfect prescription*. TEACH Services, Inc.: Brushton NY.

Hurwitz, Brian and Richardson, Ruth (1997), 'Swearing to care: the resurgence in medical oaths', *BMJ*, 315 (7123): 1671.

Ilberg, Johannes (ed.) (1927), *Vita Hippocratis secundum Soranum*. CMG IV, Berlin: Teubner.

Israelowich, Ido (2015), *Patients and Healers in the High Roman Empire*, Baltimore, MD: Johns Hopkins University Press.

Jaacks, Lindsay M. and Bellows, Alexandra L. (2017), 'Let food be thy medicine: linking local food and health systems to address the full spectrum of malnutrition in low-income and middle-income countries', *BMJ Global Health*, 2.4: 1–4.

Jackson, Robert B. (2001), 'Vis mediatrix naturae, vital force to innate intelligence and concepts for 2000', *Journal of Chiropractic Humanities*, 10: 41–7.

James, George G.M. (1954), *Stolen Legacy: The Egyptian origins of western philosophy*, New York: Philosophical Library.

Jensen, Bernard (1988), *Foods That Heal: A guide to understanding and using the healing powers of natural foods*, New York: Penguin Books.

Johnson, J. Aaron (1964), 'The vanishing oath', *Journal of the Medical Society of New Jersey*, 61: 513–4.

Johnson, Ruthie (2014), *An Abridged History: Africa and her history*, Bloomington IN: Xlibris Corporation.

Johnston, Carol S. and Gaas, Cindy A. (2006), 'Vinegar: medicinal uses and antiglycemic effect', *Medscape General Medicine*, 8.2: 61.

Jones, Robert (1925), 'Lady Jones' lecture on crippling due to fractures: its prevention and remedy', *BMJ*, I: 909–13.

Jones, W.H.S. (1923), 'General introduction' to *Nutriment* in *Hippocrates Vol. I*, ix–lxix, Cambridge, MA: Harvard University Press and London: Heinemann

Jones, W.H.S. (1923), 'Introduction' to *Nutriment* in *Hippocrates Vol. I*, 337–41, Cambridge, MA: Harvard University Press and London: Heinemann.

Jones, W.H.S. (1947), *The Medical Writings of Anonymus Londinensis,* Cambridge: Cambridge University Press.

Jordanova, Ludmilla (1989), *Sexual Visions: Images of gender in science and medicine between the eighteenth and twentieth centuries*, London: Harvester Wheatsheaf.

Jouanna, Jacques (1983), 'Littré, éditeur et traducteur d'Hippocrate' in *Actes du Colloque Emile Littré, 1801–1881. Paris, 1–9 octobre 1981*, 285–301, Paris: Eds Albin Michel.

Jouanna, Jacques (1999), *Hippocrates*, Baltimore, MD and London: Johns Hopkins University Press; Fr. original *Hippocrate* (1992), Paris: Librairie Arthème Fayard.

Jouanna, Jacques (2012), 'Egyptian medicine and Greek medicine' in Philip van der Eijk (ed.), *Greek Medicine from Hippocrates to Galen. Selected papers*, 1–20, Leiden and Boston: Brill.

Jouanna, Jacques (2012), 'Galen's reading of Hippocratic ethics' in Philip van der Eijk (ed.), *Greek Medicine from Hippocrates to Galen. Selected papers*, 261–85, Leiden and Boston: Brill.

Jouanna, Jacques (2012), 'Galen's reading of the Hippocratic treatise *The Nature of Man*: The foundations of Hippocratism in Galen' in Philip van der Eijk (ed.), *Greek Medicine from Hippocrates to Galen:. Selected papers*, 313–33, Leiden and Boston: Brill.

Jouanna, Jacques (2016), 'Regimen in the Hippocratic corpus: *diaita* and its problems', in DJR, 209–41.

Jütte, Robert (1996), *Geschichte der Alternativen Medizin. Von der Volksmedizin zu den unkonventionellen Therapien von heute*, Munich: Beck Verlag.

Jütte, Robert (1999), 'The historiography of nonconventional medicine in Germany: a concise overview', *Medical History*, 43: 342–58.

Kákosy, László (1987), 'Some problems of the magical healing statues', in Alessandro Roccati and Alberto Siliotti (eds.), *La Magia in Egitto ai tempi dei Faraoni*, 171–86, Milan: Rassegna Internazionale di Cinematografia Archeologica Arte e Natura Libri.

Kellogg, John Harvey (1928), 'The rise of bran', *Good Health* 63.5: 36–7.

Keyes, Ralph (2006), 'The quote verifier', *The Antioch Review*, 64.2: 256–66.

King, Helen (1985), 'From *parthenos* to *gynê*: the dynamics of category', PhD thesis, University of London.

King, Helen (1993), 'Once upon a text: the Hippocratic origins of hysteria' in Sander Gilman, Helen King, Roy Porter, George S. Rousseau and Elaine Showalter, *Hysteria Beyond Freud*, 3–90, Berkeley CA: University of California Press.

King, Helen (1995), 'Medical texts as a source for women's history' in Anton Powell (ed.), *The Greek World*, 199–218, London: Routledge.

King, Helen (1996), 'Review of Laurinda Dixon, *Perilous Chastity: Women and illness in pre-Enlightenment art and medicine*', *Medical History*, 40: 505–6.

King, Helen (1998), *Hippocrates' Woman: Reading the female body in ancient Greece*, London: Routledge.

King, Helen (2002), 'The power of paternity: The Father of Medicine meets the Prince of Physicians' in David Cantor (ed.), *Reinventing Hippocrates*, 21–36, Aldershot: Ashgate.

King, Helen (2007), *Midwifery, Obstetrics and the Rise of Gynaecology: Users of a Sixteenth-Century Compendium*, Aldershot: Ashgate.

King, Helen (2011), 'Galen and the widow. Towards a history of therapeutic masturbation in ancient gynaecology', *EuGeSta: Journal on Gender Studies in Antiquity*, 1: 205–35.

King, Helen (2013), 'Female fluids in the Hippocratic corpus: how solid was the humoral body?' in Peregrine Horden and Elisabeth Hsu (eds), *The Body in Balance*, 25–49, New York: Berghahn.

King, Helen (2013), *The One-Sex Body on Trial: The classical and early modern evidence*, Aldershot: Ashgate.

King, Helen (2018), 'Women and doctors in ancient Greece' in Rebecca Flemming, Nick Hopwood and Lauren Kassell (eds), *From Generation to Reproduction*, 39–52, Cambridge: Cambridge University Press.

King, Helen (2019), 'Hippocratic Whispers: telling the story of the life of Hippocrates on the internet' in Laurence Totelin and Rebecca Flemming (eds), *Medicines and Markets: Essays on Ancient Medicine in Honour of Vivian Nutton*, London and New York: Classical Press of Wales/Bloomsbury.

King, Helen and McClive, Cathy (2008), 'When is a foetus not a foetus? Diagnosing false conceptions in early modern France' in Véronique Dasen (ed.), *L'Embryon humain à travers l'histoire: Images, savoirs et rites*, Actes du colloque international de Fribourg, 27–29 octobre 2004, 223–38, Gollion: Infolio.

King, Helen and Green, Monica (2018), 'On the misuses of medical history', *The Lancet*, 7 April: 1354–5.

König, René (2013), 'Wikipedia. Between lay participation and elite knowledge representation', *Information, Communication & Society*, 16.2: 160–77.

La Berge, Ann F. (2002), 'The rhetoric of Hippocrates at the Paris School' in David Cantor (ed.), *Reinventing Hippocrates*, 178–99, Aldershot: Ashgate.

Lacey, Gerald de, Record, Carol and Wade, Jenny (1985), 'How accurate are quotations and references in medical journals?', *BMJ (Clinical Research Ed.)*, 291 (6499): 884–6.

Langholf, Volker (1990), *Medical Theories in Hippocrates: Early texts and the 'Epidemics'*, Berlin and New York: de Gruyter.

Langholf, Volker (2004), 'Structure and genesis of some Hippocratic texts' in Manfred Horstmanshoff and Marten Stol (eds), *Magic and Rationality in Ancient Near Eastern and Graeco-Roman Medicine*, 219–75, Leiden: Brill.

Lawrence, Steve and Giles, C. Lee (1999), 'Accessibility and distribution of information on the Web', *Nature*, 400 (6740): 107–9.

Le Clerc, Daniel (1699), *The History of Physick, or, an account of the rise and progress of the art*, London: D. Brown et al.

Lederer, Susan E. (2002), 'Hippocrates American style: representing professional morality in early twentieth-century America' in David Cantor (ed.), *Reinventing Hippocrates*, 239–56, Aldershot: Ashgate.

Lefebvre G. and Porge, J.F. (1966), 'La médecine égyptienne' in René Taton (ed.), *La science antique et médiévale. Des origines à 1450*, Paris: Presses Universitaires de France.

LeFevre, Edwin (1924), 'Making vinegar in the home and on the farm', *Farmers' Bulletin* 1424, U.S. Department of Agriculture.

Lefkowitz, Mary R. (1996), *Not Out of Africa: How Afrocentrism became an excuse to teach myth as history*, New York: Basic Books.

Lefkowitz, Mary R. and Rogers, Guy Maclean (eds) (1996), *Black Athena Revisited*, Chapel Hill, NC and London: University of North Carolina Press.

Lessof, Maurice H. (1992), *Food Intolerance*, London: Chapman and Hall.

Levinovitz, Alan (2015), *The Gluten Lie: And other myths about what you eat*, New York: Regan Arts.

Lichtenstein, Gary R. (2013), 'Letter from the editor', *Gastroenterology & Hepatology*, 9.9: 552.

Lieberman, Hallie and Schatzberg, Eric (2018), 'A failure of academic quality control: *The Technology of Orgasm*', *Journal of Positive Sexuality*, 4.2: 24–47.

Lifton, Robert Jay (1986), *The Nazi Doctors: Medical killing and the psychology of genocide*, New York: Basic Books, https://phdn.org/archives/holocaust-history.org/lifton/contents.shtml.

Lloyd, G.E.R. (1991), *Methods and Problems in Greek Science: Selected papers*, Cambridge: Cambridge University Press.

Lloyd, G.E.R. (2003), *In the Grip of Disease. Studies in the Greek imagination*, Oxford: Oxford University Press.

Loewy, Erich H. (2000), 'Oaths for physicians: necessary protection or elaborate hoax?', *Medscape General Medicine*, 9.1: 7.

Longhi, Vivien (2018), 'Hippocrate a-t-il inventé la médecine d'observation?', *Cahiers Mondes Anciens*, 11: 1–15.

Lonie, Iain M. (1978), 'Cos versus Cnidus and the historians: Part I', *History of Science*, 16: 42–75.

Lonie, Iain M. (1981), *The Hippocratic Treatises 'On Generation', 'On the Nature of the Child', 'Diseases IV'*, Berlin and New York: De Gruyter.

Lonie, Iain M. (1983), 'Literacy and the development of Hippocratic medicine', in François Lasserre and Philippe Mudry (eds), *Formes de pensée dans la collection hippocratique: Actes du Colloque hippocratique de Lausanne 1981*, 145–61, Geneva: Droz.

Lonie, Iain M. (1985), 'The "Paris Hippocratics": teaching and research in Paris in the second half of the sixteenth century' in Andrew Wear, Roger K. French and Iain M. Lonie (eds), *The Medical Renaissance of the Sixteenth Century*, 155–74, Cambridge and New York: Cambridge University Press.

Luauté, Jean-Pierre; Saladini, Olivier and Walusinski, Olivier (2015), 'L'arc de cercle des hystériques. Histoire, interprétations', *Annales Médico-Psychologiques*, 173: 391–8.

Luz, Menahem (1998), 'The philosophical background of Hippocrates' *On Nutriment*' in Konstantine J. Boudouris (ed.), *Philosophy and Medicine Vol. I*, 114–22, Alimos: Ionia Publications.

Lyon, Louisa (2018), '"All disease begins in the gut": was Hippocrates right?' *Brain*, 141.3: 1–5.

McCabe, Anne (2007), *A Byzantine Encyclopaedia of Horse Medicine: The sources, compilation and transmission of the* Hippiatrica, Oxford: Oxford University Press.

McDonald, Peter (2015), *Oxford Dictionary of Medical Quotations*, Oxford: Oxford University Press.

Macfie, Ronald Campbell (1907), *The Romance of Medicine*, London: Cassell and Co.

McGlone, Matthew S. (2005), 'Quoted out of context: contextomy and its consequences', *Journal of Communication*, 55.2: 330–46.

McKeown, J.C. and Smith, Joshua M. (2016), *The Hippocrates Code: Unravelling the ancient mysteries of modern medical terminology*, Indianapolis and Cambridge: Hackett Publishing Company.

MacLeod, Elizabeth and Wishinsky, Frieda (2013), *A History of Just About Everything: 180 events, people and inventions that changed the world*, Toronto, ON: Kids Can Press.

Magnus, P.D. (2008), 'Early response to false claims in *Wikipedia*', *First Monday*, 13.9.

Magnus, P.D. (2008), 'Fibs in the Wikipedia (Supplemental Data)', *Philosophy Faculty Scholarship* (University of Albany, SUNY) 9.

Maines, Rachel (1999), *The Technology of Orgasm: 'Hysteria', the vibrator and women's sexual satisfaction*, Baltimore, MD: Johns Hopkins University Press.

Mallette, Karla (2014), 'The *Seven Sages of Rome*: narration and silence' in Marion Vuagnoux-Uhlig and Yasmina Foehr-Janssens (eds), *D'Orient en Occident: Les Recueils de fables enchâssées avant les 'Milles et une nuits' de Galland*, 129–46, Turnhout: Brepols.

Manetti, Daniela (2011), *Anonymus Londiniensis*, Berlin: de Gruyter (Teubner edition).

Manetti, Daniela and Roselli, Amneris (1982), *Ippocrate, Epidemie, libro sesto. Introduzione, testo critico, commento e traduzione*, Biblioteca di studi superiori, 66, Florence: La nuova Italia editrice.

Mansfeld, Jaap (1980), 'Plato and the method of Hippocrates', *Greek, Roman and Byzantine Studies*, 21: 341–62.

Mantri, Sneha (2008), 'Holistic medicine and the Western medical tradition', *Virtual Mentor*, 10.3: 177–80.

Manuli, Paola (1980), 'Fisiologia e patologia del femminile negli scritti ippocratici dell'antica ginecologia greca' in Mirko D. Grmek (ed.), *Hippocratica. Actes du Colloque hippocratique de Paris 1978*, 393–408, Paris: Eds de CNRS.

Manuli, Paola (1983), 'Donne mascoline, femmine sterili, vergini perpetue. La ginecologia greca tra Ippocrate e Sorano' in Silvia Campese, Paola Manuli and Giulia Sissa, *Madre Materia. Sociologia e biologia della donna greca*, 147–92, Turin: Boringhieri.

Marganne, Marie-Helene (1994), *L'ophthamologie dans l'Égypte gréco-romaine d'après les papyrus littéraires grecs*, Leiden: Brill.

Markel, Howard (2004), '"I swear by Apollo" – On taking the Hippocratic Oath', *New England Journal of Medicine*, 350.20: 2026–9.

Marsh, Henry (2014), *Do No Harm: Stories of life, death and brain surgery*, Weidenfeld & Nicholson.

Martindale, Charles (1993), *Redeeming the Text: Latin poetry and the hermeneutics of reception*, Cambridge: Cambridge University Press.

Mayer, Milton (1966), *They Thought They Were Free: The Germans, 1933–45*, Chicago: University of Chicago Press.

Mazzini, I. and Flammini, G. (1983), *De conceptu: Estratti di un'antica traduzione latina del Περὶ γυναικείων pseudoippocratico l*, Bologna: Pàtron.

Micale, Mark (1995), *Approaching Hysteria: Disease and its interpretations*, Princeton NJ: Princeton University Press.

Micke, Oliver and Jutta Hübner (2009), 'Traditional European Medicine: after all, is Hildegard of Bingen really right?' *European Journal of Integrative Medicine*, 1.4: 226.

Miles, Steven H. (2004), *The Hippocratic Oath and the Ethics of Medicine*, Oxford: Oxford University Press.

Moerman, Daniel E. (1992), 'Minding the body: the placebo effect unmasked' in Maxine Sheets-Johnstone (ed.), *Giving the Body Its Due*, 69–84, Albany NY: SUNY Press.

Money, Mike (2001), 'Shamanism as a healing paradigm for complementary therapy', *Complementary Therapies in Nursing & Midwifery*, 7: 126–31.

Morgenstern, Justin (2008), 'The medical oath: honorable tradition or ancient ritual?', *University of Western Ontario Medical Journal*, 78.1: 27–9.

Morson, Gary Saul (2011), *The Words of Others: From quotations to culture*, New Haven and London: Yale University Press.

Moss, Ann (1996), *Printed Commonplace-Books and the Structuring of Renaissance Thought*, Oxford: Oxford University Press.

Most, Glenn W. (1983), 'The Hippocratic Smile: John le Carré and the traditions of the detective novel' in Glenn W. Most and William W. Stowe (eds), *The Poetics of Murder*, 341–65, San Diego, CA: Harcourt Brace Jovanovich.

Mueller, Ian (1997), 'Greek arithmetic, geometry and harmonics: Thales to Plato' in C.C.W. Taylor (ed.), *Routledge History of Philosophy, Vol. I: From the Beginning to Plato*, 249–97, London and New York: Routledge.

Nachmanson, Ernst (1918), *Erotiani vocum Hippocraticarum collectio cum fragmentis*, Upsala: Appelberg.

Nelson, Eric (2001), 'Hippocrates, Heraclids, and the "Kings of the Heracleidai": Adaptations of Asclepiad history by the author of the *Presbeutikos*', *Phoenix*, 61.3/4: 234–46.

Nelson, Eric (2005), 'Coan promotions and the authorship of the *Presbeutikos*', in Philip van der Eijk (ed.), *Hippocrates in Context. Papers Read at the XIth International Hippocrates Colloquium, University of Newcastle-upon-Tyne 27–31 August 2002*, 209–36, Leiden: Brill.

Nelson, Eric (2016), 'Tracking the Hippocratic Woozle: Pseudepigrapha and the formation of the Corpus' in DJR, 117–41.

Neuburger, Max (1944), 'An historical survey of the concept of Nature from a medical viewpoint', *Isis*, 35.1: 16–28.

Newman, David H. (2008), *Hippocrates' Shadow: Secrets from the house of medicine*, New York: Simon & Schuster.

Nomikos, Nikitas; Trompoukis, C.; Lamprou, Chris and Nomikos, G. (2016), 'The role of exercise in Hippocratic medicine', *American Journal of Sports Science and Medicine*, 4: 115–19.

Nuland, Sherwin B. (1988), *Doctors: The biography of medicine*, New York: Vintage Books.

Numbers, Ronald L. (2008), *Prophetess of Health: A study of Ellen G. White* (3rd edition), Grand Rapids MI: Wm. B. Eerdmans.

Nutton, Vivian (1995), 'What's in an oath?', *Journal of the Royal College of Physicians of London*, 29.6: 518–24.

Nutton, Vivian (1997), 'Hippocratic morality and modern medicine' in Helmut Flashar and Jacques Jouanna (eds.), *Médicine et morale dans l'Antiquité: dix exposés suivis de discussions, Genève, Vandoeuvres 1996*, Entretiens 43, 31–63, Geneva: Fondation Hardt.

Nutton, Vivian (2004), *Ancient Medicine*, London and New York: Routledge.

Nutton, Vivian (2008), 'Review of A. Anastassiou and D. Irmer, *Testimonien zum Corpus Hippocraticum*, Teil I,' *Gnomon* 80: 173–5.

Odent, Michel (1985), *Entering the World: The way to gentle, loving birth*, Harmondsworth: Penguin.

Orr, Robert D.; Pang, Norman; Pellegrino, Edmund D. and Siegler, Mark (1997), 'Use of the Hippocratic Oath: A review of twentieth century practice and a content analysis of oaths administered in medical schools in the U.S. and Canada in 1993', *Journal of Clinical Ethics*, 8: 377–88.

Osler, William (1899), 'Address to the students of the Albany Medical College', *Albany Medical Annals*, 20: 307–9.

Osler, William (1921), *The Evolution of Modern Medicine: A series of lectures delivered at Yale University on the Silliman Foundation in April, 1913*, New Haven CT: Yale University Press.

Pai-Dhungat, J.V. (2015), 'Hippocrates – Father of Medicine', *Journal of the Association of Physicians of India*, 63: 18.

Parker, Steve (2013), *Kill or Cure. An illustrated history of medicine*, London: Dorling Kindersley.

Parsons, Kelly (2014), *Doing Harm*, New York: St Martin's Press.

Paterson, Edith Bruce (1930), 'Hippocrates', *Medical Life*, 37.6: 303–8.

Paulien, Gunther B. (1995), *The Divine Prescription and Science of Health and Healing*, Fort Oglethorpe, GA: TEACH Services Inc.

Pechenick, Eitan Adam; Danforth, Christopher M. and Dodd, Peter Sheridan (2015), 'Characterizing the Google Books Corpus: Strong limits to inferences of socio-cultural and linguistic evolution', PLOS One, 7 October; https://journals.plos.org/plosone/article?id=10.1371/journal.pone.0137041 accessed 27 October 2018.

Petersen, William F. (1946), *Hippocratic Wisdom: For him who wishes to pursue properly the science of medicine*, Springfield IL: Charles C. Thomas.

Picard, Charles (1947), 'Sur l'iconographie d'Hippocrate d'après un portrait d'Ostie', *Comptes rendus des séances de l'Académie des Inscriptions et Belles Lettres*, 91–2: 317–36.

Pickett, Anthony C. (1992), 'The oath of Imhotep: in recognition of African contributions to Western medicine', *Journal of the National Medical Association*, 84.7: 636–7.

Pinault, Jody Rubin (1992), *Hippocratic Lives and Legends*, Studies in Ancient Medicine 4, Leiden and New York: E.J. Brill.

Pitman, Vicki (2005), *The Nature of the Whole: Holism in ancient Greek and Indian medicine*, Delhi: Motilal Banarsidass Publishers.

Pormann, Peter E. (2018), 'Introduction', *The Cambridge Companion to Hippocrates*, 1–24, Cambridge: Cambridge University Press.

Potter, Paul (1998), 'Why we go back to Hippocrates', Thirteenth John P. McGovern Award Lecture, 6 May 1998 (Wellcome Collection).

Powell, Owen (2003), *Galen* On the Properties of Foodstuffs, Cambridge: Cambridge University Press.

Poynter, F.N.L. and Keele, K.D. (1961), *A Short History of Medicine*, London: The Scientific Book Club.

Precope, John (1952), *Hippocrates on Diet and Hygiene*, London: Williams, Lea and Co.

Prefontaine, M. (2015), *The Big Book of Quotes: Funny, inspirational and motivational quotes on life, love and much else*, Isle of Man: MP Publishing.

Price, Campbell (2016), 'On the function of "healing" statues', in Campbell Price, Roger Forshaw, Andrew Chamberlain, & Paul Nicholson (eds), *Mummies, Magic and Medicine in Ancient Egypt: Multidisciplinary essays for Rosalie David*, 269-83, Manchester: Manchester University Press.

Prioreschi, Plinio (1998), *A History of Medicine*, Vol. III, *Roman Medicine*, Omaha: Horatius Press.

Procopiou, Hara (2014), 'Barley meal processing in the ancient world: a look at diversity' in Annelou van Gijn, John Whittaker, Patricia C. Anderson (eds), *Exploring and Explaining Diversity in Agricultural Technology*, 243-6, Oxford: Oxbow Books.

Ratner, Herbert (2011), 'Hippocrates has vital meaning for physicians' (originally 1953), in Patrick Guinan, *Hippocrates is Not Dead: An anthology of Hippocratic readings*, 7-18, Bloomington IN: AuthorHouse.

Reynolds, Edward H. (2018), 'Review Article. Hysteria in ancient civilisations: A neurological review. Possible significance for the modern disorder', *Journal of the Neurological Sciences*, 388 (15 May): 208-13.

Reynolds, Edward H. and Wilson, James V. Kinnier (2014), 'Neurology and psychiatry in Babylon', *Brain*, 137: 2611-9.

Rho, Jong M. (2017), 'How does the ketogenic diet induce anti-seizure effects?', *Neuroscience Letters*, 637.1: 4-10.

Richter, Gisela M.A. (1965), *Portraits of the Greeks*, 3 vols, London: Phaidon Press.

Robson, Barry and Baek, O.K. (2009), *The Engines of Hippocrates: From the dawn of medicine to medical and pharmaceutical informatics*, Hoboken NJ: Wiley.

Rocca, Julius (2014), 'Present at the creation: Plato's "Hippocrates" and the making of a medical ideal' in Brita Alroth and Charlotte Scheffer (eds), *Attitudes towards the Past in Antiquity. Creating Identities. Proceedings of an international conference held at Stockholm University, 15-17 May 2009* (Acta Universitatis Stockholmiensis, Stockholm Studies in Classical Archaeology, 14), 285-99, Stockholm: Stockholm University.

Roselli, Amneris (2016), '"According to both Hippocrates and the truth": Hippocrates as witness to the truth, from Apollonius of Citium to Galen', in DJR, 331-44.

Rosen, Ralph (2016), 'Towards a Hippocratic anthropology: *On Ancient Medicine* and the origins of humans', in DJR, 242-57.

Rosenfeld, Louis (1997), 'Vitamine—vitamin. The early years of discovery', *Clinical Chemistry*, 43.4: 680-5.

Rossi, Marco (2010), 'Homer and Herodotus to Egyptian medicine', *Vesalius* Congress Supplement, 3-5.

Rousselle, Aline (1980), 'Images médicales du corps. Observation féminine et idéologie masculine: le corps de la femme d'après les médecins grecs', *Annales E.S.C.*, 35: 1089–115.

Rousselle, Aline (1983), *Porneia*, Paris: Presses Universitaires de France, 1983, trans. Felicia Pheasant, *Porneia: On desire and the body in antiquity* (1988), Oxford: Blackwell.

Rush, Benjamin (1811), *Sixteen introductory lectures, to courses of lectures upon the institutes and practice of medicine, with a syllabus of the latter. To which are added, Two lectures upon the pleasures of the senses and of the mind, with an inquiry into their proximate cause*, Philadelphia: Bradford and Innskeep.

Rütten, Thomas (2002), 'Hippocrates and the construction of "progress" in sixteenth- and seventeenth-century medicine' in David Cantor (ed.), *Reinventing Hippocrates*, 37–58, Aldershot: Ashgate.

Rütten, Thomas (2010), 'Hippocrates', in Anthony Grafton, Glenn W. Most and Salvatore Settis (eds), *The Classical Tradition*, 438–9, Cambridge MA: Harvard University Press.

Saks, Mike (2003), *Orthodox and Alternative Medicine. Politics, professionalization and health care*, London: Sage Publications.

Sapp, Jan (1990), 'The nine lives of Gregor Mendel' in Homer E. Le Grand, *Experimental Inquiries*, Dordrecht: Reidel.

Sapp, Jan (1999), *Where the Truth Lies: Franz Moewus and the origins of molecular biology*, Cambridge: Cambridge University Press.

Satyanarayana, U. and U. Chakrapani (2014), *Biochemistry*, 4th edition, New Delhi: Elsevier.

Saumell, Jordi C. (2017), 'New lights on the *Anonymus Londiniensis* papyrus', *Journal of Ancient Philosophy*, 11.2: 120–50.

Sawday, Jonathan (1995), *The Body Emblazoned: Dissection and the human body in Renaissance culture*, London and New York: Routledge.

Scull, Andrew (2009), *Hysteria: The disturbing history*, Oxford: Oxford University Press.

Scurlock, JoAnn (1999), 'Physician, exorcist, conjurer, magician: a tale of two healing professionals' in Karel van der Toorn and Tzvi Abusch (eds), *Mesopotamian Magic*, 69–79, Groningen: Styx.

Scurlock, JoAnn (2013), 'Marginalia to Mesopotamian malevolent magic', *Journal of the American Oriental Society*, 133.3: 535–40.

Shackelford, Jole (2002), 'The chemical Hippocrates: Paracelsian and Hippocratic theory in Petrus Severinus' medical philosophy' in David Cantor (ed.), *Reinventing Hippocrates*, 59–88, Aldershot: Ashgate.

Scheper-Hughes, Nancy and Lock, Margaret M. (1987), 'The mindful body: a prolegomenon to future work in medical anthropology', *Medical Anthropology Quarterly*, 1: 6–41.

Schleiner, Winfried (1995), *Medical Ethics in the Renaissance*, Washington DC: Georgetown University Press.

Schommer, J.J. (1912), *Manufacture of Pure Cider Vinegar in the United States* (B.Sc. thesis in Chemical Engineering, Armour Institute of Technology).

Schultze, Quentin J. and Bytwerk, Randall L. (2012), 'Plausible quotations and reverse credibility in online vernacular communities', *ETC: A Review of General Semantics*, 69.2: 216–34.

Sellars, W.C. and Yeatman, R.J. (1930), *1066 And All That: A Memorable History of England, comprising all the parts you can remember, including 103 Good Things, 5 Bad Kings and 2 Genuine Dates*, London: Methuen.

Shackelford, Jole (2002), 'The chemical Hippocrates: Paracelsian and Hippocratic theory in Petrus Severinus' medical philosophy' in David Cantor (ed.), *Reinventing Hippocrates*, 59–88, Aldershot: Ashgate.

Shorter, Edward (1986), 'Paralysis – the rise and fall of a "hysterical" symptom', *Journal of Social History*, 19: 549–82.

Shorter, Edward (1996), 'Primary care' in Roy Porter (ed.), *Cambridge Illustrated History of Medicine*, 118–53, Cambridge: Cambridge University Press.

Shorter, Edward (2005), 'The history of the biopsychosocial approach in medicine: before and after Engel' in Peter White (ed.), *Biopsychosocial Medicine: An integrated approach to understanding illness*, 1–11, Oxford: Oxford University Press.

Shurtleff, William and Aoyagi, Akiko (2014), *History of Seventh-Day Adventist Work with Soyfoods, Vegetarianism, Meat Alternatives, Wheat Gluten, Dietary Fiber and Peanut Butter (1863–2013)*, Lafayette, CA: Soyinfo Center.

Shutt, R.J.H. (1985), 'Letter of Aristeas: a new translation and introduction' in J. Charlesworth (ed.), *The Old Testament Pseudepigrapha*, vol. 2: *Expansions of the 'Old Testament' and Legends, Wisdom and Philosophical Literature, Prayers, Psalms and Odes, Fragments of Lost Judeo-Hellenistic Works*, 7–34 London: Darton, Longman & Todd.

Silverman, Mark E., Murray, T. Jock and Bryan, Charles S. (2003), *The Quotable Osler*, American College of Physicians.

Slater, Eliot (1965), 'Diagnosis of hysteria', *BMJ*, 1: 1395–9.

Slavin, Joanne L. and Lloyd, Beate (2012), 'Health benefits of fruit and vegetables', *Advances in Nutrition* 3.4: 506–16.

Smith, Cedric M. (2005), 'Origin and uses of *primum non nocere* – above all, do no harm!', *Journal of Clinical Pharmacology*, 45.4: 371–7.

Smith, Dale C. (1996), 'The Hippocratic Oath and modern medicine', *JHM*, 51: 484–500.

Smith, G. Munro (1909), 'Vis Medicatrix Naturae: Inaugural Address at the Annual Meeting of the Bath and Bristol Branch of the British Medical Association', *Bristol Medico-Chirurgical Journal*, 27 (106): 321–36.

Smith, Wesley D. (1979), *The Hippocratic Tradition*, Ithaca and London: Cornell University Press.

Smith, Wesley D. (1990), *Hippocrates. Pseudepigraphic Writings Letters-Embassy-Speech from the Altar-Decree*, Studies in Ancient Medicine, 2, Leiden: Brill.

Smith, Wesley J. (2009), 'Defending the Hippocratic Oath; the importance of conscience in health care', *Human Life Review*, 35.1/2: 63–70.

Snider, Pamela and Turner, Roger Newman (2010), 'Nature cure in Europe: the transatlantic journey from pragmatism to principles', *Naturopathic Doctor News and Reviews*, 6.10: 8–9.

Sokol, Daniel K. (2013), '"First do no harm" revisited', *BMJ*, 347 (6426): 23.

Solomon, Jon (1995), 'The Apician sauce: *ius apicianum*' in John Wilkins et al. (eds), *Food in Antiquity*, 115–31, Liverpool: Liverpool University Press.

Stephens, Susan (2010), 'The new Alexandrian library' in Susan Stephens and Phiroze Vasunia (eds), *Classics and National Cultures*, 267–84, Oxford: Oxford University Press.

Stol, Marten (1993), *Epilepsy in Babylonia*, Groningen: Styx.

Stone, Jon; Warlow, Charles; Carson, Alan and Sharpe, Michael (2005), 'Eliot Slater's myth of the non-existence of hysteria', *Journal of the Royal Society of Medicine*, 98.12: 547–8.

Stubbs, Blaxland and Bligh, E.W. (1931), *Sixty Centuries of Health and Physick*, London: Sampson Low, Marston & Co.

Stuhmer, Rolf (2000), *The Big Book of Health*, Zurich: PSM Publishing.

Swift, Kathie Madonna and Mullin, Gerard E. (2011), *The Inside Tract: Your good gut guide to great digestive health*, New York: Rodale.

Tai, E. Shyong and Gillies, Peter J. (2007), (eds), *Nutrigenomics: Opportunities in Asia*, Basel: Karger.

Tasca, Cecilia; Rapetti, Mariangela; Carta, Mauro Giovanni and Fadda, Bianca (2012), 'Women and hysteria in the history of mental health', *Clinical Practice and Epidemiology in Mental Health*, 8: 110–19.

Taylor, Michael A. (2013), *Hippocrates Cried: The decline of American psychiatry*, Oxford and New York: Oxford University Press.

Temkin, Owsei (1973), *Galenism. Rise and decline of a medical philosophy*, Ithaca and London: Cornell University Press.

Temkin, Owsei (1991), *Hippocrates in a World of Pagans and Christians*, Baltimore MD: Johns Hopkins University Press.

Thivel, Antoine (1981), *Cnide et Cos? Essai sur les doctrines médicales dans la collection hippocratique*, Paris: Eds Belles Lettres.

Thompson, Jennifer (2014), *Green Smoothies for Dummies*, Hoboken NJ: John Wiley & Sons.

Thumiger, Chiara (2016), 'The tragic *prosopon* and the Hippocratic *facies*: face and individuality in classical Greece', *Maia*, 68: 637–64.

Tipton, Charles (2014), 'The history of "Exercise is Medicine" in ancient civilizations', *Advances in Physiology Education*, 38.2: 109–17.

Torrance, Isabelle C. (2014), 'The Hippocratic Oath' in Alan H. Sommerstein and Isabelle C. Torrance, *Oaths and Swearing in Ancient Greece*, 372–80, Berlin and Boston, MA: De Gruyter.

Totelin, Laurence (2009), *Hippocratic Recipes: Oral and written transmission of pharmacological knowledge in fifth- and fourth-century Greece*, Studies in Ancient Medicine 34, Leiden and Boston: E.J. Brill.

Totelin, Laurence (2011), 'Old recipes, new practices? The Latin adaptations of the Hippocratic *Gynaecological Treatises*', *Social History of Medicine*, 24.1: 74–91.

Totelin, Laurence (2015), 'When foods become remedies in ancient Greece: The curious case of garlic and other substances', *Journal of Ethnopharmacology*, 167: 30–7.

Trompoukis, Constantinos; German, Vasilios and Falagas, Matthew E. (2007), 'From the roots of parasitology: Hippocrates' first scientific observations in helminthology', *Journal of Parasitology*, 93.4: 970–2.

Trowell, Hugh (1974), 'The development of the concept of dietary fiber in human nutrition', *American Journal of Clinical Nutrition*, 31.10: 3–11.

Tsekourakis, Damianos (1991–3), 'Plato's *Phaedrus* and the holistic viewpoint in Hippocrates' therapeutics', *Bulletin of the Institute of Classical Studies of the University of London*, 38: 162–73.

Tsiompanou, Eleni and Marketos, Spyros G. (2013), 'Hippocrates: timeless still', *Journal of the Royal Society of Medicine*, 106: 288–92.

Vallis, Charles P. (1982), *Hair Transplantation for Male Pattern Baldness*, Springfield IL: Charles C. Thomas.

van der Eijk, Philip (1991), '"Airs, Waters, Places" and "On the Sacred Disease": two different religiosities?', *Hermes*, 119: 168–76.

van der Eijk, Philip (ed.) (2005), *Hippocrates in Context. Papers Read at the XIth International Hippocrates Colloquium, University of Newcastle-upon-Tyne 27–31 August 2002,* Leiden: Brill.

van der Eijk, Philip (2016), 'On "Hippocratic" and "non-Hippocratic" medical writings' in DJR, 15–47.

van der Linden, Johannes Antonides (1665), *Magni Hippocratis Coi opera omnia*, Lugduni Batavorum [Leiden]: Gaasbeeck.

van Dijck, José (2013), *The Culture of Connectivity: A critical history of social media*, Oxford: Oxford University Press.

Vandiver, Elizabeth (2010), *Stand in the Trench, Achilles: Classical receptions in British poetry of the Great War*, Oxford: Oxford University Press.

Veith, Ilza (1965), *Hysteria: The history of a disease*, Chicago: University of Chicago Press.
von Bönninghausen, Clemens (1834), *Die Homöopathie, ein Lesebuch für das gebildete, nichtärztliche Publikum*, Münster: Coppenrath.
von Staden, Heinrich (1966), '"In a pure and holy way": personal and professional conduct in the Hippocratic Oath?', *JHM*, 51.4: 404–37.
von Staden, Heinrich (1989), *Herophilus: The art of medicine in early Alexandria: edition, translation and essays*, Cambridge: Cambridge University Press.
Wake, William C. (1966), 'Who was Hippocrates?', *The Listener*, 29 December, 966–7.
Walker, Kenneth (1959), *The Story of Medicine*, Tiptree: Arrow Books.
Walshe, Francis (1965), 'Diagnosis of hysteria', *BMJ*, II: 1451–4.
Wanjek, Christopher (2003), *Bad Medicine: Misconceptions and misuses revealed, from distance healing to Vitamin O*, Hoboken NJ: John Wiley & Sons.
Warner, John Harley (1977–8), '"The nature-trusting heresy": American physicians and the concept of the healing power of nature in the 1850's and 1860's', *Perspectives in American History*, 11: 291–324.
Warner, John Harley (1986), *The Therapeutic Perspective: Medical practice, knowledge, and identity in America, 1820–1885*, Cambridge MA: Harvard University Press.
Warner, John Harley (2002), 'Making history in American medical culture: the antebellum competition for Hippocrates' in David Cantor (ed.), *Reinventing Hippocrates*, 200–36, Aldershot: Ashgate.
Weber, Max (1922), 'The three types of legitimate rule', transl. Hans Gerth, 1958, *Berkeley Publications in Society and Institutions*, 4.1: 1–11.
Weisz, George (2002), 'Hippocrates, holism and humanism in interwar France' in David Cantor (ed.), *Reinventing Hippocrates*, 257–79, Aldershot: Ashgate.
Weisz, George (2003), 'The emergence of medical specialization in the nineteenth century', *BHM*, 77: 536–75.
Weisz, George (2006), *Divide and Conquer: A comparative history of medical specialization*, Oxford: Oxford University Press.
Wellmann, Max (1929), 'Hippokrates des Herakleides Sohn', *Hermes*, 64: 16–21.
White, Ellen (1898), *The Desire of Ages*, Mountain View CA: Pacific Press Publishing Association, 1940.
White, Ellen (1905), The *Ministry of Healing*, Mountain View CA: Pacific Press Publishing Association, 1942.
White, K.D. (1995), 'Cereals, bread and milling in the Roman world' in John Wilkins, David Harvey and Mike Dobson (eds), *Food in Antiquity*, 38–43, Exeter: University of Exeter Press.

Whorton, James C. (1988), 'Patient, heal thyself: popular health reform movements as unorthodox medicine' in Norman Gevitz (ed.), *Other Healers: Unorthodox medicine in America*, 52–81, Baltimore, MD: Johns Hopkins University Press.

Whorton, James C. (2000), *Inner Hygiene: Constipation and the pursuit of health in modern society*, Oxford and New York: Oxford University Press.

Whorton, James C. (2002), *Nature Cures: The history of alternative medicine in America*, New York, Oxford University Press.

Willis, Ika (2018), *Reception*, Abingdon and New York: Routledge.

Wilson, Adidas (2013), *The Alkaline Diet CookBook: The alkaline meal plan to balance your pH, reduce body acid, lose weight and have amazing health* (self-published).

Wilson, Emily (2007), *The Death of Socrates. Profiles in History*, Cambridge, MA: Harvard University Press.

Wilson, James V. Kinnier and Reynolds, Edward H. (1990), 'Translation and analysis of a cuneiform text forming part of a Babylonian treatise on epilepsy', *Medical History*, 34: 185–98.

Winkler, Jack (1981), 'Gardens of nymphs: Public and private in Sappho's lyrics' in Helene P. Foley (ed.), *Reflections of Women in Antiquity*, 63–89, New York: Gordon and Breach.

Witherington, Ben (2012), *A Week in the Life of Corinth*, Downer's Grove IL: InterVarsity Press.

Withington, Edward T. (1894), *Medical History from the Earliest Times: A popular history of the healing art*, London: The Scientific Press.

Wittern, Renate (1971), 'Zum Hippokratesglossar des Erotian κατάπηροι im Corpus Hippocraticum', *Sudhoffs Archiv*, 55.1: 76–9.

Wittig, Monique and Zeig, Sande (1979), *Lesbian Peoples: Material for a dictionary*, London: Virago.

Woodruff, Robert A. (1974), 'Hysteria: an evaluation of objective diagnostic criteria by the study of women with chronic medical illnesses', *British Journal of Psychiatry*, 114: 1115–9.

Wootton, David (2007), *Bad Medicine: Doctors doing harm since Hippocrates*, Oxford: Oxford University Press.

Youngson, Robert (2000), *The Royal Society of Medicine Health Encyclopedia*, London: Bloomsbury.

Index

abortion 25, 65, 192
acacia oil 13
Acanthius 116
acupuncture 139
Adams, Francis 27, 36, 107, 118, 177, 191, 208, 210
advertising 3, 12–13, 43, 48, 111, 114, 121–3, 138
advice literature 156
Afrikan Center of Well Being, Inc. 75–6
AIDS 138
Al Binali, Hajar 124–5
Alcibiades 56
Alexa 51
Alexander the Great 47–8, 67
Alexandria, Great Library of 29–30, 173
Alive Polarity 122–3
allergies 62–3, 66
alliteration 80, 82, 86
allopathy 146, 149
alternative medicine 2, 5, 16, 37, 40, 43, 65, 66, 106, 111, 132, 134, 135–6, 138, 143, 147, 152–3, 221; *see also* chiropractic; homeopathy; naturopathy; osteopathy; reflexology
Alzheimer's disease 69
anatomy 20, 32, 33, 61, 62, 66, 190
Anaxagoras 56, 58
Andreas 30
Andromachus 25
anonymity 34, 101
Anonymus Londinensis 26, 28, 112
answers.com 12, 57, 62–3, 102, 115, 123
antibiotics 144
anti-vaccination 4, 65–6, 152
aphrodisiacs 126
Apollonius of Citium 39
apple cider vinegar 47–9, 50, 128
apples 123
Aristeas 29

Aristotle 11, 22, 26, 28, 30, 37, 86
Armour, Richard 19, 44, 64
army, Roman 3
Arnaud, Sabine 83, 200–1
aromatherapy 142, 185
Artaxerxes 39
Asclepiads 28, 172
Asclepius 28, 53, 58, 59, 74, 112, 172, 188, 191
Aspen Institute 1
ass 124
Assassin's Creed: Odyssey 10–11, 24, 38, 64, 102, 178, 208
asthma 62–3, 66
astrology 49, 73, 139, 195
Athenaeus 130
athletics 62, 81, 107, 109
autism 152
autointoxication 128, 129
Axe, Josh 115

Babylonia 89–91
Bacchius of Tanagra 25, 31
Bagnall, Roger 29, 173
balance 106, 108, 135, 144
baldness; *see* hair
BBC *Panorama* 70, 193
BBC Question Time 69
bedside medicine 25, 38, 159
beetroot 13
Bernal, Martin 75
Bible 29, 44, 57, 92, 144, 156, 188
Big Pharma 65–6, 70, 110, 138, 149, 159
bile 24, 131, 144, 155
binaries, in classification 20, 90
biochemistry 116
biographies; *see* Hippocrates, biographies of
Blair, Ann 97, 98
blood 24, 45, 46, 47, 53, 54, 126, 144, 152, 166, 217, 230

blogs 50, 61, 68, 82, 96, 98, 103, 104, 111, 116, 120, 126, 139, 140, 142, 206
bloodletting 147
body
  essentialist and constructivist approaches 88, 94
  self-healing 134–7, 152
Borland, Christine 8
Boudon-Millot, Véronique 23–4
Bower, Frank W. 121–2
bran 129–30, 218
bread 112, 127, 129–31
British Medical Association 69, 143, 221
Brown, Dan 67
Brown, Joanna viii, 68, 120
bumper-stickering 99, 101, 142
Burke, Edmund 100
Burkitt, Denis 218

cancer 66, 69, 122, 135, 142, 150, 151, 152, 161, 228; *see also* chemotherapy; Gerson, Max
Cañizares, Pilar Perez 25, 29, 34
Cantor, David viii, 3, 4, 16, 40, 190, 193
Cardenas, Diana 119–20
Carley, Rebecca 65, 152
castor oil 76, 77
cataplasms 14, 130, 131
Catholicism, Roman 6; *see also* Christianity
Cawadias, Alexander 131
celery 114, 122, 161, 212–3
Celsus 125, 130
Cham (Amédé Charles de Noé) 155–6
Charaka 52
Chaucer, Geoffrey 100
chemistry 114
chemotherapy 103, 149
chiropractic 115, 120, 140, 215
Chishti, Ghulam 119, 140–1
Christian Medical & Dental Associations 2
Christianity 19, 23, 167, 181; *see also* Bible; God (Christian)
Clement of Alexandria 93
Clement, Brian 93, 136, 149–52, 180, 215, 228
Clifton, Francis 8–9
Clinton, Bill 96
cloning 8, 65

club foot 27
Coan 'school' 24, 29, 45 112
colonic irrigation 128
comfort-eating 113
commonplace books 97, 98, 206
compassion 2
complementary medicine 141, 150; *see also* alternative medicine
computer games 3; *see also* Assassin's Creed: Odyssey
conspiracy theories 57, 67
Constantine the African 54
constipation 127–30, 218
consumption (disease) 108
contextomy 99, 206
continuity, attempts to create 5, 6, 71, 82, 83, 86–6, 88–90, 91, 94, 101, 149, 158
cookery 96, 114, 124–5
Cooter, Roger 148
Coren, Giles 105
Cos; *see* Coan 'school'
cosmetics 138
Coward, Rosalind 40, 135–6, 138
Craik, Elizabeth 3, 27, 31, 32, 33, 34, 124, 174, 175
Crates (Hippocrates) 116–7, 158
Crystal, David 50, 80, 98
Cullen, William 134, 221
cumin 12–14, 76

Da Vinci Code; *see* Brown, Dan
Daily Mail 80, 81, 85, 88
Dalby, Matthew 120
Databases, use in research 15, 103
David, Rosalie 76–7, 197
Davidson, James 177
Daya, Shamim 145
Dean-Jones, Lesley 29, 35, 109
deception 39, 109
decoding, imagery of 67, 85, 94
Demand, Nancy 35
detox diets 91–3, 122, 229; *see also* Gerson, Max
diabetes 48, 119
digestion 26, 122, 123, 129
digital literacy viii, 51, 87, 184
Dioscorides 39, 124
dissection 15, 24, 61, 62

Dixon, Laurinda 84
doctor–patient relationship 2, 20, 136, 142; *see also* patients
dosimetry 43
dropsy 131
drugs 7, 33, 96, 110, 112, 114, 116, 120, 131–2, 135, 149; *see also* Big Pharma
drumstick fingers 61
dung
    pig 198
    pigeon 13
Dusenbery, Maya 7, 15

eating disorders 140
Edelstein, Ludwig 21, 36
Edison, Thomas 96
education, medical 20, 65, 71, 103, 148
Edwin Smith Papyrus 73–4
efficacy 12, 40, 76, 123, 127, 152
Egypt 73–8, 91–3, 198
Egyptian Medicinal Plant Conservation Project 76, 91
Einstein, Albert 100
electrosmog 145
elements, four 23, 24, 63
Eleusis 11
empiricism 19, 20, 25, 38, 55
Erasmus 97
Ernst, Edzard 141–2
Erotian 25, 33
ethics 4, 37, 65, 70, 73, 93, 102, 105, 147, 159
Euclid 30
eunuchs 12
euthanasia 65, 192
excretion 119, 127, 130
exercise 7, 45, 105–9, 112, 119, 123, 135, 144–5, 146, 159
Exercise Is Medicine 106–7, 109
experience 35, 41; *see also* empiricism

face reading 69
family, in ancient medicine 24, 30, 35, 36
fan fiction 4
fibre, dietary 128–30, 157
Flemming, Rebecca ix, 23
florilegium 97

fragmentation
    of body 136
    of medicine 148, 149, 157
fragments, textual 30–1, 136
France, history of medicine in 25, 137, 146, 155
Franklin, Benjamin 100

Galen 123, 130
    Hippocratic commentaries 22, 27, 226
    interpreter of Hippocrates 22–3, 25–6, 39, 94, 106, 118–9, 157, 169
    as Hippocrates' nephew 56
    on medical history 24, 136
    as Prince of Physicians 54–5
    reception of 54, 85, 86–7, 103, 145
garlic 113, 123, 125, 127
Garrison, Fielding 38, 47, 74–5
gender 7, 15, 146
generation 32 53
genuine works 25–6, 27, 146
Germany, history of medicine in 2, 5, 129, 148
Gerson, Max 122, 123, 161
Gill, N.S. 103
glaucoma 114
God (Christian) 19, 44, 57, 58, 70, 100, 144; *see also* Christianity
gods, pagan 19, 37, 53, 56, 58–62, 70, 76, 89, 143
Goebbels, Joseph 57, 100; *see also* Nazi medicine
Google 14, 15, 64, 87, 120
Gorski, David 114
Graham, Sylvester 129–30, 219
graphology 140
Green, Monica 15, 192
Grensemann, Hermann 33
guilt 44, 151
Gundry, Steven 115
Gustavus Adolphus College ix
gymnastics 105, 107, 109
gynaecology 14, 20, 32–5, 127, 174, 175, 217

Haas, Gustave 120–1
hair 8–14, 126, 138
Hall, Lesley 84
Hankinson, Jim 24
Hanson, Ann Ellis 22, 23, 31

Hauser, Gaylord 122
head 11, 37, 74, 88, 124
　as seat of the soul 10
health 5, 10, 20, 40, 47–8, 54, 64–5, 75, 78,
　　93, 106–9, 112, 114, 116, 129, 135–8,
　　145–8, 205, 209
　public 113; *see also* body, self-healing:
　　Nature, healing power of
Health (Hygieia) 58
heat 23, 109, 118, 119, 145
Heggie, Vanessa 148, 227
helminths 78–82
Heraclitus 117
herbalism 125, 131, 135, 139, 143, 144
Herodicus of Cnidos 112
Hildegard of Bingen 5
Hip (Dr) 213
Hip (Hippocrates) 116
Hippocrates of Chios 56
Hippocrates of Cos
　appearance 8–10
　biographies of 4, 11, 35–7, 39, 44, 162
　death 12, 37, 56–7, 116
　divinity of 20, 23, 58
　education of 62
　as Father of Food Science 122
　as Father of Health 20
　as Father of Medicine 12, 16, 19, 20, 31,
　　37, 38, 48, 52–5, 64, 66, 75, 82, 85,
　　111, 122, 126, 129, 134, 140; *see also*
　　Imhotep
　in fiction 4, 47, 61
　in motivational literature 59–60, 98
　personality 21, 37–9, 71, 95, 157
　in prison 49, 51–2, 55–62, 64, 66, 140,
　　151, 159
　and Protestant work ethic 56
　as rebel 58, 134, 140, 157
Hippocrates of Cos, treatises
　　attributed to
　Affections 33
　Airs Waters Places 8, 26, 45, 112, 140
　On the Anatomy of the Veins 49
　On Ancient Medicine 112, 137, 140
　Aphorisms 25, 37, 140
　Astrology 49
　On Bones 32
　On Breaths 26
　Coan Prognoses 25, 26, 79, 171
　The Complicated Body 49, 52, 55, 56–66,
　　159
　The Cos and Effect of Disease 44–5
　Decorum 150
　Diseases 3 108
　Diseases 4 32
　Diseases of Women 14, 19, 32–3, 88
　Diseases of Young Girls/Virgins 32,
　　175
　Epidemics 25, 38, 39, 79, 102, 103–4,
　　116, 134, 147
　On the Excision of the Foetus 32–3
　Fistulas 45
　Fractures 27, 32
　Generation/Nature of the Child 25,
　　32, 53
　On Glands 32, 33
　Internal Affections 108, 131
　Joints 27, 32
　Natural Exercise 45, 159, 180
　On the Nature of Man 22, 23–4, 25, 32,
　　112
　Nature of Woman 33
　On Nutriment 117–9, 121, 122, 132
　The Oath 2, 4, 6, 7, 25, 38, 58, 66, 69–72,
　　75, 80–1, 93, 101–5, 113, 115, 142,
　　149, 155–7
　Pharmakitis 33
　On the Physician 10, 61
　On Places in Man 109
　Prognostics 26, 37, 46, 79, 81, 171, 188
　Prorrhetic 26, 81
　Regimen 1 25, 26, 106, 108, 109
　Regimen 2 109, 123, 130
　Regimen 3 106, 109
　Regimen 4 (On Dreams) 106
　Regimen in Acute Diseases 107, 159,
　　171
　Regimen in Health 108–9
　On the Sacred Disease 58
　Sight 124
　Speech at the Altar 36
　On Sterility/Barrenness 32, 33
　Superfetation 127
　On Ulcers 127
　Wounds and Traits 33; *see also* genuine
　　works
Hippocrates Health Institute 93, 123, 136,
　　150, 152, 229

Hippocrates Soup 1, 122, 159, 161
Hippocrates' Famous Green Juice 123, 159, 161; *see also* juicer
Hippocrates/hypocrite 69
Hippocratic, origins of adjective 23
Hippocratic corpus
   anonymity and 22, 25, 30, 34, 36, 72
   concept of 'author' 22, 25, 27, 31–5
   number of treatises in 31–2
   as practical handbooks 40
   women as source for 34–5
Hippocratic face 46
Hippocratic question 22, 25
Hippocratic sleeve 46
Hippocratic smile 46
history, authority of 5–6, 107
history, teaching 51, 73
history of medicine 2, 27, 37–8, 71, 75, 83, 86, 133, 143, 146, 148
Hitler, Adolf 20, 64; *see also* Nazi medicine
Holbrook, Martin Luther 114
Holby City 102, 104
holism 5, 20, 52, 66, 75, 133–53
Holmes, Oliver Wendell 103
Holmes, Sherlock 46
homeopathy 14, 146
honey 47–8, 68, 124
horseradish 12–13
horse-riding 45, 180
hospitals 15, 65, 102, 113, 125–6, 148
Houdart, M.S. 26, 31
Huebner, Sabine 86
Hughes, Jessica 136
humour; *see* jokes
humours 23–4, 79
Hygicia 58
hygiene 46–7, 58, 155
Hyman, Mark 96
hypocras 46
Hypocras, Master (Hippocrates) 187
hysteria 82–91, 94, 158

Ilberg, Johannes 30, 173
Imhotep 52, 69, 73–8, 91, 111
impact agenda 68, 76, 192
infertility 45
inflammation 116, 147
Instagram 95

internet 14, 19, 20, 44, 45, 50, 51, 55, 59, 64, 68, 75, 98, 100, 105, 127, 140, 156; *see also* digital literacy; Wikipedia
intestinal worms; *see* helminths
integrative medicine; *see* alternative medicine
Isotalo, Peter 46

Jensen, Bernard 128
Johnson, J. Aaron 72
jokes 10–11, 44, 64, 98, 127–8, 190
Joly, Robert 119
Jones, Indiana 67
Jones, Robert 148
Jones, W.H.S. 21, 30, 109, 117–8, 173
Jouanna, Jacques 23, 29, 30, 36, 73
journalism 45, 67–8, 76, 77, 80, 87, 88, 155
juicing 1, 43, 44, 115
Jütte, Robert 2

Kellogg, John Harvey 129, 219
Killgrove, Kristina 79, 81
KNH Centre for Biomedical Egyptology 76
Kutch, Rob 116–7

La Puma, John 96
Langholf, Volker 32, 34
Lasagna, Louis 70, 142, 194, 221
Latin 19, 35, 54, 55, 63–4, 97, 102–3, 134, 135, 208
Le Clerc, Daniel 11
Lederer, Susan 7
leeks 122, 127
Levinovitz, Alan ix, 44, 114, 159, 219
libraries, in ancient world 59, 73 *see also* Alexandria, Great Library of
libraries, monastic 91–2
lifestyle medicine 119, 157, 159
lilies 13
Lincoln Memorial 3
Littré, Emile 30, 31, 88, 136, 147
liver 124–5
Lloyd, G.E.R. 22, 23, 31, 40
Loma Linda University 144–5

magic 58, 74, 102, 122, 141
magnetism, animal 27
Maines, Rachel 84–5, 91

Mansfeld, Jaap 21, 26, 172
Manuli, Paola 34
Martindale, Charles 3
masturbation, therapeutic 84–5, 219
mathematics 30, 56
McCoy, 'Bones' 4
medical education; *see* education, medical
medicine, heroic 135
medicine, medieval 14–15, 32, 34, 46, 49, 57, 197, 200
Medline 15, 68, 91, 192
melancholy 24, 83
memes 44, 93, 105, 106
Mendel, Gregor 53
Menon 26–7
menstruation 33, 35
mesmerism 27
Metchnikoff, Elie 128–9
meteorology 6, 71
Micale, Mark 83
microbiota, gut 129
Miles, Steven 70, 104
milk 127
Mill, John Stuart 50
modernity 159
money, Hippocrates and 39, 59, 64
More, Thomas 97
Mukwege, Denis 2
murder 56, 70, 206
Muses 97

Nature 28, 38, 93, 121, 147, 159
    feminized 53
    healing power of 61, 134–5, 137, 143–4
naturopathy 120, 138, 139, 146, 229
Nazi medicine 7; *see also* Hitler, Adolf
Nelega, Pauline 135, 143, 146
Nelson, Eric 23, 36
neo-Hippocratic movement 146–8
Nero 25
news media 3, 12, 13, 67–94, 96, 114, 158; *see also* journalism
Newton, Isaac 100–1
night blindness 124–5
Nonnius, Ludovicus 8
Normalettes 121–2
nutritionists 1, 11
Nutton, Vivian 58, 70–1, 72, 155, 162, 193

ObamaCare 69, 101
obesity 108
observation 25, 34, 38, 54, 79, 146, 157
olive oil 13
opium 13
orgasm 84
orthopaedic medicine 108, 148
Osborn, David K. 139–42
Osler, Sir William 15, 38, 75–6, 103, 142
osteopathy 2, 16
ox 124

pain 20, 39, 63, 69, 76, 131, 151
Paltrow, Gwyneth 115
Panacea 58
papyri 68, 76–7, 85, 86, 108, 112, 124, 174; *see also* Anonymus Londinensis; Edwin Smith Papyrus
Paracelsus 25
parasites; *see* helminths
Paré, Ambroise 103
parsley 122
Parsons, Kelly 15, 102
patients 2, 7, 20, 38, 65, 69, 70, 75, 83, 84–5, 96, 104–5, 111, 113, 119, 124, 131, 145, 147–9, 152, 194, 205, 208, 216
    of Hippocrates 8, 24, 26, 38, 39, 46, 48, 59, 102, 107–8, 122, 125–6, 141–2, 146, 190, 217, 226
Patrick, Sean 59–60
patriotism 39, 102
Paul, Joanna 173
Paulien, Gunther B. 132
perfumes 13
Petronius 130
pharmaceutical industry 59, 65, 138, 149; *see also* Big Pharma; drugs
Phelps, Michael 92
Phideas of Athens 28
Philippines 66
philosophy 25, 26, 30, 43, 54
phlegm 24, 131, 144
Pinault, Jody Rubin 30, 158
pinworm 81; *see also* helminths
plague 39
plane tree 8
Plato 22, 28, 30, 136, 153, 159,
Pliny the Elder 81–2
poisoning 46, 102, 128

politics 37, 59, 62, 69, 73, 83, 99
Polonius 99
Polybus 22–3
Pormann, Peter 6
positive thinking 110
postage stamps 8
Potter, Paul 22, 33, 108, 166
priests 59, 90, 151, 188
priority disputes 53, 74, 93, 111
press releases 68, 76–7, 79, 85–87
proctoscopy 69
professionalization 1, 5, 37, 38, 52, 70, 146, 148
prose 27, 29, 33, 45
Protestant work ethic 56, 159
proverbs 101, 103, 118, 126, 129, 158
pseudepigrapha 36, 39
pseudoscience 150
psychiatry 7, 56, 138
psychotherapy 7
public health; *see* health, public
PubMed 15, 68, 91, 103, 192
purging 117–18, 147
purity 44, 93, 114, 131, 144, 152, 159

quickening 53
quotation
    culture of 98
    as found art 101
    and identity 98
    referential credibility 100

radish 14, 127
raw foods 129, 135, 137, 150, 157
reception 1, 2–5, 16, 21, 40, 43, 55, 58, 67, 72, 98, 99, 157
recipes 14, 33, 34, 92, 116, 123
reflexology 142
reiki 142
religion 1, 37, 58, 60, 66, 74, 118, 142
    language of 20, 44, 114, 151, 156
Reynolds, Edward 88–91
risk 50, 90, 102, 103–4
Rocca, Julius 1, 30
Roselli, Amneris 39
Rosen, Ralph 137
roses 13
roundworm 78, 81, 198; *see also* helminths
Rousselle, Aline 34

Rubens 8–9, 104
Rush, Benjamin 10, 40, 82
Rütten, Thomas 37, 40–1

Sapp, Jan 53
Sawday, Jonathan 53–4
science 2, 6, 20, 26, 52, 53, 86, 89, 90, 92, 94, 100, 112, 114, 123, 128, 140, 146, 169, 206
    Hippocratic 28, 31, 37, 222
    opposed to religion 58, 59, 74
scientocracy 65
Scurlock, JoAnn 90
seafood 127
Seneca 98, 206
Seventh-Day Adventist 129, 132, 144
Severinus, Petrus 25
sexual frustration 84
Shipman, Harold 70
shopping 3
Sigur, Sandra 142, 225
The Simpsons 70
sin 114
sleep 47, 108, 145
smell 13–14
Smellie, William 8
Smith, Cedric 103
Smith, Dale 72
Smith, Wesley D. 29, 30, 36, 134–5, 136, 169, 172, 177
Smith, Wesley J. 65
The Smithsonian 86–7
soap 138
social media 2, 3, 14, 15, 44, 158; *see also* Instagram, Twitter
Socrates 1, 28, 60, 64, 177
Sokol, Daniel 103, 194
Soranus 37
soul 11, 28, 109, 137, 138, 151
soup, curry 114; *see also* Hippocrates Soup
Spock, Mr 4
sports medicine 106–7, 109, 148, 227
sports nutrition 1
Star Trek 4
Steel, Karl 184
Stephens, Susan 29
Still, Andrew Taylor 2
Stoics 26
storytelling 5

Suda 37
sun 56, 58, 108, 120–2, 144
The Sun 85
superfoods 125, 131, 140, 157
surgery 9, 16, 27, 32, 70, 103, 104, 112, 113, 115, 148, 206, 216
Susruta 107
sweating 109, 119
Sydenham, Thomas 25–6, 103

Taylor, Michael A. 7, 56
tea, herbal 131
technē 35
television 4, 70, 96, 104, 145
temperaments 24, 139
Theophrastus 81
thermal imaging 145
The Times 13, 86, 92
Tipton, Charles 107–8
Totelin, Laurence ix, 14, 112–13
Tselikas, Agamemnon 92–3
Twitter 1, 73, 79, 80, 184, 192
　as a research tool 15, 68–9
Tzetzes, John 37

UltraWellness Center 96
Uwechia, Jide 77, 196

vaccination; *see* anti-vaccination
vagina 34
van der Eijk, Philip 31, 34, 58
veganism 135; *see also* raw foods
Vegetarian Times 114, 122
vegetarianism 129, 144
Veith, Ilza 85, 91, 201
vinegar, balsamic 68; *see also* apple cider vinegar
vitalism 93, 146
vitamins 114, 121, 124–5, 126, 230
von Staden, Heinrich 117, 124

Waffen-SS 5; *see also* Nazi medicine
Warner, John Harley 5, 6, 43, 65, 147

watercress 125–7
Weeks, Bradford 59, 66, 151
Weisz, George 147
Wellmann, Max 29
West, Charles · 44
whipworm 78, 81; *see also* helminths
White, Ellen G. 144–5
wholistic 133, 143–5
Whorton, James C. 2, 127–8, 129, 134, 138, 139
Wigmore, Ann 150
Wikipedia
　advertising on 12, 47–8
　attempts to sabotage 43, 44
　editors' role 14, 45, 51–2, 141, 183
　Hippocrates page 12, 47, 61, 73, 119, 141, 181–2, 187, 188, 189
　outside the academy 16, 45, 51, 67, 158
　sources 46, 51, 75
　talkpages 45, 49, 51–2, 73, 106
　use for marketing · 40, 41
　use in teaching 51, 184
　vandalism of 49–50, 55–64, 183, 186
　vis medicatrix naturae page 134–5
willow bark 63
wine 13, 46, 47, 112
Witherington, Ben 47
womb 34, 53, 82–4, 86, 88, 89, 127,
women
　bias in modern medicine 7, 84, 105
　gendered diagnoses 83
　and Hippocratic medicine 34–5, 81, 85–6
Wootton, David 27, 71
world medicine 139
wounds 33, 47, 74, 182

Xenophon 127
Xerxes 127

yoga 139, 142
YouTube 96
Yun Shui 51–2

www.ingramcontent.com/pod-product-compliance
Lightning Source LLC
Chambersburg PA
CBHW050324020526
44117CB00031B/1704